Epidemics and the Modern World

EPIDEMICS

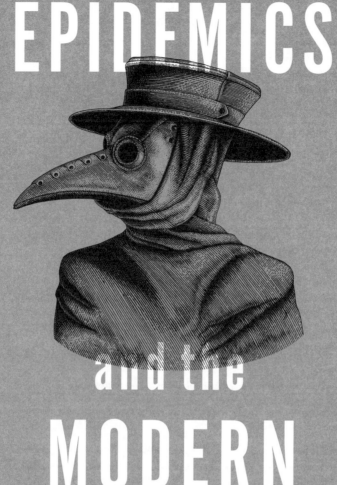

and the
MODERN
WORLD

MITCHELL L. HAMMOND

UNIVERSITY OF TORONTO PRESS
Toronto Buffalo London

© University of Toronto Press 2020

Toronto Buffalo London

utorontopress.com

Printed in Canada

ISBN 978-1-4875-9374-2 (cloth)   ISBN 978-1-4875-9375-9 (EPUB)

ISBN 978-1-4875-9373-5 (paper)   ISBN 978-1-4875-9376-6 (PDF)

Library and Archives Canada Cataloguing in Publication

Title: Epidemics and the modern world / Mitchell L. Hammond.

Names: Hammond, Mitchell L., 1967– author.

Description: Includes bibliographical references and index.

Identifiers: Canadiana 20190189428 | ISBN 9781487593742 (cloth) | ISBN 9781487593735 (paper)

Subjects: LCSH: Epidemics—History. | LCSH: Epidemics—Social aspects. | LCSH: Communicable
    diseases—History. | LCSH: Communicable diseases—Social aspects.

Classification: LCC RA649.H36 2019 | DDC 614.4/9—dc23

We welcome comments and suggestions regarding any aspect of our publications—please feel free to contact us at news@utorontopress.com or visit our internet site at utorontopress.com.

Every effort has been made to contact copyright holders; in the event of an error or omission, please notify the publisher.

University of Toronto Press acknowledges the financial assistance to its publishing program of the Canada Council for the Arts and the Ontario Arts Council, an agency of the Government of Ontario.

 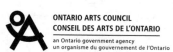

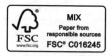

CONTENTS

IMAGES

FIGURES AND MAPS

Figures

Maps

SCIENCE FOCUS BOXES AND WORKSHOPS

Boxes

Workshops

PREFACE AND ACKNOWLEDGEMENTS

The framework for this text emerged from my teaching of an introductory class at the University of Victoria. The book is conceived as an interdisciplinary "gateway": the history of individual diseases serves as a route for students to explore key aspects of modern history and to practice strategies of historical interpretation. In particular, the text profits from scientific advances that are reframing how we understand the origin and impact of many infectious diseases in relation to other forces.

The need for a text of manageable length guided decisions concerning what would be included in the book and what would be omitted. It is not a comprehensive history of medicine, even of the Western medical tradition that is a key topic. Nor is it a comprehensive global history of disease. Many important diseases are discussed, but others such as measles, typhus, or helminth infections (such as schistosomiasis) are referenced in passing or not at all. The swift pace of research in many fields ensures that some scholarship discussed in this book may soon bear revision. To note just one example, I was unable to incorporate insights from Amir A. Afkhami's study *A Modern Contagion: Imperialism and Public Health in Iran's Age of Cholera* (Baltimore: Johns Hopkins University Press, 2019). This book is best seen, therefore, as an invitation to deeper engagement for students and also for instructors who may match this with their own expertise and pedagogical approaches to chronology, themes, and skills.

It is a pleasure to acknowledge the scholars, scientists, and media professionals who helped me write a better book. The final product was much improved by thoughtful feedback from three anonymous reviewers of the initial proposal and two more who assessed an intermediate draft. Caroline Cameron, Jason Colby, JoAnne Flynn, Sheila Lukehart, Timothy Newfield, Duane Osheim, Terry Pearson, and Chris Upton all provided comments on individual chapters. Faith Wallis and Michael Worobey shared expertise and forthcoming work; Greg Blue and Martin Bunton offered helpful suggestions, as did Jean Hammond. At the University of Toronto Press, editor Natalie Fingerhut buoyed me with her enthusiasm and expertise, and the production staff led by Christine Robertson combined the elements of the book into an engaging whole. I was ably assisted with the creation of maps and figures by Patrick Szpak of the Humanities Computing and Media Centre at the University of Victoria. Ashley Rayner helped track down images and permission to reprint various excerpts, and Eileen Eckert provided a sharp eye for copyediting. The generous attention of many professionals has contributed to this work. I am responsible for the shortcomings that remain.

It has been observed that an author's family responsibilities encourage a quality that readers appreciate: brevity. This may be less true for me than for some other writers, but my wife, Susan, my son, Zachary, and my daughter, Abigail, deserve my thanks and gratitude nonetheless. The challenges that this book explores belong not only to the past but also to our children. I dedicate this work to mine.

ACRONYMS

ADA	Americans with Disabilities Act
AIDS	acquired immunodeficiency syndrome
APHA	American Public Health Association
ART	anti-retroviral therapy
AZT	azidothymidine
BCG	Bacillus Calmette-Guérin tuberculosis vaccine
BSE	bovine spongiform encephalitis
CDC	US Centers for Disease Control and Prevention
DDT	dichloro-diphenyl-trichloroethane
DNA	deoxyribonucleic acid
DOTS	directly observed therapy, short course
EDF	Environmental Defense Fund
EPA	Environmental Protection Agency
EPI	Expanded Programme on Immunization
EVD	Ebola virus disease
FDA	United States Food and Drug Administration
FMD	foot and mouth disease
GREP	Global Rinderpest Eradication Program
GRID	Gay-Related Immune Deficiency
GRO	British General Registry Office
H/HA	hemagglutinin
HAART	highly active anti-retroviral therapy

HAT	human African trypanosomiasis
HCMV	human cytomegalovirus
HEW	United States Department of Health, Education, and Welfare
HIV	human immunodeficiency virus
HSV-2	herpes simplex virus
HTLV	human T-cell leukemia virus
IPT	isoniazid preventive therapy
IPV	inactivated polio vaccine
LAV	lymphadenopathy associated virus
MBTC	mycobacterium tuberculosis complex
MCA	Medieval Climate Anomaly
MCWA	Office of Malaria Control in War Areas
MDR-TB	multi-drug-resistant tuberculosis
MEP	Malaria Eradication Programme
MHS	United States Marine Hospital Service
MSM	men who have sex with men
N/NA	neuraminidase
NFIP	National Foundation for Infantile Paralysis
OIE	World Organization for Animal Health
OPV	oral polio vaccine
ORT	oral rehydration treatment
PAHO	Pan American Health Organization
PAS	para-aminosalicylic acid
PCR	polymerase chain reaction
PLHIV	people living with HIV
POP	persistent organic pollutant
PPS	post-polio syndrome
RNA	ribonucleic acid
SARS	severe acute respiratory syndrome
SNP	single nucleotide polymorphism
STI	sexually transmitted infection
UN	United Nations
UN-FAO	United Nations Food and Agriculture Organization
UNICEF	United Nations International Children's Fund
USPHS	United States Public Health Service
WHO	World Health Organization
YFV	yellow fever virus

INTRODUCTION

n 1972, two preeminent scientists suggested that, barring mishap, "the most likely forecast about the future of infectious disease is that it will be very dull."[1] One of these men, Frank Macfarlane Burnet, had won a Nobel Prize after decades devoted to the study of viruses and immunology. Many signs pointed toward a bright future. In the previous quarter century, vaccinations had banished polio from North America and Europe; global childhood mortality had diminished; a new antibiotic, penicillin, had transformed the treatment of many bacterial infections; and the total eradication of smallpox was within sight. Burnet had even suggested that the mid-twentieth century had reached the end of a revolution: "the virtual elimination of the infectious diseases as a significant factor in social life."[2]

This optimism now appears very distant. Beginning in the 1980s, it was cut short by the emergence and harrowing impact of acquired immunodeficiency syndrome (AIDS), a resurgence of tuberculosis and malaria, and the new visibility of other threats such as severe acute respiratory syndrome (SARS), Ebola virus disease (EVD), and Zika virus disease. Instead of a confident march toward the defeat of such scourges, researchers discovered numerous new human pathogens. They glimpsed the dawn of an era of emerging infections.[3] Lethal diseases are an old problem—they receded somewhat from Western countries but never disappeared—and they are also a new problem because the social, ecological, and environmental changes of the last several centuries have transformed the planet's landscapes of health and illness. The quickening pace of change in recent decades has served to increase the significance of disease in global affairs rather than diminish it.

The premise of this book is that diseases and the forces of modernity are mutually constitutive—in other words, diseases have both shaped and been shaped by distinctive aspects of the modern world. Or, as two recent scholars more bluntly put it: "Microbes are the ultimate critics of modernity."[4] * A study of diseases in history enables us to reflect on how the modern world took shape. Many contemporary challenges, and the tools available to meet them, have arisen from an extraordinary interplay of human, biological, and environmental forces.

At the outset, it is useful to consider what is meant by "modern," a term that provides a framework for this book but is also subject to interpretation and revision. Although some aspects of current culture may be described as postmodern, or as a reaction against modernity, the term still describes many important concepts, technologies, and social patterns. The idea of a modern world owes much to the seminal works of the German sociologist Max Weber (1864–1920). Writing in the early twentieth century, Weber contemplated the global dominance of western Europe and North America, which seemed unparalleled in human history. Weber stressed the influence of a rational, calculating approach to the natural world and human society. He further suggested that religious belief and communal solidarity had largely been replaced by regulation and technologies designed to channel, measure, and control the actions of individuals and groups.[5] Although Weber himself was ambivalent about the evolution he perceived, many Western observers adopted a concept of "modernity" as a yardstick with which to judge the achievements of societies around the world. The adoption by non-Western peoples of Western scientific medicine and public health, the spread of industrialization and economic development, and the growth of Western political institutions were all taken as signs of increasing prosperity and progress.

Weber described many dimensions of his world, but he also left aside others that were significant in his era and have only grown in importance over the last century. As critics have pointed out, beginning in the late fifteenth century many elements of modernity in the West were influenced by relationships of dependency or exploitation that Europeans forged with other peoples. Non-Western countries contain a majority of the world's population, and many societies have

---

* This book will use the term "microbe" in an expansive sense to refer to microbiological organisms including viruses and prions.

religious, political, and cultural configurations that evolved along paths that Weber and other theorists did not envision. Narratives of world history written from a Western viewpoint are only beginning to account for the many reciprocal interactions and independent developments around the globe that have shaped modernity for all.

Even more fundamental is the shift that has taken place over the last several centuries in the human relationship with nature. In a remarkably short time, human activity has become an environmental and ecological force that affects the planet as a whole. Of course, premodern societies shaped the natural world. Many environments that explorers considered pristine actually bore the influence of human manipulation that reached back thousands of years. Only in relatively recent times, however, have humans crisscrossed continents with railroads and highways or linked oceans with large canals, introduced antibiotics and vaccines into billions of people and animals, and dropped vast quantities of pesticides (as well as bombs) from the air. In particular, some historians point to the importance of a "Great Acceleration" in demographic and environmental change after World War II, when human actions increasingly shaped fundamental dynamics in the Earth's biosphere.[6] Whether we consider the last seven centuries or the last seventy years, there can be no doubt of the far-reaching consequences of this shift. Any concept of modernity must encompass human interrelationship *with* the natural world as well as the development of societies *in* the world.

From this point of view, the range of modern achievements and challenges appears very different in the early twenty-first century than what many experts perceived only a few decades ago. Medicine and public health have vastly expanded the capacity to prevent and cure disease, and, in two spectacular cases, even eradicated dangerous diseases from nature. However, the benefits of these advances must be measured against the disease-causing impact of industrial cities; the involuntary migration of millions of people, including the forced migration of slaves; the ecological transformation of vast landscapes; devastation caused by warfare; and the inequality that is a persistent feature of local communities and the world economy. The effects of such forces on human health and well-being have been mostly unintentional, and often unacknowledged, but they belong on the balance sheet when we consider how the modern world has taken shape. A fuller balance sheet suggests that Burnet's revolution may be closer to its beginning than its end.

Disease, Epidemics, and Their Historians

The human contemplation of diseases and their significance probably accompanied the earliest reflections on mortality and vulnerability. Ancient oral traditions and writings linked diseases to spirits or the ultimate forces that governed existence. The stories that became the Hebrew sacred writings (*Tanakh*, also the Christian Old Testament) describe how the god Yahweh punishes both the Hebrews and their enemies with pestilence. The opening of the Greek epic *The Iliad* recounts that the god Apollo rained down arrows of pestilence as punishment for the mistreatment of one of his priests. Likewise, Indian teachings about disease in the Sanskrit texts *Atharvaveda* and *Ṛigveda* (ca 1000 BCE) attributed disease to the actions of deities or demons. For example, the divine figure *takmán* was conceived in terms of thunder and lightning that brought fever along with the monsoon rains.[7]

By the end of the first millennium BCE, medical authors in various societies also considered health in relation to human physiology and natural forces. As city populations and trade networks expanded throughout the ancient world, observers reflected upon the causes and impact of pestilence. A famous example is *The Peloponnesian War* in which the Greek historian Thucydides (ca 460–400 BCE) describes the devastation wrought in 430 BCE by an outbreak of disease in Athens during its war with Sparta. Historians have been struck by his cool, detached analysis of the scourge's movement into Athens, its violent, deadly symptoms, and the disintegration of morality in its wake. Devoid of spiritual content, Thucydides's narrative nonetheless carries a stern message. The description of the pestilence follows a lengthy oration by the esteemed leader Pericles that proclaims the virtues of Athenian society. The juxtaposition of lofty ideals with an unsparing account of social collapse implicitly criticizes Athens's ignoble departure from its essential values as it pursued a mirage of imperial glory. Through the centuries, countless chroniclers echoed Thucydides's verdict on Athens with their own commentaries upon human frailty and fallibility in the face of war, famine, and plague.

Thucydides wrote during a pivotal era in the development of Greek medicine. He used the term for disease that was conventional in his day (*nosos*) to refer to the Athenian plague. However, in his lifetime some Greeks began to apply the term **epidemic** to contexts related to health and disease, although in a way that differed from the word's uses thousands of years later. This term combined a prefix, *epi*—meaning "upon, or among"—with *demos*, a word for "people." It carried a further connotation of a person who is "back home" or "in his country." Here it is useful to note that modern scientists use other Greek words in a similar way. The term **epizootic** combines *epi* with a Greek term for animal, *zoon*, to indicate disease among one or more nonhuman animal species. Likewise, **zoonoses**, or zoonotic infections, are diseases that are transmitted from animals to people.

The earliest known use of "epidemic" in connection with disease is as a title for seven books titled *Epidemics* that were written at different times between the late fifth century and the mid-fourth century BCE. These books were ascribed (like many Greek medical works from this period) to the shadowy figure Hippocrates (ca 460–380 BCE). Brief references to him by classical Greek authors convey an impression that Hippocrates was already well known during his lifetime, but it is not clear that he wrote any of the texts that later were credited to him.[8] Broadly speaking, the Hippocratic writings did not reject religion entirely but they focused upon environment, behavior, physiology, and psychology as factors that influenced health. The *Epidemics* grouped together clinical descriptions of diseases that seemed typical of particular seasons and regions. An epidemic might be a winter cough, a marshland fever, or a summer diarrhea; it was "that which circulates and propagates in a country."[9] The term made no claim about *how* diseases spread; indeed, the *Epidemics* were concerned with diseases that were common or characteristic in a particular setting, rather than sudden, unexpected outbreaks. Another Hippocratic text, entitled *Airs, Waters, Places*, provided further reflections on the role played by the seasons, weather, and landscape in the distinct disease environments of various regions.

Alongside other Hippocratic writings, *Epidemics* and *Airs, Waters, Places* exerted tremendous influence. In Europe, they were read for their medical content at least until the eighteenth century. Thereafter, the concepts of both "epidemic" and "disease" shifted, especially as theorists developed various concepts of **contagion** to explain how disease moved from one object or person to another. In the spirit of the Hippocratic writings, ideas concerning disease transmission at first were linked to the environment, and especially to atmospheric changes that seemed to foster or inhibit the movement of disease from place to place. Beginning in the later nineteenth century, scientific accounts of the **etiology** of disease—its causes, or manner of causation—increasingly focused on **infection** that resulted from the behavior of **pathogenic** (or disease-causing) microbes. This shift was enabled by new microscopes with sufficient power to observe many microbes and, more broadly, by the development of laboratory procedures for the investigation of cells, bacteria, and other natural forms that were invisible to the unassisted eye.

In tandem with the growth of the natural sciences, medical history—and within it, the history of disease—emerged as a subject of scholarly inquiry. Interest in the topic was particularly strong among German academics. In 1906, the first institute of medical history was founded in Leipzig under the direction of Karl Sudhoff. At universities with prominent medical schools, notably in the United States at the Johns Hopkins Institute of Medical History, the discipline established itself as a supplement or a corrective to the scientific study of diseases and cures. Several outstanding historians of this era, including Owsei Temkin, Erwin Ackerknecht, and Henry Sigerist, were immigrants to the United States who were deeply influenced by European sociology and philosophy. As investigation of the material causes of disease rapidly advanced, they argued that disease was a social construct as much as a biological reality.

The historians' intellectual thrust revolved around several basic claims. First, works such as Temkin's essay "The Scientific Approach to Disease" (1946) argued that there is no such thing as a "normal body."[10] This idea, Temkin asserted, is an intellectual construct that serves human purposes, not a natural state that exists on its own. He pointed out that individuals are unique, and their experience of disease over time—which is subjective as well as physical—is influenced by personal circumstances and events in ways that biological forces cannot explain. Second, historical works explored how communities determined which physical or mental conditions were (or were not) diseases. It was claimed that biological changes, such as physical symptoms that accompany infection with a particular pathogen, only become diseases when a society acknowledges them as such. A classic study by the Polish physician Ludwik Fleck further argued that scientists are influenced by their community just like everyone else. In his book published in 1935, and later translated as *The Genesis and Development of a Scientific Fact* (1979), Fleck traced centuries of change in the perception of syphilis and its relationship to other maladies. In Fleck's own day, scientists had identified a causal microbe, and a test that detected this microbe in the body defined who "had syphilis." Nonetheless, Fleck argued, science had not found the absolute truth of the disease. Perceptions of natural phenomena were always bound to prevailing scientific theories and methods. While such concepts might shift over time, Fleck argued that the "thought collective" among investigators usually conditioned them to accept some ideas and reject others.

How did advances in the natural sciences and historical sociology influence the concept of an epidemic and the current use of the term? Epidemics became linked to outbreaks of specific diseases that were defined by the presence of causal microbes or distinctive manifestations in individual sufferers. Today, experts in the discipline of **epidemiology** often rely on statistics: in general, they define an epidemic as a marked increase in the **incidence** of a disease (the number of reported cases in a defined population over a given time interval) above a given baseline in a designated region. Further, a disease's incidence is distinguished from its **prevalence** (the number of cases observed in a population at one particular time). An epidemic's severity may also be gauged by levels of **morbidity**—the cases of disease attributed to a specific cause—and **mortality**, or deaths attributed to a specific cause. Statistics must always be used with care and especially for disease outbreaks in the past. For events of earlier centuries, counts of the sick or dead are often unavailable, and even when such numbers are reported they often do not reflect modern conceptions of disease. Accordingly, this book will use statistics sparingly to indicate the magnitude of an event or to make broad comparisons between the disease landscapes of historical periods or geographic regions.

Other important terms require similar nuance. An example is **endemic**, which denotes a disease or condition that is considered widespread and continually present (usually at a low level) in a particular region. While this term is often used in contrast with "epidemic," in fact the distinction sometimes blurs. Some diseases, such as tuberculosis or malaria, can flare up in sudden outbreaks in some contexts and smolder over a long period in others. When we recall that the Hippocratic author used "epidemic" in a way that resembles the current use of "endemic," it is clear that the use of these terms requires a thoughtful approach. The word **pandemic** is usually reserved for great eruptions of disease that strike across continents or, in the extraordinary case of influenza in 1918–19, the entire world. But even this word is not entirely unproblematic. Some pandemics of the past may not have left traces in the historical record, either because the disease was not severe or because observers did not discern how widespread it was. And diseases may change character over time. In the mid-1980s and 1990s, AIDS was described as a pandemic disease, but in the twenty-first century it has become a continuous, steady presence at lower levels of incidence.

In writing that is addressed to a broad public, the term "epidemic" frequently evokes a crisis that is caused by an uncontrolled, spreading threat. Writers may deploy the word to raise alarm about conditions other than diseases, such as violent crime, poverty, or opioid use. The word itself tells a story: "epidemic" signals an increased incidence of a disease (a beginning); a continuation and measures to combat the problem (a middle); and an eventual decline of disease and a return to the status quo (an end). The dramatic quality assigned to this term in its modern usage has not been lost on historians. They have found outbreaks of disease, like other crises, to be a kind of laboratory for the investigation of social structures and movements. The classic example is cholera in nineteenth-century Europe: the disease marched across continents in waves, announced its arrival with violent physical symptoms, and exacerbated all sorts of social conflicts between classes, ethnic groups, and religious clans before it abated. Since the 1960s, many historians such as Charles Rosenberg, Richard Evans, and Catherine Kudlick have used the framework that cholera epidemics offered to explore class tensions and other key themes in nineteenth-century social history.[11] Scholars have applied a similar model to other diseases as well, such as Pule Phoofolo's discussion of rinderpest in southern Africa at the end of the nineteenth century.[12]

More broadly, historians have debated how to describe the interrelated biological and social factors that constitute disease. Especially from the 1960s to the 1980s, some scholars resorted to the concept of **social construction** to assert that medicine and disease were shaped at their core by contingent social factors. Studies with this approach—which were not limited to medical history—often were influenced by the French philosopher Michel Foucault (1926–1984), who popularized the claim that knowledge often becomes a tool of domination. Although the exercise of power can be diffuse, Foucault suggested that institutions frequently use technologies and classifications to marginalize certain groups or legitimize social control. To a degree, interest in this theme continues, notably among scholars such as Amy Fairchild and Alison Bashford, who explore the important relationship between public health, border control, and national identity.[13]

However, some scholars objected that the notion of social construction makes the practice of medical science seem arbitrary, or even dictated by ideological and mercenary interests. These critics pointed out that diseases can exist without any social commentary—in animals as well as people—and medical advances such as **vaccines** depend upon the manipulation of microbes and chemicals rather than social relationships. Human scientists may have a social agenda, but such natural entities do not. Charles Rosenberg's influential approach to the problem has been to suggest that the biological realities of disease are "framed" by individuals and groups who are influenced by numerous psychological, social, and cultural forces.[14] "[W]e cannot discuss the *what* of disease," Rosenberg writes, "without discussing the *when* and the *where*." A sixteenth-century physician used a different set of tools and theories than a nineteenth-century one. Likewise, a modern hospital database that relies on number codes will frame disease differently than a clinician who is talking with a patient. But Rosenberg maintains that biology matters—a pathogen's behavior and a disease's manifestations influence not only individual health but also the collective understanding of the disease within a society. Thus, nineteenth-century observers understood "the cholera," which was marked by violent spasms, diarrhea, and vomiting, quite differently than the coughing, chronic wasting, and slow loss of vitality attributed to "consumption" and later to "tuberculosis."

While the history of disease often has been exploited by social historians working in national traditions, it has also been a theme for scholars who explore developments on a transnational or global scale. As Emmanuel Le Roy Ladurie observed in an important essay, after 1300 a thickening web of communication across Eurasia and across the oceans resulted in a "unification of the globe by disease."[15] William McNeill's *Plagues and Peoples* (1976) introduced a broad audience to the claim that diseases have fundamentally shaped the interactions of different peoples. McNeill suggested that "civilized" regions such as the ancient Roman and Chinese empires developed distinctive "disease pools" of characteristic ailments. Pandemics ensued when disease pools collided. Thus, McNeill claimed, the Black Death was the result of East-West contact between Mongols and Europeans. Likewise, the decimation of Indigenous American peoples after 1500 reflected their vulnerability to diseases such as smallpox and influenza that were brought by early explorers and conquerors.[*]

In a similar vein, Alfred Crosby produced a series of works focused on the transatlantic exchange between Europe and the Americas. Crosby popularized the term "**virgin soil epidemic**" to indicate that Indigenous Americans were defenseless against European microbes to which they had no immunity.[16] As these authors and others observed, transport technology played a key role by vastly increasing the speed and scale of interregional contact. Particularly in the nineteenth century, steam-powered ships and railroads enabled the rapid global spread of diseases such as cholera, plague, yellow fever, and the cattle disease rinderpest. The early stages of modern globalization exacted a heavy toll on the health of many peoples, including islanders and inhabitants of the Arctic. Elements of this line of argument were restated in Jared Diamond's influential

---

[*] This book uses the widely adopted term "Indigenous" to refer to the pre-European inhabitants of the Americas and other regions. Terms such as "Native," "Native American," or "American Indian" are used in some circumstances and readers are encouraged to consider what is most appropriate for them.

Guns, Germs and Steel (1997), which suggested that early exposure of Eurasians to diseases contributed to their dominance in the later global balance of power.

Although aspects of these works are persuasive, critics have noted that they can lead to a distorted vision of history that rests on a false opposition of "the West and the rest." Non-Western peoples may be cast in various roles: as inevitable victims of disease because of their incomplete social (and therefore immunological) development; as the source of "tropical" diseases that strike the developed West; or, in recent decades, as the inhabitants of weak societies unable to stem the tide of suffering caused by AIDS, tuberculosis, and malaria. While the exploration of cross-cultural connections has value, such a history can flatten out the distinctive stories of cultures that are described in terms of their "progress" or "response" to the forces of a Western-led globalization. Recent historians have sought approaches that avoid this binary. With respect to early encounters across the Atlantic, David Jones and others have claimed that the presumed lack of immunity to disease among Indigenous Americans fails to explain high mortality among them after the arrival of Europeans.[17] The picture is more complex: social, economic, and political forces, which varied according to particular contexts, played a greater role than innate biological differences among peoples. Robert Peckham's *Epidemics in Modern Asia* demonstrates that "epidemic histories" provide a way to explore the interaction of local circumstances and global processes among diverse Asian communities.[18] Insights from various disciplines, including environmental history, archaeology, historical anthropology, and epidemiology, have contributed to a narrative that takes account of a wider range of historical actors and forces.

This textbook rests upon a rich intellectual tradition that has been energized by its ability to embrace insights from numerous types of studies. In particular, the book is structured to incorporate recent research in the natural sciences—in genetics, microbiology, immunology, parasitology, and climatology—that has made important contributions to our understanding of many diseases in the past and today. This research illuminates the profound influence that humans have exerted, and continue to exert, upon the circumstances of life on our planet. For thousands of years, humans have spread diseases from one place to another and created agricultural and urban environments within which diseases take hold in complex and changing ways. However, human influence now goes even deeper: by transforming landscapes on a vast scale, and by altering microbial environments, humans have irrevocably changed the pathogens that cause disease, the means by which pathogens spread, and the relationships between diseases. The forces of modernity have solved some problems, exacerbated others, and in some cases created challenges that are completely new.

The Plan for This Book—And How to Read It

Epidemics and the Modern World concentrates upon infectious diseases: pathological conditions caused by microbes that enter the body. Many infections, including the main ones discussed in this book, are also communicable, meaning that they pass between people directly—by touch or a cough, for example—or indirectly through an insect, a contaminated water supply, or some other medium. Although (apparently) noncommunicable conditions such as heart disease are now leading causes of death and are important historically, over centuries it is diseases such as plague, smallpox, cholera, and AIDS that have left the greatest imprint.

The eleven main chapters are all laid out the same way. A brief—and necessarily superficial—outline of the current scientific understanding of a disease is followed by a chronological discussion of topics that are related to this disease in modern history. Each chapter concentrates on a particular time frame to illuminate a theme that is pertinent to the development of the modern world. On occasion, the chronologies overlap and material in one chapter will contribute to the discussion in another. Words that are in bold type are included in a glossary. In addition to the notes, suggestions for further reading are provided at the end of the book.

Historians have found the "biography" of disease to be a useful means of exploring environmental, social, and scientific change over the long term. The format lends itself to comparison of the forces that have created the distinctive challenges of each disease. Following the lead of historians such as Bruce Campbell and Monica Green, this book uses recent scientific insights to help understand nature as a protagonist in history.[19] Science Focus boxes in each chapter provide expanded explanations of particular concepts and technologies, both to elaborate on a chapter's narrative and for general reference.

While this structure has its advantages, cautions to the reader are also in order. A clear focus upon one disease may serve as a starting point from which to consider interrelationships among various forces. However, the claim is not made that diseases act independently in history or that we can always tell when a particular disease as understood today was at work in the past. One reason is that, prior to the mid-nineteenth century, medical practitioners usually focused on the indications of disease that appeared in individuals rather than groups.

They categorized all sorts of maladies very differently than later scientists who focused on causal microbes. Second, microbes and their relationship to environments and other organisms change over time. Usually, this has been a gradual process, but not always—we must allow for factors that may have altered the characteristics and impact of disease-causing agents. Finally, there is often great variation in how persons perceive or experience disease. Two individuals today who contract the same influenza virus may encounter their illness very differently because of many social or biological factors. The same was true in the past, of course, which adds to the challenge of understanding how (or if) a particular disease influenced persons or groups.

An illustration may demonstrate the challenge. Tuberculosis, viewed with the tools of genetics and evolutionary biology, has a continuous human history that reaches back thousands of years or more. But the ancient Greeks referred instead to an apparently similar malady, or group of maladies, that they called **phthisis**; Europeans in 1800 described a cluster of ailments that, in English, was labeled **consumption**; only in the 1880s was a causal microbe observed and later named *Mycobacterium tuberculosis*; and today, in an era when microbial environments have been shaped by antibiotics, many cases of the disease are called multi-drug-resistant tuberculosis (MDR-TB). After all the material and conceptual shifts that have taken place, can all of these reckonings belong to the history of a single disease? Most historians believe they can; the alternative is to treat diseases of different eras or regions as entities that cannot be compared or adequately described by a human-constructed medical science. This latter perspective hardly seems more accurate and ultimately may be self-defeating. Nonetheless, we must respect the gaps in historical sources, resist the urge to apply contemporary concepts in ways that are anachronistic or unsupported by historical evidence, and not assume that the vantage point of Western medicine can always explain the experience of disease among peoples around the world.

These cautions also apply to the use of modern scientific tools to identify diseases of the past, an exercise known as **retrospective diagnosis**. As explained in chapter 1, the analysis of ancient strands of genetic material—deoxyribonucleic acid, or DNA—now allows researchers to identify some long-ago pathogens with far greater confidence than was possible only a few years ago. Some historians have proclaimed an end to a heated debate about the causes of Europe's Black Death in the mid-fourteenth century. Analysis of ancient DNA is an exciting advance but it has limits—only a few diseases have left genetic footprints that can be analyzed at present. There is always the potential that a disease was experienced differently in the past, even if the causal microbe bears a close relationship to microbes of today. Diseases are a moving target; often we must acknowledge that our ability to understand past landscapes of disease is constrained by a lack of knowledge about all the factors at work.

This book, therefore, draws freely on recent science but does not assume that our knowledge about diseases today applies equally to all times and places. Moreover, as the following chapters will explore, the creation of scientific knowledge is itself a historical process that requires explanation and critical engagement. All science will be history one day. With this in mind, we may approach current scientific explanations critically and also maintain a sympathetic approach to the insights about nature that were developed in the past.

A Note about Primary Sources

Reading an account of history can be rewarding, but the main work of historians is to investigate documents or artifacts that were produced in the past. Broadly speaking, historians distinguish the products of a past era that are their subject of interest (primary sources) from subsequent analyses and commentary that reflect on the past from a critical distance (secondary sources). A workshop at the end of each chapter invites the reader to enter into the practice of history by presenting a selection of primary sources that are related to the chapter's main themes, as well as suggestions for secondary readings.

Exploring the past through primary sources is fascinating and also often difficult. One challenge is that the stuff of history survives in many different forms. This applies not only to physical evidence, such as ruins or skeletons, but also to various kinds of written documents. Different genres of writing are intended to accomplish various objectives. In order to understand a text, one must first know something about why it was produced and the audience for whom it was written. Then there is the challenge of actual reading: the ideas of earlier writers, or the ways that they express them, may appear exotic or obtuse. Most writing, after all, is produced for an author's contemporaries and addresses concerns of the day, not the interests of a future reader. Decades or centuries later, students may be surprised or uncomfortable when they encounter people whose core beliefs concerning divine forces, women and men, "foreign" ethnic groups, or the environment differ radically from theirs. But this is inevitable—principles of equity or justice that seem fundamental today were simply not shared, or sometimes even imagined, by people of earlier times. Moral convictions often were linked to beliefs concerning human beings, the natural world, or the causes of events that later societies have radically recast or discarded altogether.

It may, therefore, seem appropriate to distance oneself from the medieval professor who believes that plague is caused by stinking clouds, the Christian moralist who suggests that cholera or syphilis are God's punishment for sin, or colonizers and slaveholders who criticize the lifestyles of "savage" or "primitive" peoples around the world. However—here is the key point—when historians read primary sources, the first goal always is to ask *why* people in the past believed and acted as they did, rather than to show how they fail to meet the standards of a later era. To understand is not to accept or agree; indeed, the best historians can develop appreciation and even sympathy for people with whom they strongly *disagree*. People of any time are complex. One of the most fascinating lessons of history is the discovery that historical actors can represent ideas that seem utterly contradictory until we investigate the mentality of their time.

Notes

1. Frank Macfarlane Burnet and David O. White, *Natural History of Infectious Disease*, 4th ed. (Cambridge: Cambridge University Press, 1972), 263.

2. Frank Macfarlane Burnet, *Natural History of Infectious Disease*, 2nd ed. (Cambridge: Cambridge University Press, 1953), ix.

3. Joshua Lederberg, Robert E. Shope, and Stanley C. Oaks Jr, eds, *Emerging Infections: Microbial Threats to Health in the United States* (Washington, DC: National Academy Press, 1992).

4. Ron Barrett and George Armelagos, *An Unnatural History of Emerging Infections* (Oxford: Oxford University Press, 2013), 1.

5. Bryan S. Turner, "The Rationalization of the Body: Reflections on Modernity and Discipline," in *Max Weber: From History to Modernity* (London: Routledge, 1993), 115–38.

6. J.R. McNeill and Peter Engelke, *The Great Acceleration: An Environmental History of the Anthropocene since 1945* (Cambridge, MA: Harvard University Press, 2014), 207–208.

7. Kenneth G. Zysk, *Medicine in the Veda* (Delhi: Motilal Bonarsidass Publishers, 1996), 34–44.

8. Vivian Nutton, *Ancient Medicine* (New York: Routledge, 2004), 55–58.

9. Paul M.V. Martin and Estelle Martin-Granel, "2,500-Year Evolution of the Term Epidemic," *Emerging Infectious Diseases* 12, no. 6 (2006): 979.

10. Beth Linker, "On the Borderland of Medical History and Disability: A Survey of the Fields," *Bulletin of the History of Medicine* 87, no. 4 (2013): 506–10.

11. Richard J. Evans, *Death in Hamburg*, 2nd ed. (New York: Penguin Books, 2005); Catherine J. Kudlick, *Cholera in Post-Revolutionary Paris: A Cultural History* (Berkeley: University of California Press, 1996); and Charles E. Rosenberg, *The Cholera Years*, 2nd ed. (Chicago: University of Chicago Press, 1987).

12. Pule Phoofolo, "Epidemics and Revolutions: The Rinderpest Epidemic in Late Nineteenth-Century Southern Africa," *Past and Present* 123 (1993): 112–43.

13. Amy Fairchild, *Science at the Borders: Immigrant Medical Inspection and the Shaping of the Modern Industrial Labor Force* (Baltimore: Johns Hopkins University Press, 2003); and Alison Bashford, ed., *Medicine at the Border: Disease, Globalization and Security, 1850 to the Present* (New York: Palgrave Macmillan, 2006).

14. Charles E. Rosenberg and Janet Golden, eds, *Framing Disease: Studies in Cultural History* (New Brunswick: Rutgers University Press, 1997); and Charles E. Rosenberg, "What Is Disease? In Memory of Owsei Temkin," *Bulletin of the History of Medicine* 77, no. 3 (2003): 496–98.

15. Emmanuel Le Roy Ladurie, "A Concept: The Unification of the Globe by Disease," in *The Mind and Method of the Historian*, trans. Siân Reynolds and Ben Reynolds (Chicago: University of Chicago Press, 1981), 28–83.

16. Alfred W. Crosby, "Virgin Soil Epidemics as a Factor in the Aboriginal Depopulation of America," *William and Mary Quarterly* 33, no. 2 (1976): 289–99; and David S. Jones, "Virgin Soils Revisited," *William and Mary Quarterly* 60, no. 4 (2003): 703–42.

17. David S. Jones, "Death, Uncertainty and Rhetoric," in *Beyond Germs: Native Depopulation in North America*, ed. Paul Kelton, Alan C. Swedlund, and Catherine M. Cameron (Tucson: University of Arizona Press, 2015), 16–49.

18. Robert Peckham, *Epidemics in Modern Asia* (Cambridge: Cambridge University Press, 2016), 15.

19. Bruce M.S. Campbell, *The Great Transition: Climate, Disease and Society in the Late-Medieval World* (Cambridge: Cambridge University Press, 2016), 21; and Monica H. Green, "The Globalisations of Disease," in *Human Dispersal and Species Movement: From Prehistory to the Present*, ed. Nicole Boivin, Rémy Crassard, and Michael D. Petraglia (Cambridge: Cambridge University Press, 2017), 494–520.

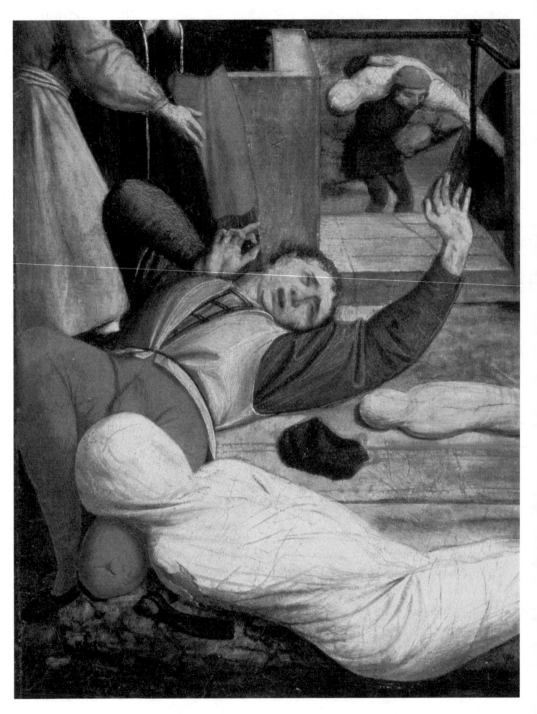

IMAGE 1.1 *St Sebastian Interceding for the Plague-Stricken*—detail (ca 1500). Signs of death attend this victim of bubonic plague. A bubo is clearly visible on his neck. The full image is reproduced on p. 32.

BUBONIC PLAGUE
AND THE MODERN STATE

I n 1345, Mongol forces led by Khan Janibeg attacked Kaffa, a fortified port on the Black Sea controlled by merchants from the Italian city-state of Genoa. Thereafter, a savage epidemic tore through the besieging army. Soldiers died as soon as telltale swellings appeared in the armpit and groin. The discouraged Mongols catapulted corpses over the walls, poisoning the air and water and filling the city with a terrible stench. As Italians fled to Genoa, Venice, and other cities they brought the pestilence with them. Death "entered through the windows" as returning sailors poisoned entire families and cities mourned in the face of God's awesome wrath.

That was how Gabriele de' Mussis, a lawyer in Piacenza, described the arrival of the great pestilence later known as the Black Death in a treatise he wrote around 1350.[1] De' Mussis was less concerned with accurate reporting than with the moral significance of the episode. To his first readers, Italians who themselves experienced horrific mortality firsthand, de' Mussis offered an archetypal tale of divine punishment for human wickedness that evoked biblical stories of the plagues of Egypt. There is little reason to doubt his description of the battle— besieging armies often used corpses as weapons—but the siege at Kaffa may not have been the only source of the pestilence that entered Europe. The conflict ended well before the pandemic reached Italy, and other maritime and overland routes probably contributed to its spread.

However, de' Mussis's apocalyptic language was entirely justified, as was his belief that great mortality had struck the entire world known to him. The Black Death followed on the heels of other challenges—cooler weather and crop failures, a massive die-off of livestock, warfare in many regions—and winnowed the European population by roughly one-third in only six years (1346–52), with a similar impact in regions of the Middle East and North Africa. Over the next 300 years, as intermittent waves of disease swept across parts of Eurasia, border control and confinement of the sick became central preoccupations for governments in small towns and vast territories. In Europe, calamity entered a world imprinted by agrarian routines, feudal hierarchies, and Christian religious unity. In the eighteenth century, it receded from lands now defined by the governments and political agendas of emergent nation-states.

As another wave of disease struck China and India in the 1890s, teams of scientists used new techniques of microbiology to identify a bacteria that caused plague. Although it killed relatively fewer people than the Black Death, and moved more slowly overland, this pandemic still destroyed millions of lives. Steamships carried it to parts of the world previously untouched by the disease, including North America, where plague persists today among rodents in the western United States.

Conventional accounts have divided plague's human impact into three pandemics: the so-called "Plague of Justinian" that appears in historical sources beginning in 541 CE; the Black Death, which began in central Asia during the 1330s and spread east and west; and the global spread of plague in the early 1890s. This framework for understanding plague's role in human history has been durable, but it has not gone unchallenged. Beginning in the 1980s, some scholars questioned the straightforward identification of plague through the centuries, suggesting instead that the Black Death might have been caused by anthrax or a deadly hemorrhagic fever. More recently, molecular genetics research has demonstrated that a pathogen akin to the bacteria that causes plague today also played a significant (but not exclusive) role in both the Plague of Justinian and the Black Death.

New research methods have also sparked other debates. How and where did the Black Death begin, and did changes in climate during the later Middle Ages influence the outbreak of disease? What is the best explanation for the periodic resurgence of pestilence in Europe between 1350 and 1650 and its almost total disappearance a few decades later? And how did the disease that caused the Black Death relate to the pandemic that killed millions of people in the early twentieth century? Recent investigations have also considered more fully the social contexts outside of Europe and how the Black Death and its aftermath may be understood in a broader continental and global history.[2]

Etiology and Early History

Researchers classify *Yersinia pestis*—named for Alexandre Yersin, one of the first scientists to identify it with a microscope—as a rod-shaped **bacillus** that belongs to a family of **enteric** (intestinal) **bacteria**. In evolutionary terms, it is considered a relative newcomer. Around 30,000 years ago, *Y. pestis* diverged from *Y. pseudotuberculosis*, a food-borne pathogen that causes mild stomach ailments. By perhaps 6,000 years ago, it had evolved into a parasite that survives in various fleas hosted by rodents, including gerbils, prairie dogs, and marmots as well as rats.[3] As fleas became a **vector** for the bacteria's spread into mammals, *Y. pestis* acquired traits that adapted it to survive in fleas and propagate through flea feeding behavior. The bacteria also developed strategies to overwhelm a mammalian host's immune system response and ensure rapid replication in the bloodstream. Transmission of bacteria may occur through flea bites, when contaminated food is eaten, or through scratches and bites from infected animals, including house pets that contract plague from wild rodents. *Y. pestis* can survive in soil for lengthy periods, and large rodent populations can maintain a reservoir of bacteria in underground burrows. Some researchers think the bacteria may inhabit soil ameba, spores, or cysts for years.[4] Future investigation may reveal that plague's persistence is enabled by soil as much as animals. In short, plague has an intricate ecology that mostly involves other animals, and human infection is incidental to its persistence.

When *Y. pestis* does enter a human, the lymphatic system drains bacteria to the lymph nodes where they cause the characteristic painful swellings (buboes) at the neck, armpit, and groin. Plague is now readily cured with **antibiotics** such as **streptomycin**, but without proper medical care the infection is often lethal after three to five days. The bacteria can also proceed to the bloodstream to cause septicemic plague or to the lungs where they cause pneumonic plague. These forms of the disease almost always result in death after less than forty-eight hours if they are left untreated. The pneumonic route of infection is especially contagious because the disease can spread rapidly among people through tiny droplets spread by coughing or sputum. Until the mid-twentieth century, when streptomycin and other antibiotics became widely available, no medicine was effective against plague.

In the late 1990s, innovations in molecular biology began to transform the debate over the nature of the Black Death. A sample of modern *Y. pestis* was genetically sequenced in 1998, and in 2000 researchers first isolated ancient plague DNA. Although early claims were disputed, evidence from numerous gravesites soon satisfied most researchers that *Y. pestis* contributed significantly to

History with Teeth: PCR, Ancient DNA, and the History of Plague

Researchers who examine samples of ancient DNA apply a technique that initially was used to diagnose modern infections: **polymerase chain reaction** (PCR). The technique has enabled them to analyze and compare the structure of ancient bacteria harvested from skeletons that are hundreds or even thousands of years old.

Where in the human body can such samples be found? Early researchers focused on bones. Some diseases left visible lesions but bubonic plague did not. Then, in the late 1990s, a research team in Marseille devised a strategy to extract ancient DNA from dental pulp, which preserved a higher concentration of genetic material from *Y. pestis* that was suitable for PCR analysis.[5]

PCR amplifies a tiny sample of DNA to enable research that otherwise would be impossible (figure 1.1). Essentially, double strands of DNA are shaped like a coiled ladder. Each rung of the ladder, or nucleotide, is formed from a pair of amino acids. In test tubes, long strands of DNA are pulled apart with heat and solvents. Researchers then cool the strands and apply primers—short sequences of single-stranded DNA—that correspond to targeted regions on the DNA ladder. An enzyme (polymerase) is then added that fills in the nucleotides between the primers to build new double strands. Each reaction doubles the number of full strands; thirty-five repetitions of the process produce billions of copies of the targeted region.

PCR helped confirm that mass burial sites in Europe did, in fact, contain numerous people who died from infection with *Y. pestis*. Evidence for the long-term presence of *Y. pestis* has continued to mount. As of 2016, eighteen burial sites had been located from western Europe to central Asia that yielded complete *Y. pestis* genome sequences.[6]

PCR also allows researchers to examine mutations in single rungs on the DNA ladder, or **single nucleotide polymorphisms** (SNPs). Over the centuries, these mutations have left an evolutionary trail that is studied with methods known as **phylogenetic analysis**. Researchers can understand evolutionary relationships among organisms in a manner similar to families that create trees of ancestors and descendants. However, guesswork is involved to estimate how frequently mutations have taken place over time and to infer relationships when physical evidence is not available.

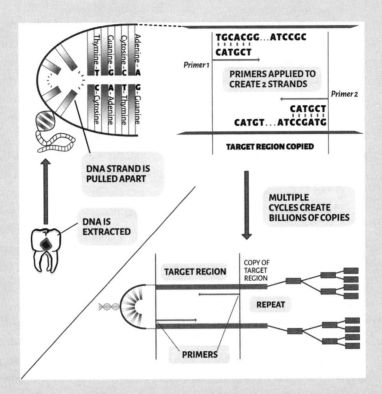

FIGURE 1.1 DNA extraction and amplification by PCR. DNA double helix strands are pulled apart. Primers and polymerase enzyme are added to create two complete strands. This enables exponential replication of DNA.

Phylogenetic analysis enabled researchers to identify a **polytomy**—a genetic divergence into several branches—that took place in *Y. pestis* before the Black Death. The same techniques also revealed astonishing similarities between the bacterial strains that caused the Black Death and those that caused the pandemic that began in China at the end of the nineteenth century. While some types of *Y. pestis* were continually present in Asia, the trail of SNPs suggests that a wave of plague moved back east from western Europe across Asia in the late fourteenth century or thereafter. The *Y. pestis* bacteria that spread out of Hong Kong in 1894 was closely related to a strain that struck London in the late 1340s.

Phylogenetic analysis contributes to public health today. Similar techniques have helped researchers understand influenza viruses and may contribute to the development of more targeted and effective vaccines. PCR has become an indispensable tool for the investigation of pathogens and other DNA from the past and in the present.

episodes of great mortality in late antiquity and the later Middle Ages. Then, in 2011, samples taken from a London burial site for Black Death victims yielded a complete *Y. pestis* genome.[7] Placed alongside modern *Y. pestis* genomes, the sample revealed that plague had actually evolved relatively slowly in the intervening six centuries. The London Black Death genome also provided a reference point that scientists could use to analyze differences among other genetic samples from both before and after the Black Death. Data drawn from more than 100 samples soon pointed to a "big bang" in plague's evolution: before the Black Death, four variants of *Y. pestis* split off from a common ancestor, creating bacterial strains that circulated in later centuries.[8]

The discovery of *Y. pestis*'s genetic divergence is a tantalizing finding but it leaves important questions unanswered. For example, the genetic branching that took place before the Black Death does not indicate that the bacteria suddenly increased in **virulence** (i.e., became more damaging to humans). The sudden polytomy, therefore, does not by itself explain why plague spread so rapidly and killed so many people during the Black Death.[9] Another question concerns the timing of plague's "big bang": while some estimates suggest that the polytomy took place around 1260–1300, dates that are a century earlier cannot be ruled out. This large time frame makes it difficult to link the polytomy to social, biological, or environmental forces that might have caused it. This is especially important when we consider the possible role of climate change in the spread of disease. As discussed later, it is clear that dramatic climate shifts in the later Middle Ages *influenced* the Black Death, but available evidence does not confirm that climate change *caused* the Black Death by affecting bacteria, mammals, or other aspects of the late medieval world.[10]

After nearly seven centuries, the Black Death has become an active arena of historical inquiry. Investigation ranges from examination of minuscule DNA fragments to analysis of long-term climate trends that span the globe. Far from establishing a single "cause" of the pandemic, recent scholarship raises numerous questions that lead us to reconsider the relationship of climatic, biological, and social forces in the later Middle Ages.

Medieval Europe before the Black Death

The swift upheaval of the mid-fourteenth century was preceded by changes that were more gradual but equally significant. Beginning in the late tenth century, European agriculture benefited from a sustained period of warmer temperatures, part of a global shift in climate patterns that is now known as the **Medieval Climate Anomaly** (MCA). For nearly three centuries (ca 950–1250 CE), farmers cleared woodlands and drained marshes. Herders extended grazing into areas that were barren in less kindly times. A vigorous Christian church provided a measure of social cohesion, and its official Latin culture introduced ancient Roman legal concepts as well as religious teachings. In the late thirteenth century, western Europe's population of 60–70 million inhabitants roughly doubled the number of three centuries earlier and approached the maximum population that the available land and farming techniques could support.

Buoyed by a growing urban population and material wealth, Europeans identified opportunities for trade and conquest abroad. After 1095, the church's leaders encouraged military campaigns against Muslim societies in the Middle East and the Iberian Peninsula (modern-day Spain and Portugal). Europeans also traded with their Mediterranean neighbors. Among other goods, they received and translated key texts of Greco-Roman antiquity from Arab scholars who had studied and elaborated on them for centuries. Merchants from Venice, Genoa, and Florence tapped into a Eurasian system of trade that was controlled by Mongol kingdoms in central Asia and anchored at the other end by the Chinese Song and Yuan dynasties. Marco Polo's three-year journey from Venice to Beijing, which he completed in 1274, is emblematic of this transcontinental network and the ascent of European influence within it.

Only a few decades later, circumstances were altogether different. In 1291, the last crusaders and their descendants were expelled from the Levant (now Lebanon and western Syria). Although central-Asian trade routes remained intact, shifting military fortunes diminished Italian trade eastward to a trickle. Rivalry between English and French ruling dynasties erupted in the so-called Hundred Years' War (1337–1453), an episodic conflict that drew in numerous European combatants and caused widespread devastation for several generations. As the MCA gave way to a less stable period in global climate, Europe was beset by an agricultural crisis caused by cooler, wetter weather. The worst effects came after 1315 when a series of bad harvests caused intermittent famine conditions across Europe for a decade. As steady rain and sodden fields became more frequent, diminishing crop yields affected the food supply for both humans and livestock.

Even before the start of the Black Death, the convergence of climate change, overland trade, and European agricultural patterns enabled another deadly threat: an animal pestilence (**panzootic**) that probably caused mortality approaching 50 per cent in the oxen and cows of northern Europe. As discussed more fully in chapter 7, most historians believe this disease was a form of rinderpest, a viral infection related to **measles** that spread among cattle through airborne secretions and water droplets. Beginning in the later 1280s, outbreaks were reported in the Mongol empires and Russia. Parts of Europe encountered the same fate after 1315. A study of manorial records in England found that, in 1319, landlords recorded appalling mortality of cows and oxen that averaged 60 per cent.[11] The overlap with poor harvests made matters worse; after a cattle plague outbreak, livestock herds did not recover for a decade or more, which reduced the availability of work animals and products such as milk and cheese.

In 1348 a writer for the medical faculty at the University of Paris noted that "for some time the seasons have not succeeded each other in the proper way." Recent climate research enables us to affirm the accuracy of such statements and to understand that many aspects of the medieval world were in upheaval in the early fourteenth century. A remarkable combination of human and nonhuman factors opened Europe to the transformative force of the pandemic.

The Black Death and Its Aftermath

As historians incorporate new research findings into their accounts, a map that accurately documents the origin and spread of plague in the thirteenth and fourteenth centuries is a work in progress. It is not unlikely that *Y. pestis* bacteria were present in several regions of central Asia for thousands of years prior to a major pandemic. One scenario for the origin of the Black Death is that, beginning around the 1260s, *Y. pestis* spread west from rodent communities near the vast Qinghai Plateau northeast of the Himalayan Mountains.[12] While this proposal relies in part upon genetic data, a more recent study has drawn attention to numerous samples of plague that were collected from rodents in the Tien Shan Mountains (modern-day Kyrgyzstan), about 1,000 miles northwest of the Qinghai Plateau.[13] Data from these recent samples suggest that plague has circulated in the region since antiquity and the region may have been a site of origin for the sixth-century pandemic. It is also possible that a wave of plague emerged from the Tien Shan region sometime after the early 1200s and progressed both east and west. No known texts from medieval China or the Mongol empires clearly describe plague, but it is likely that the disease caused devastation in central Asia during the early 1330s that was comparable to the experience of Europe fifteen years later.[14]

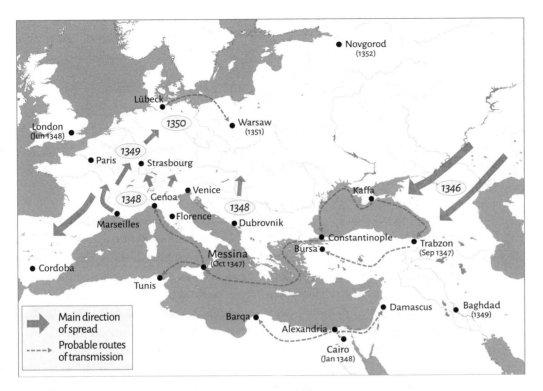

MAP 1.1 Movement of the Black Death, 1346–1352. In the 1340s, a wave of plague spread from central Asia to western Europe. After moving both overland and by ship through the Mediterranean, plague swept north and east across Europe. Ongoing research may soon refine our understanding of its emergence and spread across various regions.

While various questions concerning the start of the Black Death await more study, chronicles and other sources broadly agree about the pandemic's path in western Eurasia from the later 1340s forward. After its arrival in 1346 at the eastern edge of the Black Sea, the plague entered the Genoese trading network, probably in numerous ships over a period of months. It soon reached ports in the Aegean Sea and probably spread overland at the same time. Plague's rapid spread throughout the Mediterranean was assured after it struck Messina, a busy port on the island of Sicily, in autumn 1347. Plague also moved inland, arriving in Paris and southwestern England in the summer of 1348 and most of Ireland and the Iberian Peninsula by the winter of 1349. Thereafter, it continued a roughly clockwise progression through Scandinavia and the rest of northern Europe until the main thrust of the pandemic ebbed in Russia by 1353. In the largest cities, such as Paris and London, outbreaks lasted over a year. Rural communities suffered at least as much, although the arrival, climax, and abatement of an outbreak was often complete in a matter of weeks. The rapid spread between communities and regions was stunning: in only a few years, waves of disease traversed thousands of miles and left few areas unscathed.

Among some historians, the astonishing rate of diffusion elicited doubt that *Y. pestis* caused the Black Death.[15] Indeed, the medieval pandemic spread faster than bubonic plague in India during the early twentieth century, an era of railway travel. Although ancient DNA has now confirmed the presence of *Y. pestis*, the evidence remains puzzling: how did the Black Death spread so quickly and kill so many people?[16] Nongenetic factors have received considerable attention since researchers have found that medieval *Y. pestis* genomes resembled strains that exist today.[17] One possibility is that some medieval communities experienced the pneumonic form of plague that spread rapidly by coughing and sputum without intervening action by fleas or other insects. Although this cannot be ruled out entirely, the rapid progression of pneumonic plague reduces the likelihood that it spread widely and affected overall mortality. Researchers are more drawn to the suggestion that a broader range of skin parasites played a role in the rapid diffusion of disease. Human fleas, and perhaps even lice, may have provided a route for person-to-person transmission. Moreover, the presence of *Y. pestis* does not rule out other infections that either heightened the spread of disease or increased mortality beyond what would be caused by plague alone.

Researchers have also considered social factors that would account for shifting mortality patterns during the Black Death and afterward. In Europe, where the most evidence has survived, roughly one-third of the population died between 1346 and 1352. And the region's population continued to shrink thereafter; the number of Europe's inhabitants in 1400 may have been half the total of a century earlier. Early chroniclers confirmed the famous observations of Giovanni Boccaccio's *Decameron* (ca 1350) that "very few were ever cured" and that the disease indiscriminately killed males and females of all ages regardless of social status. However, some evidence indicates that mortality was somewhat selective, especially in later waves of pestilence. In central Italy, for example, the surviving wills in Tuscan and Umbrian cities indicate that progressively fewer people died in outbreaks from the 1360s forward, and an increasing proportion of the dead were children. It does not seem that repeated exposure to plague resulted in immunity for large populations, but historians have considered factors that may have influenced **immune competence** and susceptibility among individuals or groups. For example, the widespread lack of animal products in the late 1310s may have influenced nutrition among children in ways that, three decades later, contributed to high mortality during the Black Death. As Fabian Crespo and Matthew Lawrenz have recently outlined, food supply, climate, and coinfection with other diseases can all affect human immune response and possibly account for mortality patterns observed across Europe.[18]

Another question that has received recent attention concerns the full extent of the spread of plague into Africa during and after the later Middle Ages. Historical accounts have long cited an epidemic in Cairo in 1348, and it is believed that Egypt experienced dozens of outbreaks in the fifteenth and early sixteenth centuries. While this has been associated with plague's dispersal throughout the Mediterranean, recent studies suggest that Y. pestis penetrated further south into Africa far earlier than previously believed. Texts from Ethiopia record waves of pandemic disease that corresponded to outbreaks in Egypt beginning in the early fifteenth century.[19] This connection relies on chronicles and the biographies of saints, but some genetic evidence—although sparse—also links East African plague samples collected in modern times to a strain that circulated in central Asia in the fifteenth century. What patterns of movement could possibly connect the plague histories of these disparate eras and regions? Monica Green has proposed that sixteenth- and seventeenth-century maritime contests in the Red Sea, a gateway to trade for the Ottoman Empire and its rivals, connected the Black Sea region to East Africa in ways that may have disseminated Y. pestis. Some bacterial strains were introduced later through Indian Ocean trade and imperialism, and plague has persisted in some African environments down to the present day. An important lesson of recent plague research is that Africa's experience with plague is much more complex and multilayered than past historical accounts have shown.[20]

Although events in Africa merit further study, it is already clear that many communities in Europe and elsewhere crossed a demographic threshold in the late fourteenth century and never reverted to pre-Black Death patterns. In the 1350s and 1360s, death and profound social disruption depressed economic activity of all kinds. Prices of food and other goods remained high despite the shrinking population. As dynamics of supply and demand reasserted themselves later in the century, in western Europe landlords struggled to maintain work forces and rent income from a smaller, more mobile group of workers. One response to this challenge was to repurpose less fertile land from farming to less labor-intensive uses such as pasturing sheep. As wages rose in some areas to more than double the pre-Black Death level, another tactic was to pass laws prohibiting demands for increased pay. The late fourteenth century was marked by peasant uprisings large and small, including a major revolt among English peasants in 1381, as lords and laborers competed for advantage in a changed demographic environment. While 90 per cent of western Europe's population remained on farms, immigration into cities increased as newcomers replaced tradesmen and clergy who had vacated their positions. Overall, changes in urbanization were selective: before 1500, while the proportion of city dwellers either stagnated or fell in Italy and Spain, cities in the Low Countries of northwestern Europe experienced marked increases. This growing urban vitality presaged the emergence of the United Provinces as a global maritime power by the end of the sixteenth century.

Across western Europe, in general the demand for relatively scarce labor contributed to the erosion of feudal relationships and their replacement by more flexible arrangements of land rental and tenant farming. However, population declines did not always foster peasant prosperity or autonomy, as examples from other regions indicate. In the Nile River delta, where the plague struck as fiercely as in Europe, repeated outbreaks of disease damaged an agricultural system that depended on labor-intensive canal dredging and dike repair. According to Stuart Borsch, after the Black Death wages fell and, by the time Ottoman rule replaced the Mamluk Sultanate in the early sixteenth century, agricultural productivity was less than half the level of the early fourteenth century.[21] Despite the political change, Egypt continued to experience outbreaks of plague every decade or so until the late nineteenth century. Peasant prospects also dimmed in the region that lay east of the Elbe River in northern Europe. Here landlords controlled large tracts of land in a vast, flat plain that offered few cities or alternatives to the conditions of serfdom. These great estates positioned themselves as suppliers of grain, lumber, and other raw materials for communities further west, ensuring profits for lords and harsh servitude for isolated subjects. Thus, disease-related depopulation did not have the same impact everywhere. A range of factors influenced a slow and halting process of recovery with contrasting outcomes among Eurasian communities.

Medicine and Faith in the Era of Plague

Nearly a century ago, in a book first translated under the title *The Waning of the Middle Ages* (1924), the Dutch historian Johan Huizinga described a late-medieval Europe scarred by suffering that hovered between desperate celebration and quiet despair. Later popular accounts, notably Barbara Tuchman's *A Distant Mirror: The Calamitous Fourteenth Century* (1962), reinforced a gloomy image of Europeans who were suffused with religious guilt and pessimism. Although historians have now called attention to the cultural harvest that this era yielded for later centuries, the contrast with the more confident secularism of recent times still poses a challenge of interpretation. It is tempting to regard both the religious and medical responses to plague with skepticism, or even suspicion. The overbearing influence of Christianity seems clear, not only from innumerable references to God's wrath but also in the violent attacks on Jews that some communities perpetrated. The impotence of medieval medicine—when compared with a swift cure by antibiotics—contributes to a perception that authorities were helpless against the Black Death and other diseases.

But such judgments do not reflect the perspective of Europeans who faced calamity in the fourteenth century. In comparison with earlier times, the resources available to counter disease in 1300 were greater than they had ever been. In universities, which began to be founded around 1200, both medicine and theology (as well as law) were advanced disciplines, although medicine was theology's junior cousin in terms of social prestige and learned pedigree. The church was Europe's largest employer and the chief sponsor of literate culture in monasteries and among Latin-trained officials. The Christian Bible, composed of the ancient Hebrew Old Testament and Greek New Testament, had been translated into Latin, and learned commentaries on it had accumulated over centuries.

In contrast to theology, medicine in the West had a practical bent until the end of the eleventh century, when translated texts introduced concepts from Greco-Roman antiquity and medieval Arabic scholarship. In the south-Italian city of Salerno, numerous texts were translated from Arabic into Latin at the monastery of Monte Cassino. These included works derived from Galen of Pergamum (ca 130–200), a Roman imperial physician who had adapted and expanded Hippocratic medicine in numerous writings. Although Galen served the Roman elite, his texts were composed in Greek and only later were translated to serve the purposes of Latin-trained students and scholars. A core anthology of treatises (called the *Articella* or *Little Art of Medicine*) coalesced in the twelfth century and formed the basis for medical curricula in some early universities. Scholars in twelfth-century Toledo, a Spanish city previously under Muslim control, also translated *The Canon on Medicine* (*Kitāb al-Qānūn fī al-tibb*) that was composed in Arabic by the Persian philosopher and physician Avicenna (ca 980–1037). This was a sprawling synthesis of medical learning and natural philosophy that drew inspiration from Galen, the classical Greek philosopher Aristotle (384–322 BCE), and other Greco-Roman and Arabic authorities. Much of what later was known as "Western" medicine was rooted in translations or original contributions to theory and practice from Arabic sources.

In the later Middle Ages, Europe's physicians emulated lawyers and theologians by casting the "art" of medicine as a theoretically rigorous discipline that imparted life lessons as well as healing techniques. Many variations of this art, later known as humoral medicine, dominated medical culture until the eighteenth century and remained influential thereafter. The approach was rooted in an ancient conception of the natural world which held that all earthly matter was composed of earth, air, fire, and water. Within the body, four corresponding **humors**—blood, phlegm, yellow bile, and black bile—determined an individual's constitution or temperament. Health was conceived as a proper balance of the humors, which existed in relation with external conditions such as temperature, wind, and the seasons. Food, drink, and behavior could also influence the humors, and internal medicines such as herbs or potions attempted to counterbalance their excesses or deficiencies. The key concepts of this medical system were simple, but they enabled infinite elaboration by Latin-educated physicians for the benefit of well-to-do clients who appreciated a learned approach to well-being.

Although humoral medicine enabled careful attention to individuals, it was less well-equipped to explain poisonous forces that seemingly moved from one person or region to another. Maladies were thought to reflect individual humoral imbalances, and they were not considered to be "cases" of a disease that might have an identical underlying cause. The mechanics of disease transmission received less attention in elite medicine than the factors that predisposed some individuals to fall ill and others to remain healthy. This did not mean, however, that the concept of spreading diseases had no place at all. Since antiquity, writers had recognized that some diseases apparently passed by skin contact or breath, and Galen's voluminous treatises referred to "seeds" of disease on a few occasions.[22] Outbreaks of pestilence were often explained as the result of **miasmas** or airborne poisons that arose from fetid sources such as unburied corpses, swamps, or air that was fouled by influence from the stars. It is likely that experience with malarial infections, which were widespread in the Mediterranean during antiquity, provided many observations that supported this concept. From the Greco-Roman perspective, harmful miasmas affected people in different ways according to their humoral balance or temperament. The relative lack of interest in contagion among elite physicians sometimes led to conflict as government officials sought to protect public health by limiting the movement of disease from one location to another.

Humoralism stressed the impact of natural forces on human life, and neither Galen nor his predecessors were Christian. We might, therefore, expect conflict between this approach to medicine and the Christian belief that the universe was controlled by an all-powerful God. In fact, during the later Middle Ages Christianity and humoral medicine coexisted peacefully and were usually considered complementary. Religious authorities attributed the Black Death, like other great misfortunes, to God's wrath over human willfulness, which was represented in the story of Adam and Eve's original sin of disobedience in the Garden of Eden. Where great pestilence was concerned, divine punishment had less to do with individual misdeeds than with humanity's innate weakness. Epidemics, like famines or floods, were tests of faith and continual reminders to rely on God. Natural forces such as comets, heat waves, or floods were considered secondary causes of disaster that God set in motion.

While theologians stressed God's absolute power as a matter of doctrine, they also contended that human actions and medicines were not futile. Writers approvingly quoted a passage from Syrach, a book of ancient wisdom that was read alongside the Bible: "Honor the doctor for his service, for the Lord created him; his skill comes from the Most High, and he is rewarded by kings."[23] In general, church leaders did not discourage medicine but they also admonished that immoral habits or a conscience burdened by sin could cause disease. For this reason, Christians were instructed to confess their sins to a priest prior to consulting a doctor. Medieval Christian teaching also endorsed the notion that saints could intercede with God on humanity's behalf. During and after the Black Death numerous shrines, church altarpieces, and statues evoked the protective power of Jesus's mother Mary. Artists depicted the martyr St Sebastian pierced with arrows or St Roch afflicted with buboes in hopes that they might offer atonement for human iniquity. Prayers and other observances promoted spiritual well-being just as medicines promoted physical and mental well-being; indeed, there was no rigid distinction between the two. In the diverse culture of medieval Christianity, the overall approach to pestilence was not as baleful as descriptions of God's wrath might suggest.

Nonetheless, the years of the Black Death tested religious authorities. The calamity signaled to some Christians that extreme responses were required. Many witnesses reported roaming troupes of "cross bearers" who conducted ritual processions of penance. Some stripped to the waist and flailed themselves with cords knotted with sharp metal. "They beat and whipped their bare skin," one

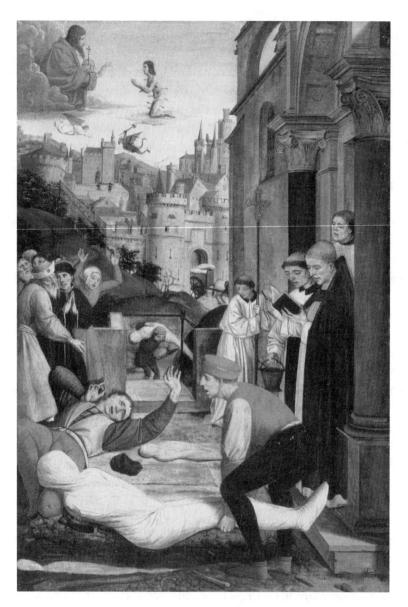

IMAGE 1.2 *St Sebastian Interceding for the Plague-Stricken* (ca 1500). This painting, attributed to Josse Lieferinxe, presents both an earthly and spiritual reality of deadly pestilence. In the lower section, a procession of bodies leads to the gravedigger stacking corpses in a grave. He is flanked by a dying man and a priest. At the top, St Sebastian, pierced with arrows, pleads for mercy on behalf of the community below. Beneath Sebastian and God, an angel and a demon duel for a corpse. Death is both a physical inevitability and a contest for the soul. In the sixteenth century, supporters of the Protestant reform movement rejected such depictions of saintly intercession.

German chronicler wrote, "until their bodies were bruised and swollen and blood rained down, spattering the walls nearby."[24] Church leaders considered these gruesome displays a troubling distortion of Christian ritual. Angry criticism by Pope Clement VI from his residence in Avignon soon dampened enthusiasm for the flagellants in many parts of Europe. Other people focused their fear and anger on outsiders, especially Jewish inhabitants who occupied separate districts in many cities and were targets of suspicion for some Christians long before the Black Death. Allegations swirled that Jews had poisoned wells or paid others to do it, and some confessions were extracted by torture. Despite protests from Clement (in July and September 1348) and secular rulers that Jews were innocent and should not be harmed, the accusations were sufficiently widespread that some municipal officials traded reports of malicious acts in search of damning proof. Other local leaders, such as those in the German city of Cologne, announced their intention to ignore the rumors and suggested that others do the same. Efforts at restraint often did not succeed. In Cologne, Strasbourg, and elsewhere throughout Europe, popular uprisings destroyed Jewish neighborhoods and murdered adult males or even entire families. Violence and persecution revealed an enduring gap between popular beliefs and elite doctrines.

Islamic authors also considered the causes and significance of the Black Death in various Arabic and Persian texts. As noted earlier, scholars in centers such as Damascus and Baghdad preserved and elaborated upon ancient medicine. Doctrines that were linked to the early history of Islam and the teachings of the prophet Muhammad (ca 570–632) also created some contrasts with Europe. Long before the Black Death, Muslims had experienced a deadly pandemic during the seventh century when followers of Islam expanded their territory northward out of the Arabian Peninsula. Death from plague was equated with martyrdom because of its association with this conquest. Prophetic traditions from this period prohibited leaving or entering a plague-stricken area. Muhammad's own statements and early Islamic doctrine did not provide a consistent explanation for the spread of disease. While at least one tradition attributed to Muhammad seemed to rule out contagion that moved from one person to another, other passages indicate that the topic was debated among his associates. What can be said with certainty is that the notion of a human "original sin" is absent from Islam. Although Muslims sometimes described pestilence as a punishment (at least for non-Muslim "infidels"), it did not inspire guilt or penitential fervor as it sometimes did among Europeans.

Such considerations led Michael Dols to draw sharp distinctions between Christian and Islamic approaches to plague during and after the Black Death. While Christians were preoccupied with sin and punishment, Dols claimed,

Muslim responses to plague were marked by "reverent resignation" all the way down to the nineteenth century.[25] To more recent historians, Dols's view is reminiscent of a long-running European stereotype of the "fatalistic Turk" whose responses to social problems were passive and ineffective. Justin Stearns has instead drawn attention to the debate about contagion after the Black Death, especially among elites in the Iberian city of Granada. In the later fourteenth century, the powerful overlord Ibn al-Khatib (ca 1313–1374) insisted that plague was contagious and that it was a spiritual obligation to avoid plague-stricken areas, although some of his contemporaries apparently disagreed. His associate, Ibn al-Khatima (ca 1310–1369), cited evidence in support of the transmission of disease in terms that were more congenial with prophetic teaching. With these examples and others, Stearns suggests that no absolute distinctions can be drawn between Christian and Muslim approaches to divine power and disease.[26] Members of both religious traditions drew on the natural explanations of ancient medicine while emphasizing the absolute sovereignty of God or Allah. Moreover, many surviving texts are moral prescriptions that do not show the full diversity of how people thought and behaved. Much remains unknown, and it is misleading to overstress either Muslim fatalism or Christian guilt in the response to plague.

The discussion of religious culture and plague relates to another broader historical question: how to explain an emergence of vigorous bureaucratic states in Europe that was not matched by developments in North Africa or the Middle East. While many factors were at work, European observers attained a consensus concerning the role of contagion and, even when the source of disease was in doubt, the importance of government power for responding to it. Over the long term, this had important consequences for both public health measures enforced by magistrates and widespread notions concerning the purpose of government.

Plague, Quarantine, and Public Health in Early Modern Europe

There were few years between 1350 and 1650 when all of Europe was free from plague. Although its demographic impact never again approached the level of the Black Death, it exerted a modest but consistent check on population growth until the early seventeenth century. The inhabitants of most major cities could reckon with at least one serious outbreak—if not of plague, then of **typhus** or measles— during their lifetime.

Various studies have explored how plague persisted in Europe and Asia Minor over such a long period. Some twentieth-century research focused on the influence of large cities. Metropolitan hubs such as Paris distributed plague to various trade routes and may have harbored rodent populations where the bacteria was endemic for lengthy periods. Nükhet Varlik's recent investigation of plague in the Ottoman Empire suggests that Istanbul's significance as a plague hub increased after it assumed the role of an imperial capital in the later sixteenth century.[27] However, recent scholars have also considered forces that created epidemic "spillover" from rodent reservoirs in rural areas or outside of Europe. As Anne Carmichael has shown, officials both north and south of the Swiss Alps perceived a persistent threat of plague in highlands that resemble the Asian regions where *Y. pestis* remains endemic today. While the Black Death initially arrived from Italian and French port cities, thereafter plague may have lingered and spread from areas where herdsmen and livestock crossed paths with alpine marmots.[28] Highland regions west of the Caspian Sea and mountainous areas of western Iran, northern Iraq, and southeastern Turkey have also been suggested as areas where plague persisted for long periods. Alternatively, Boris Schmid and others have focused attention on climate fluctuations in central Asia that presumably influenced rodent and flea populations. Some evidence suggests that outbreaks of plague in Europe lagged several years behind episodes further east, and that plague was reintroduced across the continent on multiple occasions.[29] These theories require further investigation, but they indicate how research has broadened beyond the role of trade routes and other human activity to include ecological factors that influenced much of Eurasia.

Within Europe, it is likely that more than one dynamic was at work as communities faced waves of pestilence that were regular but never completely predictable. In the Mediterranean and northwestern Europe, periodic reinfection from ship traffic caused severe outbreaks that were concentrated in large cities. It was different in Bohemia and the German lands of central Europe where, especially between 1560 and 1640, one wave of plague gave rise to the next, and rural areas experienced mortality as severe as in larger communities.[30] The contrasting patterns of these regions were probably related—particularly after the early seventeenth century, when outbreaks were separated by longer intervals—but no meaningful connections could be made by observers. And sometimes the usual patterns shifted, especially when military forces spread disease and violence caused social disruption for civilians as well as soldiers. In 1629, during the Thirty Years' War (1618–48), German and French forces carried plague south to the

Italian city of Mantua. Over the next two years, hundreds of thousands of Italians died from disease in Milan, Venice, and smaller communities.

No matter what doctors counseled about miasma, leaders usually responded to the threat of plague by restricting movement and commerce, especially in busy Mediterranean ports. Many towns performed border control during the Black Death, but Dubrovnik is usually considered the pioneer of an ongoing maritime **quarantine** system. In 1377, this port on the eastern Adriatic coast began to detain ships and crew that were suspected of infection for thirty days before release. In the next decades, north-Italian cities followed suit and established boards of health that were led by local political elites and physicians. Many authorities eventually mandated a forced isolation of forty days—*quaranta giorni* in Italian, *quarantine* in French—in imitation of ritual isolation described in the Christian Old Testament.[31]

By the mid-seventeenth century, the Italian peninsula had well-developed networks of informants that monitored trade conditions in the Adriatic and Mediterranean. Upon news of a disease outbreak, health magistrates suspended trade or banned ships from suspicious ports. To a degree, the common interest in disease control among trading partners overrode competitive pressures and the desire for political independence. To cite one significant example, in 1652 the rival cities Florence and Genoa agreed to align their quarantine procedures and to include a representative from each city at the main ports to ensure fair enforcement. The arrangement did not last, but such collaboration presaged the national and international quarantine regimes that would take shape in later centuries.

As ports further north imitated Italian models, many inland cities also refined strategies for treating victims and forestalling the spread of disease. By the mid-sixteenth century, most sizeable communities had a building outside the walls to isolate individuals, especially the poor, when their health was deemed a risk to others. City leaders resisted opening such facilities as long as possible—often to placate merchants who feared bad rumors and a loss of trade—but when danger was revealed, a train of disaster measures was set in motion. Public works offices hired barber surgeons, stretcher carriers, and grave diggers; large funerals and other gatherings were forbidden; public places were disinfected with vinegar solutions; and the belongings of plague victims were fumigated or burned. Street by street, individuals were appointed to monitor the spread of disease and sometimes to visit the sick. The infected who could remain at home were often ordered to isolate themselves for a period of weeks. Neighboring cities exchanged information not only about impending waves of disease but also sanitary regulations for trades that were considered noxious or foul, such as tanning and butchery.

Plague outbreaks could be devastating but, because they were intermittent, leaders could reflect on the factors that apparently contributed to the start of an epidemic. It was possible, for example, to identify patterns in the time of year that outbreaks took place—for much of Europe it was late summer—and, more importantly, to consider what social groups were most affected. Mortality statistics, in evidence for German cities from at least the 1530s, enabled reckonings that could be compared across the decades. Beginning in the 1660s with English writer John Graunt, such records were analyzed with increasing statistical precision. Unlike the broad impact of the Black Death, authorities found that urban outbreaks in the fifteenth and sixteenth centuries tended to concentrate in poorer neighborhoods or suburbs. As one later English observer put it, plague inhabited "the back lanes and remote places" of a city.[32] It was, therefore, increasingly viewed as a social problem that elites could attack alongside other social ills such as begging or vagrancy. In Italy, this trend began in the fifteenth century, as Florence instituted policies that aimed to control the movements of the poor as much as to halt disease.[33] Across Europe in the next two centuries, measures against plague and other diseases coincided with broader efforts to curb begging, expel vagrants, and impose punishments for various types of social disorder, such as drunkenness.

Most religious leaders agreed that people should do all they could to fight the plague or avoid it by flight. As the unity of Christianity broke down in the sixteenth century, leaders of the **Protestant** religious movement offered various perspectives on the crises and suffering caused by plague. The leading German reformer Martin Luther (1483–1546) left no doubt about his support of orthodox medicine. In December 1527, as plague approached his home town of Wittenberg, Luther published a German tract entitled *Whether One May Flee from a Deadly Plague* (*Ob man vor dem Sterben fliehen möge*) that eventually was translated and reprinted numerous times. Luther acknowledged the impulse to flee but urged Christians to fulfill social obligations and care for their neighbors. The use of medicine was a sacred duty, as Luther warned: "he who does not use it [medicine] when he could do so without harming his neighbor injures his body, and must beware lest he be deemed a suicide in God's eyes."[34] A generation later, Theodore de Bèze, a follower of the French Protestant John Calvin, also acknowledged the need to meet social obligations but stressed that Christians should flee when possible.

As divides deepened between Protestant and **Catholic** religious factions, writers sought to reconcile human agency with the belief in a sovereign, omnipotent God. Most Christian authorities had never rejected medicine, but Catholic rituals also continued to invoke the power of saints to intercede on behalf of humanity. Protestant leaders dismissed such appeals, which they considered an insult to God's absolute power and the goodness of the divinely created natural order. The Protestant focus on responsible conduct by ordinary Christians encouraged many to look to earthly measures they could undertake in times of crisis. A few more radical dissenters, whose ideas concerning theology and society differed from most other Protestants as well as Catholics, rejected medicine and relied exclusively upon God's sovereign power to heal. In later centuries, some of their followers would form separatist Amish and Mennonite communities that would continue to reject public health measures such as vaccination.

Over the long term, a broad religious consensus concerning the value of plague controls served to legitimize the authority of national and imperial governments. The importance of coordinated, rigorous measures was underscored in 1720 by a disastrous outbreak at the southern French port of Marseille, which killed tens of thousands of inhabitants and sparked a Europe-wide panic. Although the port had observed quarantine procedures since the late fourteenth century, plague breached the defenses after merchants colluded with local officials to allow a contaminated ship to unload before an upcoming trade fair. As the scourge spread north, a delegation of physicians rushed to the city from the medical faculty of Montpellier, only to conclude that poor food and living conditions (not contagion) were mostly to blame for the outbreak. City doctors argued otherwise and the French national government agreed: tens of thousands of army troops formed a ***cordon sanitaire*** that ringed Marseille and the surrounding territory. Trespassers were warned to turn back or face gunfire. Sections of the stone wall constructed to keep them in still dot the French countryside.

This was not the last that Europe saw of plague—epidemics struck Messina (Sicily) in 1748 and Moscow in 1771—but its influence in the region subsided while outbreaks in Egypt and the Levant continued into the nineteenth century. Historians have considered various factors that might account for the difference. After 1770, a permanent *cordon sanitaire* prevented plague from passing the military frontier between the Austro-Hungarian and Ottoman Empires. This fact, and the absence of plague from England after 1665, lend support to the claim that maritime quarantine and border control exerted a significant influence over the long term. Interactions between humans and rodents may also have changed over time, either because of human innovations (such as different building materials), or because of changes in rodent population and ecology. Some clues have come from ancient DNA gathered from a mass grave that was dug during the Marseille outbreak. The evidence indicates that the responsible *Y. pestis* strain descended directly from a strain that circulated in England nearly four centuries earlier during the Black Death.[35] This strengthens the likelihood that a source of plague infection persisted in southern Europe or western Asia before its impact ebbed after the early eighteenth century.

For leaders around Europe, protective measures against epidemics highlighted the desirability of effective "police," a Latin-derived term that initially referred to rules and practices that fostered a well-regulated city or state. In 1616, the German author Ludwig von Hörnigk published a Latin treatise entitled *Medical Police* (*Politia Medicina*), one of the first blueprints for the role of medicine in government. Voicing a sentiment that others echoed, von Hörnigk claimed that medicine was the greatest and most useful gift of God. As protectors of the body—as well as the soul—magistrates were empowered to act in the common interest, even when this came at the expense of individual liberties.

The Global Spread of Plague

Historians have often separated the Black Death and its centuries-long aftermath from the "third pandemic" of the 1890s that broke out in China, devastated India, and spread to ports around the world. Despite the gaps in time and distance, the division is not absolute. Analyses of dated DNA samples from numerous sites indicate that the strain of Y. *pestis* that diffused most widely in the late nineteenth and early twentieth centuries descended from a strain that spread across Europe in the late 1340s. This evidence suggests that after plague completed its sweep of Europe in 1352, a strain traveled back east into central Asia where several other foci of plague had long persisted. Beginning in the mid-eighteenth century, observers recorded epidemics in China's southern Yunnan Province, where profitable copper mines brought numerous immigrants, animals, and road construction. A rebellion of the region's Muslims against the ruling Qing dynasty and growth in the sale of Yunnan opium further disrupted ecological balances in the region. Tens of thousands of people died in outbreaks of pestilence that apparently included plague alongside other human and animal diseases. In 1894 plague reached Hong Kong, a port that served as a gateway to maritime arteries of global commerce.

The British navy had wrested control of Hong Kong Island from the Qing dynasty in 1841, and after 1860 it controlled a portion of the adjoining Kowloon Peninsula. The outbreak of plague thus provided an opportunity for Westerners to observe a scourge they now associated with a distant medieval world. As we will see in chapter 5, European scientists armed with microscopes had articulated germ theories beginning in the 1860s. In Hong Kong, the inquiry into the causes of plague was a focus of intense competition among visiting French, Japanese, and British researchers. Although the Japanese team led by Kitasato Shibasaburō (1853–1931) published its report first, a solitary Swiss researcher named Alexandre Yersin (1863–1943) successfully isolated the microbe, described it with greater precision, and drew attention to the role of rats in spreading the disease. Much excitement accompanied these findings, but neither Yersin nor Shibasaburō thoroughly explained how the bacteria circulated among different animals. Many investigators believed that human and rodent excreta were a means of transmission. In 1898, Paul-Louis Simond (1858–1947), a Frenchman at work in the city of Karachi (now in Pakistan), first suggested that fleas or other parasites spread the bacteria among rodents and to humans. But his experimental results were difficult to replicate and they remained contested for another decade. This was especially true in India, where Britain had instituted formal colonial rule in 1858. British medical officers clung to the stereotype of an unsanitary "barefoot Indian" who would be infected by bacteria that lay on dung-covered floors.

The continued confusion over plague transmission proved costly. In 1897, at an international health congress held in Venice, many leading nations agreed to an array of surveillance and quarantine measures. These efforts may have limited mortality but they did little to halt the transoceanic movement of disease. Steamships leaving Hong Kong spread plague to distant islands and an entire American continent that had never encountered plague before. The new locations included the French-controlled island of Madagascar, where plague established a lasting presence among highland rodents. Busy ports such as San Francisco, Cape Town (southern Africa), and Santos (Brazil) were especially vulnerable. In San Francisco, several bouts with plague between 1900 and 1908 resulted in 113 deaths. The outbreak aggravated racial tensions between the city's dominant white population and recent Asian immigrants who were concentrated in the Chinatown district. Local officials imposed harsh quarantines until the Chinese residents successfully opposed them in federal court.[36] Plague also worked its way inland to create reservoirs among prairie dog colonies and other rodents in arid regions of Colorado and New Mexico. In South America, the port city Santos experienced a relatively minor outbreak while plague also caused roughly 500 deaths in Brazil's capital city, Rio de Janeiro.[37]

Imperial Crises in India, Southern Africa, and Manchuria

The resurgence and global spread of plague confronted imperial rulers and their subordinate peoples with grave challenges. For administrators in the far-flung British Empire, especially in India, the disease endangered not only lives but also the foundations of an economic order that was based on the free circulation of goods. For the Chinese Qing dynasty, plague undermined imperial sovereignty in the contested borderland of Manchuria. The measures taken against the pandemic illustrate how these governments attempted to put public health regimes in the service of imperial objectives.

After plague reached India in 1896, it exacted a terrific toll. Before 1914, the disease killed an estimated 180,000 people in the western port city of Bombay (now Mumbai), and plague-related mortality in the entire subcontinent may have exceeded 10 million by 1921. Although smallpox and malaria also caused high mortality, it was bubonic plague that most seriously threatened Britain's governance of the vast colony.[38] In the late 1890s, the identification of Y. pestis, and the recent finding that cholera was also caused by bacteria, transformed the perception of epidemics among elites. Now the cause of disease was located within the human body rather than an unhealthy landscape or atmosphere. For colonial officials, therefore, international pressure to control plague corresponded to a desire to assert control over the inhabitants of India's largest cities. Accordingly, in February 1897 the government granted public health officials almost unlimited power to search homes and segregate individuals, suspend religious pilgrimages, or even raze the dwellings of impoverished Indians to the ground. In cities such as Bombay and Pune, the houses of plague victims were drenched in carbolic acid solution and sewers were flushed with vast quantities of carbolic acid and water. During a mass exodus from urban centers, railway and road travelers were inspected and detained. Corpses were handled in ways that violated traditional burial norms.

British officials were unprepared for the violent backlash among Indians, to whom the intrusions by the state seemed completely new and unjustified. Thousands rioted to protest the destruction of property, the violation of caste requirements, and, perhaps above all, the disrobing and touching of women by male examiners. Among many violent episodes, in Pune the head of the Plague Committee was assassinated in June 1897 and Bombay's hospitals were attacked by angry mobs in March 1898. Fear of hospitals led many of the sick to conceal their condition. The colonial government soon retreated from the most extreme measures such as body searches and forced segregation. They also turned to

Indian volunteers and troops for house inspections and sought the moral support of influential middle- and upper-class Indians. This shift in colonial plague policy marked a turning point for the role of Western public health in India. In the early 1900s, many people sought to apply the new lessons of science and sanitation to serve diverse communities, although later Indian leaders such as Mohandas Gandhi (1869–1948) would be selective in their appropriation of Western science.

In southern Africa, the appearance of plague in February 1901 sparked actions in the British Cape Colony that had far-reaching consequences for the history of racial subjugation in the region.[39] Prior to the outbreak, colonial administrators had considered proposals to create residential reserves that would make black Africans available for labor but separate their living quarters from whites. When several dockworkers died of plague in Cape Town, racial ideology framed colonial fears concerning public health and a potential loss of trade. In March, under the authority of a Public Health Act passed in 1883, colonial officials ordered the forced relocation of more than 6,000 Africans from Cape Town to Uitvlugt, the environs of a sewage farm several miles out of town. Initially considered a temporary move, Uitvlugt became the site of the township Ndabeni. The episode laid ideological and institutional foundations for more thorough segregation regimes in the unified South Africa later in the twentieth century. We will see that similar motivations influenced imperial regimes elsewhere, notably in the 1900s among US administrators in the Caribbean and the Philippines after the Spanish-American War (chapter 4).

In November 1910, the convergence of public health imperatives, political tensions, and local conditions also created conflict when plague struck Harbin, a Manchurian city near the border of Russia and China.[40] Apparently, this outbreak was not directly related to China's earlier epidemics further south. It was sparked by thousands of amateur trappers who were attracted to the steppes and mountain slopes northwest of Vladivostok by a sharp increase in the market value of Siberian marmot pelts. Unbeknownst to the newcomers, the burrowing marmots, also called tarbagans, harbored plague and had caused continual small outbreaks in the region's sparse human population. The trappers experienced pneumonic symptoms and the disease passed rapidly among them as they slept close together in crowded hostels. Railway travel then brought the disease southwest to Harbin, Changchun, and Shenyang, where officials recorded nearly 44,000 deaths between November 1910 and February 1911. The crisis carried broader political implications since Russia and China contested political control over the region.

Harbin's response was overseen by a young physician, Wu Lien-teh (1879–1960), whose background uniquely qualified him to adapt Western medicine to the

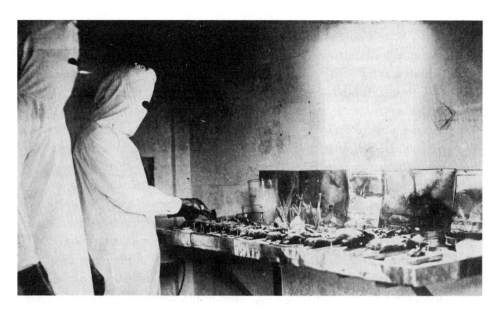

IMAGE 1.3 "In the laboratory: searching for infected rats." Photographs of the Manchurian plague outbreak, such as this one taken at Harbin in 1911, were not intended solely to document events. Chinese officials, mindful of competition with Russia, wished to demonstrate the superiority of their scientific response. To this day, images of protective suits and face masks symbolize medical authority and government intervention against epidemic diseases. Early-twentieth-century field work in Harbin and elsewhere also cemented the rat's reputation as the bearer of dangerous pathogens. See Christos Lynteris, *Ethnographic Plague: Configuring Disease on the Chinese-Russian Frontier* (London: Palgrave Macmillan, 2016).

circumstances of Pacific Rim countries. Born to Chinese parents in Penang, a British colony on the Malay Peninsula, Wu completed medical school at the University of Cambridge and eventually joined the Chinese Imperial Army College. In December 1910, imperial officials dispatched Wu to Harbin where he identified pneumonic plague and discovered the causal role of tarbagan pelts. Under his direction, hundreds of soldiers and police conducted searches for the sick, monitored people who were fleeing the city, and isolated the infected in railway freight cars. Like many other educated Chinese, Wu considered rural Manchuria a primitive backwater, and his methods boldly overstepped the boundaries of traditional custom. Postmortem examinations deeply offended local inhabitants, and, because Harbin's frozen ground prevented burials, Wu secured permission from the imperial government for a mass cremation of over 2,000 corpses. The imperial edict that consigned bodies to the flames also signaled a willingness among China's elites to adopt some Western public health practices. Thereafter, Wu's stature as an authority on plague enhanced China's prestige in international health gatherings. After the Qing dynasty was replaced by a republic in 1912, Wu led the organization of several public health agencies and advocated for Western medicine in general.

The Indian pandemic and the smaller Manchurian outbreak differed in scale, but they offer a useful comparison of how subordinate societies were subjected to Western public health. In both regions, local inhabitants considered the new measures to be disruptive exercises of state power rather than scientifically advanced strategies of disease control. In addition to the division (in India) between rulers and colonial subjects, Western disease-control measures widened the gap between educated, relatively wealthy groups and poorer classes who often were considered the source of disease. Isolation of the sick and disinfections may have saved lives—their effectiveness is hard to assess—but the programs also served various political objectives within nations and for international diplomacy. In China, as in Europe centuries before, public health measures provided a vehicle for the consolidation of state control.

Conclusion

In the twenty-first century, cases of plague are more geographically dispersed than they were in the fourteenth century. The pandemic of the 1890s spread the bacteria globally, including to the Pacific coast of the United States where they were carried inland from ports such as San Francisco. Roughly half a dozen cases still occur in the United States each year, mostly in the open lands of the Southwest that supports large populations of squirrels and prairie dogs. The bacteria's pervasive presence in rodents, fleas, and soil rules out any immediate prospect that plague can be eradicated.

Individual cases usually do not pose a major public health threat since plague can be identified by a blood test and effectively cured with streptomycin. The exceptions arise when humans are not separated from the usual transmission of plague among rodents and rapid antibiotic treatment is not available. Since 2010, the impact of plague has been concentrated in Madagascar, where the **World Health Organization** (WHO) reports an average of about 600 cases annually that cause dozens of deaths.[41] Much of this large island is sparsely populated and mountainous, and plague is endemic among rodents that live in upland areas. There is a potential for a wider outbreak when plague reaches a large city that lacks effective sanitary infrastructure or has enclosed facilities, such as prisons, where numerous people live in close proximity to rodents. In a recent outbreak of more than 800 cases in the fall of 2017, researchers documented the spread of pneumonic plague in the island's large cities including its capital, Antananarivo. Pneumonic plague's rapid transmission and high mortality have aroused fears of a broader outbreak in neighboring islands or mainland Africa.

A relationship between poverty and susceptibility to plague was already noted by some observers in the later fourteenth century, as European cities linked anti-plague measures to the control of people who were deemed marginal, disorderly, or dangerous. Plague outbreaks justified state measures to compel isolation, disinfect or destroy private property, regulate the work of various trades, oversee medical examinations and burials, and manage the safe passage of people and goods. Such actions became integral to the modern notion of a functioning state that assumed responsibility for the protection of borders and the preservation of health among its citizens.

As later chapters in this book will explore, the third plague pandemic broke out just as laboratory-based medicine was assuming a lead role in the public health policies of some nations. The great contrast between relatively small death tolls in more developed regions and high mortality in India and China revealed inequalities in public health that would grow through the twentieth century.[42] Large plague epidemics also fed stereotypes against Asian immigrants to the Americas and reinforced notions concerning the superiority of Western science and sanitation. In India, by contrast, coercive anti-plague measures by the British revealed the profound gap in perspective between colonial administrators and the average city dweller.

Other aspects of plague's cultural imprint developed over the centuries. The dramatic symptoms, high mortality, and intermittent character of plague outbreaks created a paradigm for epidemics and the destruction they could cause. The image of a wave of disease that moves from place to place, rising and ebbing within individual communities, seemed especially instructive to observers in the nineteenth century when cholera outbreaks followed a similar trajectory. Plague outbreaks have prompted reflections about human survival and integrity in the face of divine or ultimate forces. While much of this discourse has been carried out in religious terms, plague has also been deeply symbolic for secular writers. For example, in *The Plague* (*La Peste*, 1947), a novel by the existentialist writer Albert Camus (1913–1960), an outbreak of the disease in a North African city forces its protagonists to seek meaning in a world that is ultimately irrational.

Plague outbreaks have most often been framed as a communal crisis that demands a collective response. Syphilis, in contrast, has often been depicted and experienced as a disease caused by individual misdeeds. The encounter with this disease has deeply influenced Western beliefs about individual morality and the role of the community in policing sexuality.

WORKSHOP: FAITH, REASON, AND PLAGUE IN FOURTEENTH-CENTURY EUROPE

An enduring stereotype of the Middle Ages is that the dominant Christian religious culture prevented a scientific or "rational" response to the Black Death and later waves of plague. One popular history of the period, for example, suggests that medieval people were "drilled by their theological and their scientific training into a reaction of apathy and fatalistic resignation."[43] To the contrary, most recent scholars have emphasized that medicine and faith were complementary. A belief in God's ultimate power was not incompatible with efforts to cure disease or halt its spread. Statements concerning sinfulness tended to emphasize collective sin and human imperfection rather than punishment for a person's individual misdeeds. Moreover, the relationship that people discerned between disease, medicine, and faith depended on their intellectual priorities and the social context.

Although observers of the fourteenth century did not attribute the spread of disease to microbes, it was often perceived that epidemic disease spread from one person or object to another. How "contagion" was understood depended on a person's social and intellectual vantage point. While the concept of contaminated air, or miasma, was the most frequent explanation, more philosophical accounts attributed disease to a hierarchy of divine, astral, and material causes. This did not prevent city officials from focusing on the role of physical proximity in disease transmission.

> **"Ordinances against the Spread of Plague"** (Pistoia, 1348)
>
> *These regulations are from a city near Florence that had a population of roughly 11,000 in 1348. An estimated one-quarter of the population died in the Black Death. City councils across Europe drafted similar regulations to monitor travel and trade, as well as to control certain occupations that were believed to spread filth or disease, such as butchers and tanners. Burial of victims and the observance of religious rituals were also of great concern. Note that some ordinances were revised or amended after they were first adopted.*

[*The initial ordinances were dated 2 May 1348.*] In the name of Christ Amen. Herein are written certain ordinances and provisions made and agreed upon by certain wise men of the People of the city of Pistoia ... concerning the preserving, strengthening and protecting the health of humans from various and diverse pestilences which otherwise can befall the human body. And written by me Simone Buonacorsi notary....

First. So that no contaminated matter which presently persists in the areas surrounding the city of Pistoia can enter into the bodies of the citizens of Pistoia, these wise men provided and ordered that no citizen of Pistoia or dweller in the district or the county of Pistoia ... shall in any way dare or presume to go to Pisa or Lucca or to the county or district of either. And that no one can or ought to come from either city or their districts ... to the city of Pistoia or its district or county ... And the gatekeeper of the city of Pistoia guarding the gates of the city shall not permit those coming or returning to Pistoia from Pisa or Lucca, their districts or counties to enter the gates....

[*An amendment revoking the first article was added on 23 May.*]

Chapter 1 to be entirely revoked.

II. Item. The wise men have ordered that no person shall dare or presume to bring ... to Pistoia, its district or county, any used cloth, either linen or woolen, for use as clothing for men or women or for bedclothes.... Citizens who are returning to Pistoia, its district and county will be allowed to bring with them the linen or woolen cloths they are wearing and those for personal use carried in luggage or a small bundle weighing thirty pounds or less....

III. Item. They ordered that the bodies of the dead, after they had died, shall not be removed from the place in which they are found unless the body has first been placed in a wooden casket covered by a lid secured with nails, so that no stench can issue forth from it; nor can it be covered except by a canopy, blanket or drape.... Likewise, such dead bodies must be carried to the grave only in the same casket, subject to the same penalty. And so that city officials may note this, rectors of Pistoia's districts in which there is a death are obliged to announce it to the podesta and captain [*these were Pistoia's chief officials*] of the city.... And the officials who have received such an announcement immediately must send an official to the location to insure that these statutes and others concerning funerals are being observed and to punish anyone who is culpable [*i.e., who disobeys the ordinances*]....

IV. Item. In order to avoid the foul stench which the bodies of the dead give off they have provided and ordered that any ditch in which a dead body is to be buried must be dug under ground to a depth of 2 1/2 braccia [*about six feet*] by the measure of the city of Pistoia....

VI. Item. They have provided and ordered that any person who has come for the burial or to bury any dead person shall not be in the presence of the body itself nor with the relatives of such a dead person except for the procession to the church where it will be buried. Such persons shall not return to the house where the deceased person lived or enter that house or any other house on this occasion....

[*The text then includes another revision. It is possible that it was added after associates of deceased persons requested a change.*]

June 4. When the corpse has been carried to the church, everyone who accompanied it there ought to withdraw, and when the next of kin leave no one ought to accompany them except their spouses and the neighbors, and also the dead man's next of kin on his mother's side. These people may go to the house of the dead man, or wherever the body is but may not enter the building. 'Neighbors' are to be understood as people who lived within 50 arms-length of the dead man during his lifetime....

X. Item. So that the sounds of bells might not depress the infirm nor fear arise in them, they [*the wise men*] have provided and ordered that the bellringers or custodians in charge of the belltower of the cathedral of Pistoia shall not permit any bell to be rung for the funeral of the dead, nor shall any person dare or presume to ring any of these bells on the said occasion....

[*Here follows another amendment that reflects changing practice later in the epidemic.*]

Revision of June 4. Whenever someone is buried no bell is to be rung at all; rather, people are to be summoned and their prayers invited only by word of mouth....

XIV. Item. They have provided and ordered that butchers and retail vendors of meat shall not maintain near a tavern or other place where they sell meats ... any stable, pen or any other thing which will give off a putrid smell, nor can they slaughter meat animals or hang them after slaughter in any stable or other place in which there is any stench....

XXII. Item. So that stench and putrefaction shall not be harmful to men, henceforth tanning of hides cannot and must not be done within the walls of the city of Pistoia....

"Report of the Paris Medical Faculty" (1348)

This academic commentary, written at the behest of the French king Philip VI, was considered authoritative in the fourteenth century and was extensively translated and cited. It illustrates how Galenic medicine combined arguments about the environment and human physiology to explain disease. Elite theorists attributed the Black Death to a hierarchy of causes: the influence of an astral convergence, corruption spread by prevailing winds, and actions among the humors within individual bodies. The concluding paragraph illustrates a typical attitude concerning medicine and faith that prevailed in many contexts during the later Middle Ages.

We say that the distant and first cause of this pestilence was and is the configuration of the heavens. In 1345, at one hour after noon on 20 March, there was a major conjunction of three planets in Aquarius [*the three planets were Saturn, Mars, and Jupiter*]. This conjunction, along with other earlier conjunctions and eclipses, by causing a deadly corruption in the air around us, signifies mortality and famine—and also other things about which we will not speak here because they are not relevant. Aristotle testifies that this is the case in his book *Concerning the causes of the properties of the elements*, in which he says that the mortality of the races and the depopulation of kingdoms occurs at the conjunction of Saturn and Jupiter, for great events then arise, their nature depending on the trigon in which the conjunction occurs.... [*The book that is cited was a paraphrase of Aristotle's works. It is now attributed to the medieval philosopher Albert the Great (ca 1200–ca 1280).*]

What happened was that the many vapors which had been corrupted at the time of the conjunction were drawn up from the earth and water, and were then mixed with the air and spread abroad by frequent gusts of wind in the wild southerly gales. And, because of these alien vapors which they carried, the winds corrupted the air in its substance and are still doing so. And this corrupted air, when breathed in, necessarily penetrates to the heart and corrupts the substance of the spirit there and rots the surrounding moisture, and the heat thus caused destroys the life force, and this is the immediate cause of the present epidemic…. The [*human*] bodies most likely to take the stamp of this pestilence are those which are hot and moist, for they are the most susceptible to putrefaction. The following are also more at risk: bodies clogged with evil humors because the unconsumed waste matter is not being expelled as it should; those following a bad life style, with too much exercise, sex and bathing; the thin and weak, and persistent worriers; babies, women and young people; and corpulent people with a ruddy complexion. However, those with dry bodies, purged of waste matter, who adopt a sensible and suitable regimen, will succumb to the pestilence more slowly.

We must not overlook the fact that any pestilence proceeds from the divine will, and our advice can therefore only be to return humbly to God. But this does not mean forsaking doctors. For the Most High created earthly medicine, and although God alone cures the sick, he does so through the medicine which in his generosity he provided. Blessed be the glorious and high God, who does not refuse his help, but has clearly set out a way of being cured for those who fear him.

"A Description of Plague in Florence"—Marchione di Coppo Stefani (ca 1380)

These excerpts are taken from the Florentine Chronicle, *a manuscript that is an important source for the history of fourteenth-century Florence. Similar to other chroniclers, Stefani emphasizes that the pestilence of 1348 severed the normal bonds between citizens and family members and that some people attempted to profit from the high mortality. His account of burial practices may be compared with the Pistoia ordinances.*

Rubric 643. Concerning a mortality in the city of Florence in which many people died.

In the year of the Lord 1348 there was a very great pestilence in the city and district of Florence. It was of such a fury and so tempestuous that in houses in which it took hold previously healthy servants who took care of the ill died of the same illness. Almost none of the ill survived past the fourth day. Neither physicians nor medicines were effective…. There was such a fear that no one seemed to know what to do. When it took hold in a house it often happened that no one remained who had not died. And it was not just that men and women died, but even sentient animals died. Dogs, cats, chickens, oxen, donkeys and sheep showed the same symptoms and died of the same disease. And almost none, or very few, who showed these symptoms were cured.

The symptoms were the following: a bubo in the groin, where the thigh meets the trunk; or a small swelling under the armpit; sudden fever; spitting blood and saliva (and no one who spit blood survived it). It was such a frightful thing that when it got into a house, as was said, no one remained. Frightened people abandoned the house and fled to another. Those in town fled to villages. Physicians could not be found because they had died like the others.... They inspected the urine from a distance and with something odoriferous under their nose. Child abandoned the father, husband the wife, wife the husband, one brother the other, one sister the other.... Many died unseen. So they remained in their beds until they stank. And the neighbors, if there were any, having smelled the stench, placed them in a shroud and sent them for burial. The house remained open and yet there was no one daring enough to touch anything because it seemed that things remained poisoned and that whoever used them picked up the illness.

At every church, or at most of them, they dug deep trenches, down to the waterline, wide and deep, depending on how large the parish was. And those who were responsible for the dead carried them on their backs in the night in which they died and threw them into the ditch, or else they paid a high price to those who would do it for them. The next morning, if there were many [*bodies*] in the trench, they covered them over with dirt. And then more bodies were put on top of them, with a little more dirt over those; they put layer on layer just like one puts layers of cheese in a lasagna.

The beccamorti [*literally "vultures," those who carried or buried the dead*] who provided their service, were paid such a high price that many were enriched by it. Many died [*from bearing the dead*], some rich, some after earning just a little, but high prices continued. Servants, or those who took care of the ill, charged from one to three florins per day and the cost of things grew. The things that the sick ate, sweetmeats and sugar, seemed priceless.... Priests were not able to ring bells as they would have liked since [*the government*] issued ordinances discouraging the sounding of bells, sale of burial benches, and limiting expenses. They could not sound bells, sell benches, nor cry out announcements because the sick hated to hear of this and it discouraged the healthy as well. Priests and friars went [*to serve*] the rich in great multitudes and they were paid such high prices that they all got rich. And therefore [*the authorities*] ordered that one could not have more than a prescribed number [*of clerics*] of the local parish church.

"Medical Treatise"—John of Burgundy (ca 1365)

Medical practitioners recommended potions and syrups (or electuaries) according to the patient's individual characteristics or "complexion." But the most frequent therapy was to release poisonous or corrupt matter by bloodletting (phlebotomy), lancing buboes, or other types of purging. The treatise containing the following text was attributed to an English physician and was widely copied in the later Middle Ages. In addition to the suggestions for therapy, the passage suggests that ancient writers, although important, were not the final authority on pestilential disease.

I say that these pestilential illnesses have a short and sudden beginning and a rapid development, and therefore in these illnesses those who wish to work a cure ought not to delay; and bleeding, which is the beginning of the cure, should not be put off until the first or second day. On the contrary, if someone can be found to do it, blood should be taken from the vein going from the seat of the diseased matter (that is, in the place where the morbidity has appeared) in the very hour in which the patient was seized by illness. And if the bleeding cannot be done within the hour, at least let it be done within six hours, and if that is not possible then do not let the patient eat or drink until the bleeding has been done.... But if it is delayed until the illness is established and then done, it will certainly do no harm, but there is no certainty that it will rescue the patient from danger—by then the bad blood will be so clotted and thickened that it will scarcely be able to flow from the vein.

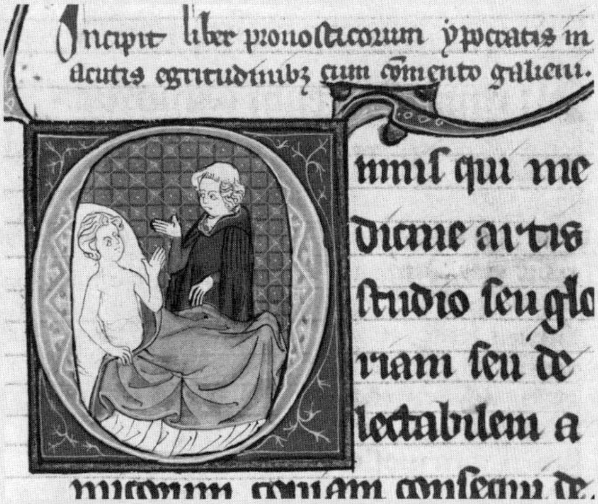

If, after the phlebotomy, the poisonous matter spreads again, the bleeding should be

IMAGE 1.4 Detail from a medieval medical dictionary. This manuscript was produced in late-fourteenth-century Italy. In the Middle Ages, European medical theory was mostly written in Latin and available to few people. Scribes created digests and anthologies of the most significant authors. Writings on the Black Death in the fourteenth century were recopied and edited for centuries thereafter. As this image illustrates, conversation between patient and practitioner was considered an essential aspect of diagnosis. Physicians also inspected urine and considered the effects of diet, behavior, and environment.

repeated in the same vein or in another going from the seat of the diseased matter. Afterwards three or five spoonsful of the herbal water, made as above, should be administered. [*The water recipe contained plants including dittany, pimpernel, tormentil, and scabious.*] And if less than that is available, let one spoonful be given morning and evening, and one spoonful should always be given after consumption of the electuary described above, whether by day (when it can be given at any hour) or by night. [*The electuary, or syrup, included sandalwood, a natural gum called tragacanth, and candied rose petals.*] ... I have never known anyone treated with this type of bleeding who has not escaped death, provided that he has looked after himself well and has received substances to strengthen his heart. As a result I make bold to say—not in criticism of past authorities but out of long experience in the matter—that modern masters are more experienced in treating pestilential epidemic diseases than all the doctors and medical experts from Hippocrates downward. For none of them saw an epidemic reigning in their time, apart from Hippocrates in the city of Craton and that was short-lived.

INTERPRETING THE DOCUMENTS

1. Make a list of the various explanations for the spread of disease in these documents. What ideas recur or overlap? How do more immediate causes (touch, air) relate to more indirect ones?

2. How would you characterize the relationship of religious beliefs and practices to public health objectives? Do these documents present a consistent picture or does one contradict another?

3. What are the principal means that are recommended for curing or treating the plague? Given the prevailing understanding of the body, why were these measures considered effective?

MAKING CONNECTIONS

1. We might expect that the lack of success in treating the plague would lead to a loss of faith in religious or medical institutions. But this was usually not the case. How can we explain this?

2. Fourteenth-century explanations of the Black Death invoked multiple natural causes. Modern explanations of bubonic plague do as well, albeit from a very different perspective. What principal similarities and differences do you see between current and medieval approaches to plague and the natural world?

3. Like Stefani's chronicle, the author Giovanni Boccaccio famously wrote that "brother was forsaken by brother, nephew by uncle, brother by sister, and oftentimes husband by wife: nay, what is more, and scarcely to be believed, fathers and mothers were found to abandon their own children, untended, unvisited, to their fate, as if they had been strangers." How should we evaluate such claims? To what extent do you think the Black Death destroyed the fabric of medieval European society?

For further reading: Justin K. Stearns, "New Directions in the Study of Religious Responses to the Black Death," *History Compass* 7, no. 5 (2009): 1363–75.

Notes

1. Rosemary Horrox, ed. and trans., *The Black Death* (Manchester: Manchester University Press, 1994), 18–19. Fourteenth-century Europeans did not commonly refer to a "Black Death." The term was popularized centuries later by a popular German history of the pandemic, *The Black Death* (*Der Schwarze Tod*), published in 1832 by J.F.C. Hecker.

2. Monica H. Green, ed., *Pandemic Disease in the Medieval World: Rethinking the Black Death*, first issue of *The Medieval Globe* (Leeds, UK: Arc Medieval Press, 2014), https://scholarworks.wmich.edu/medieval_globe/1/.

3. Simon Rasmussen et al., "Early Divergent Strains of *Yersinia pestis* in Eurasia 5,000 Years Ago," *Cell* 163, no. 3 (2015): 571–82.

4. David W. Markman et al., "*Yersinia pestis* Survival and Replication in Potential Amoeba Reservoir," *Emerging Infectious Diseases* 24, no. 2 (2018): 6–8.

5. M. Drancourt et al., "Detection of 400-Year-Old *Yersinia pestis* DNA in Human Dental Pulp: An Approach to the Diagnosis of Ancient Septicemia," *Proceedings of the National Academy of Sciences* 95 (1998): 12637–40.

6. M. Drancourt and D. Raoult, "Molecular History of Plague," *Clinical Microbiology and Infection* 22, no. 11 (2016): 911–15.

7. Kirsten I. Bos et al., "A Draft Genome of *Yersinia pestis* from Victims of the Black Death," *Nature* 478 (2011): 506–10.

8. Yujun Cui et al., "Historical Variations in Mutation Rate in an Epidemic Pathogen, *Yersinia pestis*," *Proceedings of the National Academy of Sciences* 110, no. 2 (2013): 577–82.

9. Anne G. Carmichael, "Plague Persistence in Western Europe: A Hypothesis," in *Pandemic Disease*, 157–62.

10. John Brooke and Monica Green, "Thinking Big about the Plague," *Inference* 4, no. 2 (2018): https://inference-review.com/letter/thinking-big-about-the-plague#endnote-5.

11. Timothy P. Newfield, "A Cattle Panzootic in Early Fourteenth-Century Europe," *Agricultural History Review* 57, no. 2 (2009): 155–90.

12. Bruce M.S. Campbell, *The Great Transition: Climate, Disease and Society in the Late-Medieval World* (Cambridge: Cambridge University Press, 2016), 246–52.

13. Galina Eroshenko et al., "*Yersinia pestis* Strains of Ancient Phylogenetic Branch 0.ANT Are Widely Spread in the High-Mountain Plague Foci of Kyrgyzstan," *PLOS One* 12 (2017): e0187230.

14. George D. Sussman, "Was the Black Death in India and China?" *Bulletin of the History of Medicine* 85, no. 3 (2011): 319–55.

15. Samuel Cohn, "The Black Death: End of a Paradigm," *American Historical Review* 107, no. 3 (2002): 703–38.

16. John Theilmann and Frances Cate, "A Plague of Plagues: The Problem of Plague Diagnosis in Medieval England," *Journal of Interdisciplinary History* 37, no. 3 (2007): 371–93.

17. Carmichael, "Plague Persistence," 160.

18. Fabian Crespo and Matthew B. Lawrenz, "Heterogeneous Immunological Landscapes and Medieval Plague: An Invitation to a New Dialogue between Historians and Immunologists," in *Pandemic Disease*, 229–58.

19. M.-L. Derat, "Du lexique aux talismans: occurrences de la peste dans la Corne de l'Afrique du XIIIe au XVe siècle," *Afriques* 09 (2018), https://doi.org/10.4000/afriques2090.

20. Monica H. Green, "Putting Africa on the Black Death Map: Narratives from Genetics and History," *Afriques* 09 (2018), https://doi.org/10.4000/afriques.2125.

21. Stuart Borsch, "Plague Population and Irrigation Decay in Medieval Egypt," in *Pandemic Disease*, 125–56.

22. Vivian Nutton, "The Seeds of Disease: An Explanation of Contagion and Infection from the Greeks to the Renaissance," *Medical History* 27, no. 1 (1983): 1–34.

23. The Book of Jesus Ben-Sirach, chapter 38, verses 1–2. Quoted in John Efron, "A Perfect Healing to All Our Wounds: Religion and Medicine in Judaism," in *Quo Vadis Medical Healing: Past Concepts and New Approaches*, ed. Susanna Elm and Stefan N. Willich (New York: Springer Publishing, 2008), 66 n. 20.

24. Horrox, *Black Death*, 150.

25. Michael Dols, *The Black Death in the Middle East* (Princeton: Princeton University Press, 1977), 281–302.

26. Justin K. Stearns, *Infectious Ideas: Contagion in Premodern Islamic and Christian Thought in the Western Mediterranean* (Baltimore: Johns Hopkins University Press, 2011).

27. Nükhet Varlik, *Plague and Empire in the Early Modern Mediterranean World: The Ottoman Experience, 1347–1600* (New York: Cambridge University Press, 2015).

28. Carmichael, "Plague Persistence," 168–71.

29. Boris Schmid et al., "Climate-Driven Introduction of the Black Death and Successive Plague Reintroduction into Europe," *Proceedings of the National Academy of Sciences* 112, no. 10 (2015): 3020–25.

30. Edward A. Eckert, *The Structure of Plagues and Pestilences in Early Modern Europe: Central Europe, 1560–1640* (Basel: Karger, 1996).

31. Ron Barrett and George Armelagos, *An Unnatural History of Emerging Infections* (Oxford: Oxford University Press, 2013), 51.

32. Paul Slack, *Impact of Plague in Tudor and Stuart England* (London: RKP, 1985), 195.

33. Ann Carmichael, *Plague and the Poor in Renaissance Florence* (Cambridge: Cambridge University Press, 1986).

34. Martin Luther, "Concerning Whether One May Flee from a Deadly Plague, 1527," in *Luther's Works*, vol. 43, *Devotional Writings II*, ed. Gustav K. Wiencke, trans. Carl J. Schindler (Philadelphia: Fortress Press, 1968), 131.

35. Kirsten Bos et al., "Eighteenth Century *Yersinia pestis* Genomes Reveal the Long-Term Persistence of an Historical Plague Focus," *eLife*, no. 5 (2016), https://doi.org/10.7554/eLife.12994.

36. Guenter B. Risse, *Plague, Fear and Politics in San Francisco's Chinatown* (Baltimore: Johns Hopkins University Press, 2012).

37. Myron Echenberg, *Plague Ports: The Global Urban Impact of Bubonic Plague, 1894–1901* (New York: New York University Press, 2007), 161–62.

38. David Arnold, *Colonizing the Body: State Medicine and Epidemic Disease in Nineteenth-Century India* (Berkeley: University of California Press, 1993), 200–39.

39. Alexandre I.R. White, "Global Risks, Divergent Pandemics: Contrasting Responses to Bubonic Plague and Smallpox in 1901 Cape Town," *Social Science History* 42 (2018): 135–58.

40. William C. Summers, *The Great Manchurian Plague of 1910–11: The Geopolitics of an Epidemic Disease* (New Haven: Yale University Press, 2012).

41. World Health Organization, "Plague Outbreak in Remote Madagascar Puzzles Investigators," 2017. http://www.who.int/hac/crises/mdg/sitreps/plague-2017/en/.

42. Myron Echenberg, "Pestis Redux: The Initial Years of the Third Bubonic Plague Pandemic, 1894–1901," *Journal of World History* 13, no. 2 (2002): 433–34.

43. Philip Ziegler, *The Black Death* (London: Collins, 1969), 39.

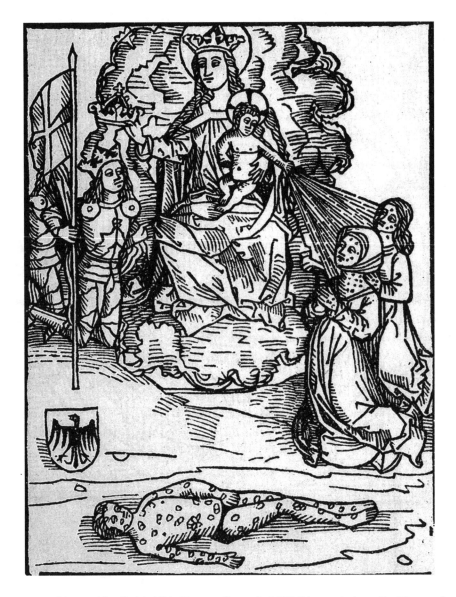

IMAGE 2.1 Mary and the Christ child with pox sufferers. In 1496, this woodcut was the title page for one of the first printed tracts to discuss the origins and treatment of "the evil French disease" (*mala de Franzos*). The woodcut commented on recent events. The German prince Maximilian Habsburg had assumed the title of Holy Roman Emperor in 1493, but warfare in Italy between his allies and a French army prevented him from visiting Rome to be crowned by the pope. The depiction of his crowning by the Virgin Mary suggests that his reign has, in fact, received divine sanction.

Late-medieval Christians considered divine forces to be the ultimate cause of both disease and healing. The gesture of the infant Jesus is enigmatic: are the rays meant to heal pious Christians or inflict punishment on Maximilian's opponents?

SEX, GENDER, AND THE POX OF MANY NAMES

2

I n 1519, a young German humanist named Ulrich von Hütten (1488–1523)
published a Latin tract about his experience with a malady that he called
"the French disease" and others called "the great pox," the "evil of Naples,"
"wild warts," or simply "the pox." By all accounts, this scourge erupted in
the fall of 1495 as an army of French soldiers and mercenaries dispersed
after a campaign in the kingdom of Naples. Thereafter, chroniclers recorded
its swift spread across all of Europe and then into Asian cities linked to the
Indian Ocean trade. Von Hütten himself submitted to painful treatments
containing mercury before he found a remarkable new remedy: potions and
salves made with **guaiac** wood brought from the exotic islands of the
Caribbean.

According to von Hütten's vivid description, the first sufferers endured
burning black-green pustules and boils the size of acorns that oozed secretions
with a sickening stench. He believed, as many others did, that the pestilence arose
from a malevolent planetary conjunction of Saturn and Jupiter, and that for some
years the disease spread through corrupted air as well as by contagion. Thereafter,
von Hütten thought, the scourge had weakened somewhat; the odor was not as
strong, and the boils were not as firm, but its venom still worked its way into the
body to cause many ailments. Now, von Hütten claimed, the French disease
spread principally by sexual intercourse. Beware of women, he warned: as an
English translation of his text (1536) put it, the pox "resteth in theyr secret places,
havynge in those places litel pretty sores full of venemus poison, being very
dangerus for those ye unknowingly medle with them."[1]

To medical historians, von Hütten's memoir stands out as one of the first self-portraits of illness ever to appear in print. In addition to his praise of guaiac, von Hütten presented two ideas that run through the history of the pox (as this book will refer to it) and the disease that might be called its descendant, syphilis. First, the malady that von Hütten described had lessened in potency and caused different symptoms after some years. To many of von Hütten's contemporaries, likewise, the pox seemed to shift from one form to another or assume the guise of other ailments. Centuries later, the leading Canadian physician William Osler (1849–1919) labeled syphilis "the great imitator" because its clinical symptoms resembled those of so many other diseases. Second, von Hütten cautioned of the danger of sex, particularly for males who might be infected unwittingly by a contaminated woman. His wariness reflected a widely held suspicion of sexuality in the culture of early modern Europe, and it was indicative of the privileged place of male sexuality in that era and in much of modern history.

Plague inspired reflection on human sinfulness and calls for repentance; the pox evoked suspicion about immoral behavior and pollution. In Europe, the pattern was firmly established by the early seventeenth century, when poets and playwrights exploited the dramatic nexus of sex, disease, and concealment. The intertwining of moral and scientific concepts continued into the twentieth century, as Europeans encountered non-Western peoples and their maladies.

The Etiology of the Pox and the "Columbian Exchange"

Observers have debated the origins of the pox ever since alarms sounded about the malady in 1495. The many names used for it at first—the "evil of Naples" by the French, the "French disease" by the Germans, or the "Canton itch" by the Japanese— reflected a universal desire to label the pollutant as foreign. Among the origin stories that linked sex and defilement, in 1526 a Spanish chronicler (Gonzalo Fernandez de Oviedo) suggested that sailors from Christopher Columbus's Atlantic voyage brought the disease to the city of Naples in 1494. Versions of this claim have endured, especially among historians who view the question through the prism of Europe's relationship to other parts of the world. According to the influential historian Alfred Crosby, the pox's arrival exemplified a "**Columbian exchange**," the ecological fallout of contact among populations that had developed in isolation for millennia.[2]

However, it now seems that Europe's pox outbreak cannot be explained as a simple transfer of disease from one continent to another. This fascinating riddle begins with a group of closely related bacteria, known together as *Treponema pallidum*, that includes the pathogen that causes venereal (sexually transmitted) syphilis. *T. pallidum* bacteria are classified as spirochetes because of their spiral shape. Humans have encountered treponemal infections for thousands of years and possibly much longer—similar bacteria have been collected from African baboons and gorillas. Many bacteria have tails—or *flagella*, from the Latin word for whip—that protrude into the environment. The *T. pallidum* flagella, however, wrap around the main body underneath a thin membrane. Effectively, **treponemes** are spinning corkscrews that burrow into tissue.

T. pallidum's high motility—its ability to move itself, and especially to move through various types of tissue—helps to explain the many symptoms of infection that are observed today and were recorded in historical sources. In cases of venereal syphilis, the variant identified as *T. pallidum* subspecies *pallidum* usually enters the body through genital contact and leaves a hard-edged lesion called a chancre. (No evidence today confirms sixteenth-century claims that the pox spread through the air.) Syphilis may now be cured with injections of **penicillin**, but if it is not treated the bacteria can migrate almost anywhere in the body: through the intestinal lining, across the placenta that protects the fetus (where they cause congenital syphilis), and even into the brain. In most cases, the initial chancre disappears but is followed several weeks later by a rash that may cover the whole body. Thereafter, syphilis enters a latent stage that is often permanent. Years later, roughly one-third of untreated sufferers eventually progress to late-stage (or tertiary) syphilis and face severe symptoms: impairment of internal organs, bone deformities—including a collapsed nose bridge, and hard nodules known as gummata—and damage to the brain and nervous system that can cause memory loss, blindness, or partial paralysis.[3] The most severe neurological damage, labeled **general paresis**, causes erratic or schizophrenic behavior and was often fatal in the era before reliable treatment was available.

While the clinical course of modern syphilis is relatively clear, researchers have puzzled over *T. pallidum* subsp. *pallidum*'s relationship to other *T. pallidum* subspecies and the diseases they cause. The maladies include **yaws** (caused by *T. pallidum* subsp. *pertenue*), a disease usually passed by skin contact among children in tropical regions of Africa and Asia, and **bejel** (caused by *T. pallidum* subsp. *endemicum*), which currently is limited to arid regions of Africa and the Middle East. The symptoms of yaws and bejel can overlap with syphilis—all of them cause skin lesions and can result in bone or cartilage damage—and some researchers have suggested that yaws, like syphilis, may pass congenitally from mother to child. However, syphilis is the only treponemal infection that spreads primarily by sexual intercourse.

Because *T. pallidum* bacteria are fragile, researchers have barely begun to successfully isolate usable DNA from ancient remains. Instead, they have used other archaeological evidence to explore how Europe's pox might have evolved in relation to the treponemal diseases that are distinguished today. Lesions in American skull and leg bones indicate that many people suffered from treponemal infections before Europeans crossed the Atlantic. Crosby and others viewed this as confirmation of the Columbian hypothesis. It was claimed that Europeans encountered a pathogen, possibly related to yaws, when they met Caribbean peoples in the early 1490s. Sexual transmission became prevalent, possibly because European clothing provided few opportunities for casual contact. However, not everyone has found this scenario convincing. Although the bone evidence for treponemal infections is more scant in Eurasia than in the Americas, some researchers have claimed that syphilis emerged from bejel during antiquity. A treponemal infection (or more than one) may have been prevalent in Europe or North Africa for centuries. Moreover, it is possible that references to the pox in the 1490s may simply reflect greater attention to an old disease rather than the emergence of a new one, although the textual evidence gives the impression that an epidemic broke out in dramatic fashion.

Genetic data from recent bacterial samples (as opposed to the ancient plague DNA discussed in chapter 1) add to our picture of how treponemal infections have evolved, but this evidence answers few questions with certainty. One study compared genetic sequences from twenty samples of *T. pallidum* isolates to estimate a rate of evolution for treponemal bacteria. The results suggested that treponemes evolve relatively slowly, and that *T. pallidum* subsp. *pallidum* emerged on the order of 5,000–16,500 years ago, well before Columbus's Atlantic voyages.[4] Other research suggests that factors other than genetic composition account for the different manifestations of syphilis and yaws. Whole genome sequences have shown that *T. pallidum* subsp. *pallidum* (venereal syphilis) and *T. pallidum* subsp. *pertenue* (yaws) share approximately 99.8 per cent of their DNA, and samples of intermediate strains have also been collected. The diseases caused by each probably reflect the influence of climate, age of the human host, and the physical opportunities for infection.[5] The situation today applies to the late fifteenth century as well: changes in the environment may have influenced the spread of a new scourge as much as changes in a pathogen's genetic signature.

The many variables and lack of ancient DNA samples cast a shadow over explanations of how one bacteria or disease evolved from another. However, the interdisciplinary detective work has reshaped our overall view of treponemal infections in history. These diseases have accompanied human societies around the world. In most times and places they have not spread through sexual contact or been associated with sinful behavior. In the later fifteenth century, a pathogen related to yaws or bejel may have arrived in Iberia from the Caribbean, entered Europe along trade routes from North Africa or western Asia, or circulated more widely after centuries in Europe. Regardless, Europe's interconnected, increasingly urbanized milieu offered fertile ground for the swift spread of a virulent scourge. Thereafter, as European explorers, soldiers, and missionaries traveled the world they carried with them both the disease and the concept of an infection that spread mainly through sexual contact.

What about the relationship between the pox of the sixteenth century and modern syphilis? Earlier historians tended to assume that these diseases were the same, but an unequivocal retrospective diagnosis is now fraught with difficulty. Sixteenth-century reports that the pox broke out suddenly and then waned in severity coexist uneasily with indications from genetic data that treponemes have evolved very gradually. Moreover, the manifestations of syphilis and other treponemal infections that are observed today vary among individuals and over a lifetime. Certainly, this was also true in the more distant past, especially since early modern medical writers relied on concepts of disease that differ fundamentally from the theories that guide inquiry today. Until the early nineteenth century, clear distinctions did not exist between syphilis, **gonorrhea**, and other genital infections, meaning that references to the pox embraced a range of conditions that later clinicians would classify as separate diseases. For various reasons, then, our histories of the pox and of syphilis are continuous but not without fault lines. Over five centuries this disease, by any name, is a moving target to us just as it seemed to Ulrich von Hütten.

The Renaissance Debate over Contagion and Cures

The outbreak of the pox posed a troubling conundrum for European physicians. In addition to their work with patients, physicians were deeply influenced by **humanism**, the attempt to renew European culture by reaping insights from a growing trove of recovered ancient texts. Just as other intellectuals emulated classical authors such as the Roman senator Cicero or the poet Ovid, learned physicians applied principles and methods that had roots more than a thousand years earlier. In doing so, they attempted not only to improve care for patients but also to assert that medicine was a learned discipline that deserved high status at universities and among government officials.

SCIENCE FOCUS

Humoral Medicine and Life in the Balance

Humoral medicine—sometimes called "Galenic medicine" after its most famous architect—often suffers in comparison to the scientific medicine that prevailed after the mid-nineteenth century. Viewed historically, however, its success is astonishing. For over 2,000 years, from Greek antiquity until the eighteenth century, the doctrine of the humors provided the main framework through which Western and Middle Eastern societies understood anatomy, physiology, and pathology. Both intuitive and at times highly complex, humoral medicine provided a foundation for learned medicine and meaningful everyday concepts about the body and its ills.

There was no single humoral medicine with a defined beginning or end. From its first clear articulation in the Hippocratic writings, it was a loose assembly of related concepts and practices that later theorists continued to adapt. As noted in chapter 1, at its center lay the concept of four humors with distinct bodily functions: blood, phlegm, yellow bile, and black bile (figure 2.1). Ancient theorists held that the humors were produced in the stomach and liver as food was "concocted" and then separated into four fluids. The humors corresponded to four elemental forms of matter (earth, air, fire, and water) and, in turn, to qualities that predominated in each type of matter.

Physicians applied the framework of humors and qualities to their observations of both individual organs within a body and to a person's overall temperament or complexion. Because humors varied among people and changed in response to various forces, theories concerning their effects in the body could be very complex.

Broadly speaking, an individual's balance of humor and qualities was thought to be a key to personality or to one's predisposition to certain afflictions. For example, "sanguine" people, in whom blood predominated, tended toward good health and cheerfulness. "Phlegmatic" people, in whom phlegm predominated, tended to retain viscous fluid that made them sluggish and susceptible to ailments caused by the retention of disease-causing matter. This also explained differences between men and women in ways that reinforced broader assumptions about gender. Males were considered innately more sanguine and vigorous; their body's natural heat enabled them to expel or burn off impurities. Females were thought to be relatively phlegmatic, cool, and prone to retention. For this reason, it was believed, after females reached maturity their bodies required periodic expulsion of putrid matter by menstruation. Humans could influence their humoral balance through lifestyle choices—called the "non-naturals"—which included sleep, food and drink, exercise, and sex. Observers also believed that heredity contributed to a person's complexion.

This focus on dynamic, internal conditions also influenced the general understanding of normal and pathological states. Health was characterized in ancient Greek terms as *eukrasia*, or proper balance of the humors, while illness resulted from *dyscrasia*, an overall lack of humoral balance or dysfunction in a particular organ. Although writers recognized that external forces (such as putrid odors or heat) influenced the body, they emphasized the primacy of internal forces. Theorists named various diseases—or pathological conditions such as "fever" that they construed as diseases—but they did not discern rigid boundaries between them. And they did not assume that external forces would cause the same disease in different persons. To cite two brief examples, a fever might evolve from relatively benign to "pestilential" because of individual circumstances, or a person was said to develop "a [form of] consumption," not to contract a disease that affected all sufferers in a similar way. This individualized approach to pathology also applied to the pox. Although some theorists speculated about the role of small particles that might spark the malady, it was agreed that conditions within bodies played a decisive role in one's health or sickness. Theorists did not attribute disease to the influence of tiny, invasive organisms.

The flexibility of the humoral framework gave learned physicians, in particular, great latitude to offer diagnoses and prescriptions that matched particular circumstances. Therapy was mostly governed by the principle that "contraries cure." Practitioners tried to restore the balance of humors by purging excess or

Humor	Combined Primary Qualities	Element
Blood	Hot and moist	Air
Phlegm	Cold and moist	Water
Yellow Bile	Hot and dry	Fire
Black Bile	Cold and dry	Earth

FIGURE 2.1 Ancient humors, qualities, and elements

putrid matter and by replenishing deficiencies. Actions such as bloodletting (venesection), vomiting (emesis), and sweating (sudification) removed excesses. A similar approach applied to local skin complaints. Lancing a boil, for example, involved drawing toxins out to the body's surface before breaking the skin. Nourishing food and tonics replenished deficient humors. Practitioners also assigned qualities to herbs and other medicinals to indicate which ones could counteract a perceived imbalance. For example, in the sixteenth century, potions brewed with guaiac wood brought from the Americas were an important remedy. Practitioners ascribed guaiac's apparent effectiveness against the pox to warm, drying qualities in the wood that removed cold, noxious matter that accumulated in pustules and sore joints.

Although the specifics of humoral theory no longer influence medicine, its legacy persists today. Any dietary supplement or remedy that purports to purge toxins or impurities owes at least some of its appeal to ancient concepts. And the notion of balance, either in one's body or one's whole life, remains one of the most powerful images of well-being in the modern world.

Further reading: Nancy G. Siraisi, *Medieval and Early Renaissance Medicine* (Chicago: University of Chicago Press, 1990), 78–114.

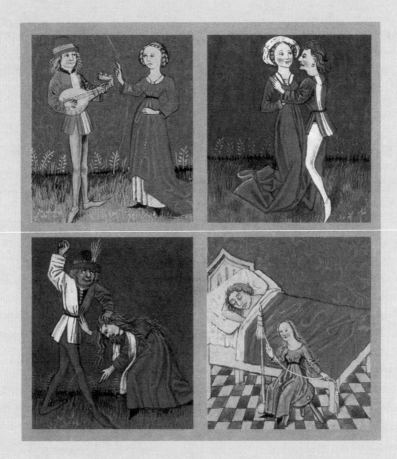

IMAGE 2.2 The four humors in everyday life. This late-fifteenth-century illustration is in the Schürstab Codex, a manuscript commissioned by a wealthy couple in the city of Nuremberg. It depicts a popular understanding of the humors and ideal types of people that prevailed for centuries. Top left: phlegmatic people tended to pensiveness and artistry; top right: sanguine individuals were vigorous and lustful; bottom left: choleric individuals were irritable; bottom right: melancholic individuals were lethargic and depressed.

As discussed in chapter 1, physicians were loyal to the writings of Galen and his successor, Avicenna, whose synthesis of Galen's medicine and Aristotle's philosophical method in the *Canon* was greatly admired during the later Middle Ages. Physicians believed, in principle at least, that all significant diseases had been discussed in antiquity. However, the pox's sudden emergence as a seemingly new, distinct malady fueled debates concerning the respective merits of Greek, Roman, and Arabist approaches to medicine. In the 1490s, physicians at several

European courts and universities debated hypotheses concerning the pox's nature and essence. For example, a leading supporter of ancient Greek medicine, a professor at the University of Ferrara named Nicolò Leoniceno (1428–1524), argued that Hippocrates had described the pox in a discussion of a "disease of summer" in the *Epidemics*. Leoniceno rejected a claim made by other scholars that the pox had been described by the ancient Roman natural historian Pliny the Elder (23–79 CE). By pointing to Hippocrates instead of the later Roman author, Leoniceno gave the pox the oldest possible pedigree and struck a blow for classical Greek as the best vehicle for explaining the natural world.

In larger cities, efforts focused on controlling the spread of the pox and treating its manifestations. Particularly in the Italian and German lands, which faced growing problems with urban poverty, the pox's sudden arrival and worrisome persistence amplified the fears of elites. The afflicted terrified passersby in the streets; their stench was as frightening as their appearance, especially since the spread of disease in general was associated with putrid air as well as physical contact. Observers sometimes considered the pox to be akin to **leprosy** because of the superficial resemblance of some symptoms and the lustful disposition that was attributed to sufferers with either disease. In many communities, the first makeshift shelters for pox sufferers occupied locations where lepers had been exiled in previous centuries.

As the pox's lasting influence became more apparent, cities devised more formal institutions where treatment of the pox was a main focus. In 1515, Pope Leo X approved the recommissioning of a large hospital in Rome, named San Giacomo, to serve poor pox-ridden individuals, who were called *incurabili* (incurables). Under the leadership of the Company of Divine Love, a confraternity of devoted lay Catholics, other Italian cities either founded independent sites for treatment or set up dedicated wards within existing facilities. The term "incurables" notwithstanding, thousands of people received medical treatment and departed after stays of forty days or less.[6] Much the same was true in German towns where local governments established numerous facilities before 1530. In some communities influenced by Protestant religious reforms, such as Zürich and Strasbourg, the closure of monasteries and convents freed up funds that were diverted to poor relief and health care schemes. These measures were especially important because the pox, unlike plague, was a chronic, long-term ailment. The costs of treatment were beyond what many individuals and families could afford.

Galenic medicine did not rigidly distinguish between "care" and "cure," but the attempts to treat the pox with medicine went beyond regimens of healthy food, drink, and rest that the sick traditionally received in medieval hospitals. Initially, many practitioners treated the pox with topical ointments containing mercury compounds such as cinnabar (a mercury sulfide) or calomel (a mercury chloride). These remedies were powerful but less toxic than elemental mercury, and they had a long history among medical writers throughout Europe and Asia. Already in the second century BCE, Chinese medical recipes included mercury formulas to treat skin conditions. More than a thousand years later, in the eleventh century CE, Avicenna prescribed mercury chloride compounds as topical remedies for scabies, chronic itching, lice, and nits. European authors suggested similar salves for leprosy accompanied by heat, which caused the mercury to evaporate so that it could be inhaled. By the early sixteenth century, pox sufferers applied mercury salves to their skin and inhaled fumes from mercury compounds poured into a hot pan. The goals of these treatments were always more or less the same: to burn off surface lesions or to internally purge the body of noxious material through profuse sweating, salivation, and vomiting.

As everyone recognized, mercury treatments were risky and painful. Excessive doses caused mouth ulcers, weakened the gums so that teeth fell out, or caused brain damage. Thus, it was of great interest when news circulated in southern Europe of a gentler remedy brought back from the Indies. So enticing was its reputation that, in 1517, the Holy Roman Emperor Maximilian dispatched several physicians on a fact-finding mission to Spain. Their writings, followed soon after by Ulrich von Hütten's treatise, were the first published accounts of guaiac, sometimes called "holy wood" or "wood of life." As it was later described, the guaiac treatment lasted a minimum of four to six weeks and required several pounds of wood. Fresh guaiac shavings were boiled for hours; patients drank the resulting potion at regular intervals and sat for sessions of profuse sweating. They also applied foam that was skimmed from the boiling liquid directly to their pustules.[7]

At first, guaiac fell outside the purview of orthodox medicine, but Latin-trained physicians and botanists soon found ways to justify its use. Because of its hardness and dark color, guaiac was often considered a type of ebony, a wood that ancient writers had recommended to treat eye ailments and long-lasting ulcers.[8] Physicians also (somewhat arbitrarily) assigned guaiac warm and dry qualities. According to the Galenic logic that "contraries cure," guaiac would, therefore, counter the effects of "cold" ailments such as arthritis or gout as well as the pox. Physicians soon distinguished their judicious use of guaiac from mercury treatments offered by unlearned healers who, so the physicians claimed, practiced a barbarous medicine governed by trial and error. In time, guaiac and the pox were linked as New World products, although, as we have seen, guaiac was in use before Oviedo and others popularized the claim that the disease had American

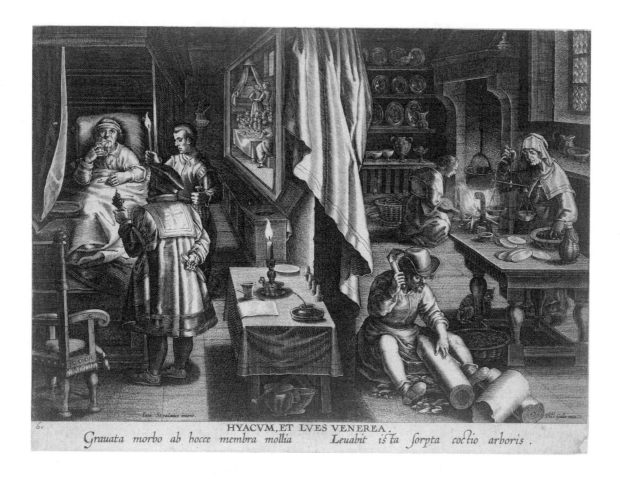

IMAGE 2.3 *Treating the Pox with Guaiac* (ca 1570). This engraving by P. Galle and Jan van der Straet combines actions that usually took place in two or more locations. To the right, guaiac bark is chopped, weighed, and simmered. To the left, a patient is attended by a servant and a surgeon as he consumes a guaiac potion. The picture on the wall facing the patient depicts revelry and fornication—an oblique reference to the pox's association with sexual misdeeds.

origins. Especially among authors who stressed the goodness of God's providence, it seemed fitting that disease and cure would spring from the same place.

However, not everyone agreed that guaiac was useful. The debate over it tapped into theoretical discussions concerning the nature of contagious disease and the ability of ancient medicine to explain it. The contrasting ideas of two theorists, Girolamo Fracastoro of Verona (ca 1478–1553) and the itinerant mage Theophrastus von Hohenheim (1493–1541), provide an effective illustration. Fracastoro was a physician with wide-ranging humanist interests. In 1530, he published a lengthy Latin poem in classical epic style that was entitled *Syphilis, or the French Disease* (*Syphilis, sive morbus gallicus*). The fanciful narrative attributed the pox to the punishment of Apollo, the sun god, upon a rebellious shepherd. In the poem's last section, which he added to satisfy an elite patron, Fracastoro described a miraculous, curative wood that explorers on a distant island were about to bring home to Europe. This enigmatic ending apparently referred to guaiac's arrival from the Indies, but Fracastoro stopped short of any suggestion that Europe's pox had foreign origins. Among humanists, the poem earned Fracastoro acclaim for literary merit; the work also introduced the term "syphilis," which physicians applied to the disease itself after the late eighteenth century.

In 1546, Fracastoro published a more sedate theoretical treatise, *On contagion* (*De contagione*), which explained the spread of disease in terms of invisible forces that he perceived throughout the natural world. The turn of a compass needle to the pole, the movement of iron toward a magnet, rot that spreads among apples— Fracastoro believed all were examples of attraction, or "sympathy," that were akin to the contagious spread of disease. Sympathy enabled disease to spread in several ways: by contact, through particles known as *fomites* (Latin for "tinder"), or even at a distance. Fracastoro considered both the pox and plague to be diseases that spread through fomites that could remain infective for long periods. He believed the pox's fomites, or seedlets, created the foul, thick phlegm found in pustules and the deforming gummata. Similar to Ulrich von Hütten, Fracastoro believed the pox initially had astrological causes, and he further thought the disease was weakening, like an aging animal or person, as time went on. Where treatment was concerned, Fracastoro did not reject the use of mercury but he praised the warming and drying effects of guaiac and provided his own version of the instructions for the cure. To readers centuries later, Fracastoro's discussion of seedlets seemed to be a prescient formulation of germ theory. In fact, as Vivian Nutton has explained, Fracastoro looked to the ancients for inspiration as other humanists did, and his ideas had much in common with other theorists of his time.[9]

The same cannot be said for Theophrastus von Hohenheim, also known as Paracelsus (ca 1493–1541), who caused an uproar as he sojourned in south-German and Swiss cities during the 1520s and 1530s. Everything about him annoyed the learned elite. Paracelsus lectured and wrote in German rather than Latin, brusquely rejected ancient medical authority, and denounced anyone who disagreed with him. His targets included Catholic healing rituals and saints, which led some people to associate him with the religious reformer Martin Luther. Paracelsus produced a remarkable number of texts that combined alchemy, medicine, biblical commentary, and speculative philosophy. While these writings were not always consistent, in general he advocated a new approach to the natural world based around three chemical principles (salt, sulfur, and mercury) instead of the four elements proposed by Aristotle (earth, air, fire, and water). Beginning two decades after his death, Paracelsus's alchemical writings enjoyed a great vogue. From 1565 forward, they were published in great numbers, and the investigations of his followers influenced the early development of chemistry.

During Paracelsus's lifetime, however, it was his combative approach to medical authority that caused the most controversy. His writings on the "French disease," which he published in 1529, served as a springboard for a comprehensive attack on the medical profession. Paracelsus favored mercury as a remedy for the pox; he rejected guaiac as useless; and he even suggested that the merchants who imported the wood were to blame for the deaths of numerous pox sufferers. He lambasted medical "imposters," physicians who subverted the true art of healing with their slavish reliance on ancient writings. The old texts were "honeyed chatter," Paracelsus claimed—the peasants of Bavaria could cure a German disease more effectively than the ancient Greeks. Some conventional physicians also criticized exotic imports, but Paracelsus's polemic went beyond expressions of solidarity with common folk and local remedies. Effectively, he denied that the words of Greek or any other language were intrinsically superior as a means of describing the world. His basic claim about the relationship of words and things struck at the heart of the humanist enterprise, which assumed that ancient languages created the best framework for human knowledge.[10]

Guaiac never replaced mercury treatments entirely—indeed, mercury-based ointments and eventually injections were used into the twentieth century—but treatments with the wood were tried for at least two centuries. How did therapeutic experiences contribute to guaiac's popularity? When we consider the stages of syphilis that have been observed in recent times, we might guess that many people credited guaiac for the natural easing of symptoms that took place as the disease entered a latent phase. Even if guaiac did not demonstrably cure the pox as we would judge today, its physical effects probably reinforced the perception that it did. Modern researchers do not regard guaiac as an antibacterial agent, but its usefulness as an expectorant to assist discharge of phlegm has never been questioned. The United States Food and Drug Administration (FDA) approved a compound derived from guaiac resin for this purpose in 1952, and a synthetic version, guaifenesin, remains a frequent ingredient in cough remedies. Since sixteenth-century medicine treated most diseases by encouraging the body to expel morbid material, it is not surprising that doctors and patients used guaiac for the pox and other ailments.

Guaiac was only one of several woods that practitioners touted as pox remedies or cure-all panaceas in a growing global trade of medical products. Soon after the arrival of the pox in East Asia, Chinese remedies included teas and inhaled vapor from the boiled root of *tu fu ling*, several related species of plants that European writers named "China root." In the second half of the sixteenth century, authors in India and Persia described this treatment, and by the mid-seventeenth century tons of the plants were shipped to ports in Japan. By the 1540s, China root arrived in Europe, where it soon competed with varieties of sarsaparilla from New Spain (Mexico) and sassafras from New England. In the West, China root eventually waned in popularity but sarsaparilla and sassafras continued to serve as medicinal ingredients and, in recent times, as the defining ingredient in some soft drinks and teas. While none of these remedies cured the pox or prevented its spread, many sufferers believed in their healing properties and experienced a sensation of relief.[11] The spread of such remedies indicates the growing willingness of European consumers to embrace exotic therapies, while learned elites adapted traditional theories to accommodate a growing list of medicinal herbs.

Although the demographic impact of the pox was not as profound as the changes wrought by plague, it created novel challenges for theorists, practitioners, and public officials. The pox's chronic effects demanded sustained attention, and the widespread belief that it was curable motivated civic health programs and the sale of new medical products. Its cultural imprint contrasted with that of plague. Whereas plague invited communal soul-searching, over time the pox provoked suspicion—and satire—about individual actions. Especially in commentary concerning women, the pox became a potent symbol of immorality as well as a threat to physical health.

The Pox, Prostitution, and Morality in Early Modern Europe

For a few short years, public responses to the pox echoed many of the themes of collective repentance inspired by plague. In 1495, the Holy Roman Emperor Maximilian issued an edict suggesting that the scourge was punishment for blasphemy. Other writers soon announced that the pox was God's just punishment for humanity's misdeeds, including nonsexual sins. However, as the sexual spread of the disease became more obvious, suspicion focused on soldiers, vagrants, and people whose sexual conduct was held in suspicion.

Among the early commentators was the humanist Erasmus of Rotterdam (1466–1536), a preeminent scholar of classical languages whose writings combined a moral sensibility with scathing wit. Beginning in 1519, Erasmus published editions of *Colloquies*, exercises and short texts for his Latin students that evolved into lighthearted dialogues on social issues. "The Unequal Match" (1529) depicted the horror of a young girl compelled to marry a pox-ridden older man. As the "scabby wedding" commenced, the groom made his entrance: "nose broken, one foot dragging after the other ... scurvy hands, a breath that would knock you over, lifeless eyes, head bound up, bloody matter exuding from nose and ears."[12] Erasmus's sad vignette criticized the forced marriage of incompatible people but also gave voice to a growing anxiety about illicit sex and the danger of disease. Although the *Colloquies* were published in Latin, vernacular printed works also grew rapidly in popularity, including medical tracts that commented on the symptoms and treatment of the pox.

As patients and medical practitioners realized, it was far easier to rail against immoral pox-spreaders in print than to deal with actual sufferers. Throughout the sixteenth century, most physicians agreed that the disease usually spread through sexual intercourse. But some evidence, especially the troubling incidence of disease in small children, suggested that other means of transmission must also be possible. Observers suggested that shared utensils, unwashed bedsheets at an inn, or even a lingering kiss might be to blame. On occasion, women hurled accusations at midwives who attended them; the operators of public baths sometimes faced charges that bloodletting cups were contaminated. Given the sanitary conditions of the time, and the potential for infection to pass through nongenital contact, some of the claims may have been true. In any case, the uncertainty over transmission benefited individuals who protested that they were infected innocently rather than through illicit sex.

Not all sufferers were held responsible for their infections, but, from the later sixteenth century forward, long-range social forces contributed to a hardening of attitudes toward pox sufferers. One key factor in many cities was a shift in the approach to prostitution that accompanied Europe's religious reform movements. Traditional Christian teachings upheld the ideals of virginity for unmarried young women and celibacy for priests, monks, and nuns as markers of moral purity. However, most church and city leaders had not objected to the sale of sex by women to adult men. For centuries, authorities had suggested instead that the evil of prostitution was preferable to the male lust that would be unbridled if brothels were closed. The legalistic bent of medieval theology blunted the sharp edge of disapproval. For example, the leading authority Thomas Aquinas (ca 1225–1274) suggested that prostitution caused lustful fornication, but the exchange of cash for sex that took place afterward was not in itself sinful.[13] From a medical standpoint, moreover, (male) sexual release was considered important to maintain good health. Accordingly, city leaders usually found it both morally acceptable and socially desirable to tolerate, or quietly encourage, a defined sexual outlet for men on the outskirts of town. During social crises, including outbreaks of disease, leaders often closed brothels temporarily to limit activities that they considered morally and physically contaminating. The initial response to the pox mostly fit this pattern; many people linked sexual activity and infection but these observations did not translate into widespread efforts to limit prostitution.

The religious reform movements of the sixteenth century (see chapter 1) upended the social acceptance of the sex trade. In particular, Luther vigorously denied that clerical celibacy had any value and he encouraged pastors to take wives and have children. At the same time, Luther and his followers discouraged sexual activity outside of marriage and prescribed a domestic role for women under male authority. Much the same was true for communities inspired by Calvin, which relied on church courts called consistories to discourage and punish offenses that included sexual misconduct. Many city brothels were shut down in the German lands beginning in the 1530s and in France during the 1550s and 1560s. In Italian cities that remained Catholic, many brothels remained open, but illicit sex was increasingly discouraged and church officials enforced clerical celibacy more strictly. As sex workers were forced to vacate specified locations to work in city streets, they increasingly were perceived as an uncontained, pervasive threat of disease and moral corruption.

Changes in Europe's urban populations also encouraged transmission of the pox and anxiety about disease in general. The growth of overseas trade and government bureaucracies created metropolises of a larger scale than medieval cities. Between 1550 and 1650, the population of Paris grew from 275,000 to nearly 450,000 despite a decline in French population during civil wars in the late sixteenth century. Amsterdam, the epicenter of northern Europe's rising merchant economy, grew tenfold from roughly 15,000 inhabitants to 175,000. In such centers, many social contacts were fleeting and young immigrants from rural areas were freed from constraints they faced at home. Port cities supported the demand for sexual services from the growing traffic of sailors and merchants. City dwellers in general tended to die young, meaning that families and networks of intimate relationships were often disrupted and refashioned. Finally, rising populations and worsening economic conditions throughout Europe forced many people to live as transients and city officials across Europe complained that they were beset by vagrants and beggars.

Recent analyses of AIDS and syphilis have confirmed that inequality, social instability, transient populations, and a double standard of sexual behavior for men and women all hasten the spread of sexually transmitted infections (STIs). Much the same was true in early modern cities, although experts debated the precise role of sexual activity, and the concepts of infection and disease were not articulated as they would be in the twentieth century. No community presented greater opportunities for the spread of the pox than London. As it became a port city of global stature, London's population mushroomed from around 120,000 inhabitants in 1550 to over 350,000 a century later. The sex trade grew to meet demand, propelled by large numbers of poor young women who came in search of work. In the Middle Ages, bathhouses and brothels had concentrated near the south bank of the Thames River. These "stews" were closed after a proclamation by King Henry VIII in 1546, but this measure and other short-lived reform efforts mostly had the effect of dispersing sex workers throughout the city. By the turn of the seventeenth century, London sex workers of all social levels numbered in the thousands and many women combined sex work with other money-making ventures. The city's numerous alehouses hosted encounters of every sort; as a comment in a play of the time put it, "a cup of Ale without a wench, why, alasse, 'tis like an egge without salt, or a red herring without mustard."[14]

How pox-ridden were the residents of early modern European cities? Rough estimates suggest that, in most cities, about one adult in ten contracted a venereal disease. For example, Simon Szreter's study of Chester, an English city of about 15,000 inhabitants in the 1770s, suggests that roughly 8 per cent of both men and women sought treatment for the pox by age 35 in facilities or privately with practitioners (and others probably concealed their maladies altogether).[15] Certainly, London's residents encountered signs of the disease everywhere, in blemishes, bald patches, damaged noses, and the odor of infection. Cosmetic products such as heavy makeup and wigs provided concealment but also offered reminders that beneath the surface not all was as it appeared. The image of the devious whore with a painted face represented the pitfalls of casual sex and further symbolized an unfettered merchant economy in which anything could be bought and sold. The didactic writer Barnabe Rich made the moral and physical dangers explicit in *My Ladies Looking Glass* (1616): "As the harlot destroieth his soule that doth frequent her, so she is a plague to the flesh ... and carries more diseases about her, then is in an hospitall."[16]

This conception of personal contamination, rooted in Christian beliefs as well as medical theory, exerted a lasting influence upon Western culture. We may compare this approach to sex and disease with the moral conventions of early modern Japan, which unified politically in the late sixteenth century after centuries of factional warfare. During the long-running Tokugawa dynasty (1603–1868), the government approach to the sex trade superficially resembled the medieval European practice of creating an isolated zone for activities that were unacceptable elsewhere. In large cities, ruling elites created *yukakū*, enclosed "pleasure districts" that were formally segregated by gates, ditches, and moats. The largest of these, the Yoshiwara district in Edo (later Tokyo), housed hundreds and eventually thousands of dancers, geishas, and prostitutes of both sexes until the late nineteenth century. As urban populations expanded, from the later seventeenth century forward government officials also tolerated "serving girls" who combined domestic service and sex work in tea shops and inns.

Venereal disease was an acknowledged health risk in early modern Japan, as evidenced by medical treatises with mercury-based recipes not unlike Chinese and European remedies. However, the pox and other ailments did not bear the same type of moral stigma as in Europe, nor was the same value placed on long-term monogamy.[17] Among elites in the stratified society of early modern Japan, improper contact with people of lower social status was a more salient concern than sex with a prostitute. Although transactional sex did not have the same stigma in Japan as in Europe, Japanese sex workers did not enjoy higher status or better conditions, and they routinely suffered from sexually transmitted diseases. In the absence of any system of poor relief, the attempted cure of these diseases mostly remained a private matter and there were no government-sponsored treatment facilities.

In Europe, by contrast, as governments expanded in the eighteenth century, the fight against sexually transmitted diseases merged with broader efforts to sustain healthy, vigorous populations. As noted in the previous chapter, many states invested increasing resources in quarantine and border control to counter the threat of plague. Various authors considered administrative measures that would foster health and the prevention of disease. Beginning in 1779, the Austrian physician Johann Peter Frank (1745–1821) sketched out an influential system of medical regulation that touched almost all aspects of life, including child-rearing, inspection of food and water, protection from epidemic disease, and the regulation of prostitutes. While the full ambitions of Frank's scheme were not realized, elites across Europe increasingly accepted that the promotion of social hygiene was an important function of the state.

European countries adopted bolder methods to control the poor and diseased. In England, the intervention took the form of workhouse clinics and so-called **lock hospitals** that were founded in several cities after 1747. The latter institutions often were funded by private donations and combined treatment for venereal diseases with moral instruction in a rigidly controlled atmosphere. In France, revolutionary upheaval in 1789 was followed by determined efforts to put rational principles into social practice. In 1792, Parisian officials gathered adult pox sufferers from various facilities into a single center for venereal patients, the Hospice des Vénériens. By 1810, the facility treated roughly 3,000 people annually with a combination of mercury and other remedies. On the Continent, more so than England, the main focus of antidisease measures shifted to prevention and especially the control of prostitutes. In the first decade of the nineteenth century, the French government took steps to require registration and regular medical inspections of prostitutes. These measures spread in the wake of Napoleon's brief occupation of much of Europe. City police officials often exercised discretion over enforcement measures such as weekly or biweekly physical examinations, a requirement to carry an identity card, or detailed rules concerning the times, locations, and clothing that prostitutes could wear when they solicited customers.

The attempts to apply enlightened principles were not always successful or even-handed, as illustrated by the Vaugirard hospital for pox-ridden infants, which was founded in 1780. In a Paris chateau that housed the facility, physicians attempted a distinctive method of mercury treatment: because infants were too weak to withstand direct exposure, destitute young mothers who already had the pox were dosed with mercury and trained to nurse the babies. Hundreds of women nursed about 2,000 infants before the results were deemed a failure. Although the facility was closed in 1790, the experimentation with infants and poor women did not end. For decades thereafter, numerous physicians helped families with infected children to hire wet nurses and dose the women with mercury without their knowledge. Remarkably, dozens of women eventually sued physicians for withholding information. After 1868, when a court ruled in a wet nurse's favor, some of them received punitive damages and physicians were forced to confront the ethical considerations of the practice more explicitly.[18] Women's bodies had long been considered the chief source of venereal infection; it would not be easy to use them as instruments of cure.

Syphilis and Its Treatments after 1850

In the later nineteenth century, the European approach to sexually transmitted diseases had much in common with that of earlier times. Government officials usually accepted that unmarried males required a sexual outlet. Prostitutes were to be tightly controlled and various forms of surveillance and confinement accompanied treatment of the poor. Alongside these continuities, evolving standards of conduct aggravated the pressures that young adults encountered. Polite society avoided discussion of sex almost entirely: men were expected to delay marriage until they reached financial independence, women were to remain "pure" for their husbands, and masturbation was considered a graver sin than premarital intercourse. These mores were not without critics. In 1881, Norwegian playwright Henrik Ibsen (1828–1906) published *Ghosts* (*Gegangere*), a scathing commentary on European bourgeois hypocrisy that depicted the destructive impact of syphilis on family ties.

The work of Jean Alfred Fournier (1832–1914), a Paris physician and university professor who devoted his career to venereal diseases, reflected a more conventional approach to such issues. In 1875, Fournier identified the relationship between early syphilis infection and its eventual effects on some sufferers, which included a stumbling gait and paralysis caused by nerve damage in the spinal cord. He urged sexual abstinence, both in numerous lectures and in the book *Syphilis in Marriage* (*Syphilis et mariage*), which was published in 1880 and soon translated into English and German. At all costs, Fournier suggested, men should avoid infecting their wives and causing the horror of "pox in the cradle."[19] Such statements fueled a fear of physical and moral degeneration that would persist across the generations, although scientists soon attributed syphilis in infants to congenital infection rather than inheritance.

As chapters 5 and 6 will discuss, advances in microscopes and staining procedures yielded insight into the causes of anthrax, tuberculosis, and other diseases. For so-called venereal disease that included syphilis, the initial results from these new methods were both enlightening and disheartening. In 1879, a German researcher in Breslau, Albert Neisser (1855–1916), identified the bacterial agent of gonorrhea, while in Naples the cause of **chancroid** was found by Augusto Ducrey (1860–1940) in 1889. These discoveries confirmed that venereal disease was, in fact, several distinct infections, but they also showed that the ailments were harder to diagnose and more widespread than physicians had realized. Although the syphilis-causing spirochete was identified in 1905, this disease also remained elusive, particularly since late-stage symptoms mysteriously appeared in some sufferers and not others. Knowledge of microbes did little on its own to relieve fears about the spread of disease, and as clinicians gathered information about the effects of late-stage syphilis it seemed that no organ was safe from its ravages.

However, scientists influenced by the German bacteriologist Robert Koch (1843–1910) soon developed more practical tools to combat venereal infections. There were several angles of attack: researchers investigated the feasibility of a vaccine or vaccine-like procedures, devised new chemical disinfectants to apply after sexual contact, or investigated ways of destroying the bacteria after an infection had ensued. One preliminary step was to find a method for determining who had infections and required treatment. At Neisser's suggestion, in 1906 a team led by August von Wassermann (1866–1925) developed a test for **antibodies** in blood that indicated the presence of syphilis bacteria. Although the test occasionally yielded false positives, for decades it was used to confirm diagnoses or to detect infection in patients with no symptoms. The premarital blood test to rule out (or discover) syphilis and other diseases soon became a ritual for betrothed couples throughout the Western world.

Even more exciting was the work of Paul Ehrlich (1854–1915), who first earned fame in the early 1890s when he helped develop a therapy for **diphtheria** (an infection of throat and nasal mucous membranes that often afflicted children). As discussed in chapter 6, Ehrlich also pioneered a technique for staining microbes that greatly assisted efforts to identify and combat tuberculosis infections. He reasoned that drug treatments could act similarly to chemical dyes, either to bind with cells—and thereby block the action of microbes—or to destroy the microbes themselves. At an institute in Frankfurt, Ehrlich tested hundreds of arsenic compounds to find a combination that could kill bacteria without damaging human organs. Research on this scale was impossible with humans, but Ehrlich collaborated with a Japanese scientist, Sahachiro Hata (1873–1938), who developed a method of reproducing syphilis in rabbits that could be used as subjects. After numerous trials, a treatment named Salvarsan—or "that which saves by arsenic"—went on sale with great fanfare in 1910. Ehrlich famously called Salvarsan a "magic bullet" for syphilis. But it soon became clear that the drug and its successor, Neosalvarsan, had limits. Multiple injections were required, and the side effects included vomiting, diarrhea and, in a few cases, sudden coma and death.

Despite their drawbacks, Ehrlich's drugs were the most effective syphilis treatment for roughly a quarter century. Thereafter, researchers borrowed techniques from industrial chemistry to create a new group of drugs based on a synthetic chemical compound, sulfonamide. In the decade after 1935, when a product sold as Prontosil was released to the public, numerous **sulfa drugs** successfully treated a wide range of bacterial infections, including syphilis. They were the most widely used antibacterial agents until the end of World War II, and they remain in use for some infections today. Sulfonamides have been credited with beginning the era of "miracle drugs" that accelerated research and raised expectations for medical care.[20]

In the mid-1940s, however, the treatment of syphilis and other bacterial diseases was revolutionized again by an entirely different kind of drug, penicillin. Derived from some types of *Penicillium*, a common mold that inhabits soil, penicillin is a natural molecule that disrupts the ability of many bacteria to build cell walls as they divide. Several nineteenth-century researchers had observed the mold's microbe-killing properties. In 1928, a team in London led by Alexander Fleming (1881–1955) isolated the active compound. Fleming's "mould juice" proved to be fussy and unstable; while he was unable to produce it on a useful scale, researchers at Oxford University in Britain resumed the work a decade later under the leadership of two scientists, Howard Florey (1898–1968) from Australia and Ernst Chain (1906–1979) from Germany. A third researcher, Norman Heatley (1911–2004), devised a procedure that used ether to extract penicillin from the mold in sufficient quantities to enable animal testing of its properties.[21] During World War II, a remarkable collaboration among Allied scientists, government officials, and pharmaceutical companies developed methods to manufacture penicillin on an industrial scale. In 1943, the drug was first made available to the public in Australia. Supplies were ready for the D-Day invasion of France in June 1944, and the following year penicillin went on sale in US pharmacies. Penicillin proved remarkably effective against skin infections, boils, abscesses, pneumonia, and other ailments. It was also highly effective against gonorrhea, and syphilis could be cured with only a few intramuscular injections.

Ehrlich's success with Salvarsan had underscored the value of methodical testing. The prospect of great gain from such projects was seductive. By this time, the success of smallpox vaccination (see chapter 3) had indicated that diseased material could cause a powerful resistance response in the body. As at Vaugirard, however, the price of knowledge was sometimes paid by unsuspecting and vulnerable people. Some investigators used human subjects with methods that are rejected today. The history of syphilis, in particular, illustrates how researchers who work without clear ethical standards may override the interests of powerless people.

Syphilis, Medical Experimentation, and Informed Consent

From the 1850s forward, scientists in Europe and the United States tested syphilis treatments and vaccines by injecting subjects with diseased material. Before Ehrlich's chemical breakthrough, a syphilis vaccine seemed within reach and well worth investigation. Researchers sometimes sought volunteers but more often used orphans, hospital patients, prostitutes, or prison inmates. It is true that some scientists were troubled by the use of human subjects. Already in 1851, Fournier's mentor, the prominent venereal disease researcher Philippe Ricord (1800–1889), had urged his colleagues to avoid human experiments regardless of the eagerness of volunteers. Nonetheless, for another century most researchers believed the value of human subjects outweighed the ethical pitfalls.

In 1899, controversy erupted in Prussia over Albert Neisser, who injected blood serum from syphilis patients into thirty-six individuals. His unknowing subjects included three young girls and five prostitutes. None of them was diagnosed with syphilis initially, but at least four of them developed the disease after the injections. After Neisser was criticized in newspapers, the Prussian Parliament discussed the case in March 1899. The following year, the government directed hospitals and clinics to obtain informed consent for any procedure other than therapy, diagnosis, or vaccination. A disciplinary court fined Neisser for his conduct with the young girls because he had not consulted their parents. However, his treatment of the prostitutes was not reprimanded; it was legal to force sex workers to undergo treatment, and the court considered Neisser's injections an attempt to help individuals who were at high risk of infection.[22] The Prussian directive was a landmark requirement of informed consent in medical research, but sex workers were excluded from its protections. The regulation also fell short of a criminal law to be enforced with clear penalties and did little to reform practices in Europe or elsewhere. As explained in chapter 4, in 1900 US Army officers conducted a yellow fever experiment in Cuba that established a similar precedent for informed consent, but this episode, too, exerted little influence on the overall research environment.

In some instances, neurosyphilis sufferers were likely prospects for medical research because their dementia made consent (or refusal) impossible, and the disease's severe, stigmatizing effects encouraged their advocates to allow desperate measures. In Vienna during the 1910s, psychiatrist Julius Wagner-Jauregg (1857–1940) tested the effects of high fever on numerous individuals at the Asylum of Lower Austria. The idea behind "fever therapy"—that a short bout of high fever might cure a pre-existing illness—had ancient origins. Nineteenth-century practitioners rarely attempted it, but Wagner-Jauregg had observed a woman whose psychotic symptoms disappeared after an episode of high fever. After conducting various experiments, in 1917 he turned to a mild form of malaria as a means of inducing a series of feverish episodes. Wagner-Jauregg collected blood from malaria-stricken soldiers at a nearby hospital and injected the samples into over 200 neurosyphilitic individuals. He later reported that fifty had recovered sufficiently to return to work. These findings were met with great excitement, particularly since Salvarsan had proven ineffective against neurosyphilis. Wagner-Jauregg even received the Nobel Prize for Medicine in 1927. Enthusiasm for fever treatment diminished after penicillin was introduced, but, through the early 1940s, numerous researchers attempted to replicate Wagner-Jauregg's success or raise body temperature by other methods.

The legacy of such trials was certainly ambiguous. Thousands of people benefited from treatment for a devastating disease that otherwise was almost incurable. Wagner-Jauregg's findings also demonstrated that mental illnesses could have a biological basis. This important idea stimulated drug research and the discipline of biological psychiatry. On the other hand, many mentally ill patients certainly did not understand the malaria infection procedure, and some individuals experienced little or no benefit from the treatment. Eventually, Wagner-Jauregg's reputation was tarnished by revelations that he sympathized with some objectives of the Nazi regime, and many scientists and historians sidelined his achievements.[23]

In the decades after World War I, national governments considered information about STIs to be of strategic interest for public health and the effectiveness of the armed forces. Public health authorities fretted over the nagging prevalence of syphilis, which in the United States was estimated to range between 5 and 10 per cent with substantially higher rates among lower-class populations. In 1937, US Surgeon General Thomas Parran called syphilis "a shadow on the land," and he dramatically called for a "Wassermann dragnet" to identify cases of the disease with blood testing.[24]

In this context, two initiatives coordinated by the United States Public Health Service (USPHS) merit closer attention: the Tuskegee Syphilis Experiment (1932–72), and research concerning STIs in Guatemala (1946–48).[25] At Tuskegee, in Macon County, Alabama, a research study recruited 399 poor African American farmers who had been diagnosed with late-stage syphilis in order to collect data for six months and then provide them with treatment. However, when the funding for treatment was withdrawn, the project was reconceived as a "study in nature": researchers would withhold all treatment and monitor the long-term effects of syphilis until the men died. At a time when racial differences in health were of interest, the study tested the claim that African Americans would suffer less severe effects from late-stage syphilis than whites. Test subjects were not told that they had syphilis—instead, the researchers used the vague label "bad blood"—and many men received misleading information suggesting that the researchers were providing treatment. In fact, for decades researchers subjected the men to painful spinal taps that provided cerebrospinal fluid for tests but offered no therapeutic benefit. Investigators also discouraged the subjects from receiving penicillin or other therapies from public health programs. When some of the subjects joined the armed forces in World War II, researchers even contacted military officials to prevent the men from receiving treatments that were provided to other soldiers free of charge. Even after penicillin came into widespread use, numerous professionals remained complicit with the project, and some defended it from critics through the 1960s.

Some writers have claimed that the Tuskegee study's moral failings appear worse in hindsight than they were in the social milieu of the 1930s and 1940s.[26] Initially, several important points were unclear: whether penicillin would be effective for individuals with late-stage, latent syphilis; if the drug might actually cause harm in such cases; or whether latent syphilis should be treated at all when patients did not experience symptoms. In 1948, a study conducted at Stanford University in California published results from hundreds of men who had opted not to receive treatment for years. However, the most critical ethical lapse at Tuskegee concerned the lack of informed consent among the experiment's participants during the lengthy study. At Stanford, the test subjects (who were white) elected to forgo treatment, and they were informed that medical procedures connected to the experiment provided research data but no health benefits for them.[27] Likewise, for a gonorrhea experiment conducted in 1942–44 at a federal prison in Terre Haute, Indiana, USPHS researchers secured the consent of inmate "volunteers" before the men were inoculated with gonorrhea's causal bacteria. (This was to test the effects of sulfa drugs taken prior to inoculation and chemical agents that were applied after inoculation.) The Terre Haute experiment violated ethical standards that are accepted today—prison inmates cannot give consent free of coercion—but at least the nature of the study was disclosed to its participants. At Tuskegee, deception continued for four decades, despite an international consensus, which emerged in response to abuses during World War II, that informed consent was necessary to conduct human medical experiments. Moreover, in the early 1950s health officials began to recommend penicillin to treat all stages of syphilis, but Tuskegee's researchers withheld the drug from their test subjects anyway.[28] The study's ethics were questionable when it began and unacceptable for many years before it ended.

The Tuskegee study recruited subjects who had contracted syphilis prior to the start of the study. Its procedures did not involve the intentional infection of test subjects. However, between 1946 and 1948, USPHS officials also conducted research with individuals in Guatemala whom they exposed to syphilis, gonorrhea, and chancroid.[29] A Guatemalan physician initially proposed the research during a visit to New York City in 1945. Some of the American researchers who were involved had participated in the gonorrhea infection study at Terre Haute. In Guatemala, the test subjects included soldiers in the Guatemalan Army, prisoners at a penitentiary, and inmates at a psychiatric hospital. Since commercial sex work was legal in Guatemala, researchers employed sex workers to expose test subjects to pathogens. Prior to sexual encounters, cotton swabs were used to expose the sex workers' genitals to the causal bacteria of gonorrhea or syphilis. Similar to the Terre Haute study, researchers wished to investigate the value of chemicals that were to be applied topically after "normal exposure" (the researchers' term for intercourse). In some cases, to increase the chance that infection would take place, test subjects were exposed to diseased material directly, often on more than one occasion. In all, a reported total of 1,308 individuals, ranging in age from 10 to 72 years, were involved in the exposure experiments. Thousands more provided blood and spinal fluid samples; the latter were often obtained with a cisternal puncture (removal of fluid from the back of the skull). No evidence indicates that the project was explained or that consent was ever sought from sex workers, soldiers, or prisoners, let alone from psychiatric patients who often were incapable of understanding or assenting to the procedures. Some test subjects received treatment after they were infected while others apparently did not.

The Guatemala experiments ended quietly in 1948, although data collection from the subjects continued for several years. The project largely escaped attention until historian Susan Reverby brought it to light in 2010.[30]

In contrast, the ongoing Tuskegee Syphilis Experiment concluded abruptly in 1972 when a concerned official exposed it to a journalist and touched off a storm of negative publicity. Although the study was then condemned, by this time numerous test subjects had already died (in most cases from conditions that were not directly related to syphilis). Public outcry prompted a thorough assessment of research practices. In 1981, the United States government adopted a requirement for independent ethical review of all studies with human subjects. However, the revelations also laid bare a systemic bias against African Americans in medicine. For a generation of Southern black men, reports about the study discouraged trust in public health authorities. The Tuskegee Syphilis Experiment remains a symbol of racism in United States health care.

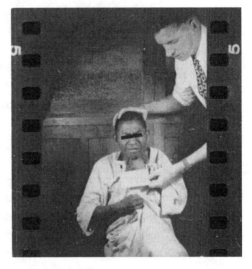

IMAGE 2.4 Guatemalan syphilis experiment subject (ca 1947). A large number of the test subjects in the Guatemala project were of Indigenous descent. This male psychiatric patient was exposed to syphilis twice and treated with penicillin. Why he was admitted to the psychiatric hospital is unknown. One researcher (who worked in the prison) suggested that it was unnecessary to explain the experiments to "Indians" since "they are only confused by explanation and knowing what is happening."[31]

The United States government has now formally apologized for both the Guatemala experiments and the Tuskegee Syphilis Experiment. The research projects have been judged indefensible according not only to twenty-first century ethical standards but also to the widely accepted conventions of the mid-twentieth century. Not only were the individuals involved treated with profound disrespect—as a mere means to an end for the researchers—but also the test subjects experienced harm that was disproportionate to any humanitarian benefit that would be gained from the investigations. The researchers believed that the goals of their study took precedence over the well-being of subjects with low social status and minimal education. In the end, the scientific knowledge gained from the projects was negligible. The Tuskegee study was compromised by a poorly conceived research program and inadequate recordkeeping, and researchers never published results from the intentional exposure experiments in Guatemala. Although hidden from public view, both projects were carried out by well-regarded scientists with the knowledge and approval of high-level officials in the federal government.

These projects reflected systems of values and institutional structures that both had far-ranging impact. As later chapters will explore, other studies investigated treatments and vaccines—notably for polio—with children, residents of mental health facilities, and other vulnerable groups. Moreover, the Tuskegee and Guatemala studies illustrated the attitudes toward non-Western peoples that consolidated among Europeans and Americans in an era of colonization and global war. Many soldiers, missionaries, and colonizers shared the perception that "Africans," "Negroes," or "Indians" were more sexualized and less intelligent than light-skinned peoples. These assumptions, combined with Western approaches toward sexuality in general, exerted a powerful influence through most of the twentieth century.

Syphilis, Colonization, and Global War

Where sexually transmitted diseases are concerned, the historical influence of Western expansion is not fully understood. For large parts of Asia and Africa, no records survive that indicate how prevalent the diseases were before the mid-twentieth century. While colonial officials sometimes attempted to gauge their impact, at least selectively, such statistics are often highly suspect. As explained at the start of the chapter, treponemal infections related to yaws and bejel closely resemble venereal syphilis, and they were often mistaken for syphilis by European doctors. The prevalence of diseases with syphilis-like manifestations, combined with the common Western view that other peoples were morally lax, encouraged colonial physicians to overestimate the prevalence of sexually transmitted diseases in local populations. At the same time, there is no doubt that venereal syphilis and gonorrhea were common in trading centers and military bases by the late nineteenth century. Western medicines had some success in treating these infections, but, in the short run, the new arrivals introduced pathogens and created social conditions in which many diseases spread more rapidly.

In Britain, the leading colonial power, a debate over "street walkers" in the late nineteenth century markedly influenced approaches to venereal diseases in colonies around the globe. Prior to 1860, British authorities had not regulated sex workers as intensively as other European nations. However, after the Crimean War (1853–56) revealed the damaging effect of venereal diseases on the armed forces, between 1864 and 1869 Parliament authorized several Contagious Disease Acts that established medically regulated prostitution in districts containing ports and army facilities. In these zones, police were empowered to detain suspected prostitutes and force them to undergo medical examination. Infected women could then be coerced to undergo treatment in lock hospitals where inmates were confined for several months or longer. The Acts soon faced a storm of protest. Some observers objected that the police targeted the lower classes. Others, including the noted feminist reformer Josephine Butler (1828–1906), noted that only women were punished. Butler called for an end to regulated prostitution. While officials in continental Europe generally agreed that regulated prostitution was the best way to limit the impact of illicit sex, the issue remained contentious in Britain and also in the United States.

Although the Contagious Disease Acts were repealed in 1886, their legacy endured in British imperial outposts. Colonial elites hoped that control of sex workers would help avert venereal diseases among soldiers and maintain social boundaries between British and non-British populations. In India, where officials had long considered prostitution a problem, the military sponsored brothels and the compulsory inspection of women until World War I. Lock hospitals, sponsored by either civilian or military authorities, were an especially common imperial import that lasted into the twentieth century. These facilities often shared precincts with prisons and resembled them in many respects. For example, in 1873, the lock hospital in the island city of Penang (Malaysia) was created from an insane asylum that adjoined the main hospital and the jail. In the city of Brisbane (Australia), the hospital's venereal ward for women was moved in 1913 from the main hospital to the prison grounds. Beginning in 1908, Australian authorities also used islands near Western

Australia and Papua New Guinea to detain Aborigines suspected of venereal infection. This set a precedent for offshore health clearance and detention centers that Australia has followed in recent times for asylum seekers and refugees.[32]

What about the actual prevalence of venereal diseases in Asian and African communities? As noted earlier, sexually transmitted diseases were sufficiently widespread in China to attract the attention of medical authors by the later sixteenth century. Likewise, city dwellers in Japan were well acquainted with venereal diseases before European and American ships began routine visits in the later 1850s. As the scale of international traffic increased, foreign visitors urged Japanese officials to test prostitutes for diseases. In 1867, a treatment clinic focused on infected prostitutes was founded in Yokohama. Six years later, Tokyo established several examination centers for prostitutes, and the brothel keepers of its Yoshiwara district sponsored a treatment clinic in 1879.[33] Elsewhere in Asia, venereal syphilis apparently was either rare or nonexistent among Indigenous groups before sustained contact with Europeans began in the later nineteenth century. Early observers in the Indochinese peninsula (Vietnam) noted, in 1868, that syphilis was rare in provinces that had infrequent contact with Europeans. Milton Lewis has suggested that Australian Aborigines probably did not experience venereal disease before the first European settlers arrived in 1788.[34] Here and elsewhere, Europeans transplanted infections as well as institutions.

In sub-Saharan Africa, the prevalence of yaws and bejel complicated attempts by Western physicians to assess the disease landscape. In southern Africa, after the discovery of diamonds in 1867 and gold deposits in 1886, European and African mineworkers flocked by the tens of thousands to camps near Kimberley and Pretoria. Venereal syphilis undoubtedly spread among laborers and sex workers, but nonsexually transmitted treponemal infections were also common. Mineworkers wore few clothes and worked at close quarters underground; poor sanitary conditions in camps enabled the spread of infections through surface contact and workers then carried the diseases to rural villages. Some medical officials noted that "syphilis" was frequent among young children, but their observations may have conflated various treponemal infections or included other diseases altogether.

Although several related diseases apparently were at work, colonial officials viewed treponemal infections through the prism of venereal syphilis. Their medical explanations were a racially tinged amalgam of concepts concerning hierarchy and heredity. It was claimed that black Africans were naturally more promiscuous than whites and, therefore, syphilis would spread rapidly among them once the disease was introduced. Another argument was that exposure to civilization had a degenerative effect on the African "race" as it moved away from traditional practices that restrained behavior. In 1910, two physicians named E.N. Thornton and D.C. MacArthur explained yaws as a milder forms of syphilis. Africans were already "syphilised" by heredity, they claimed, and therefore Africans would experience less severe symptoms than whites when they became infected. (Such claims served as inspiration for the Tuskegee Syphilis Experiment.) As Karen Jochelson suggests, the notion that black South Africans were inherently diseased or culturally susceptible to venereal syphilis lent support to racial segregation policies that culminated in South Africa's era of legalized apartheid between 1948 and 1994.[35]

Colonial authorities framed "venereal disease" as a consequence of inappropriate sexual encounters, especially among nonwhite men and white women of low morals. However, as two brief examples will show, Indigenous elites also influenced public health campaigns and used them to meet their own social objectives. In Egypt during World War I, the arrival of thousands of troops from Britain and its allies raised concerns among both military and civic leaders. British generals worried about the moral climate of Cairo and Alexandria; conversely, Islamic leaders of these cities angrily demanded relief from the drugs and prostitution that accompanied the influx of young soldiers. In the spring of 1916, a Cairo Purification Committee was convened to recommend reforms. In contrast to wartime Europe, where many local leaders supported licensed brothels, the Cairo committee suggested measures to make illicit sex as unappealing as possible: punishment of anyone who knowingly spread venereal disease, the arrest of pimps and forced treatment of infected women, the prohibition of "indecent dances," a ban on the evening sale of alcohol, and a crackdown on hashish smoking. In both Alexandria and Cairo, locals and soldiers were tried by military courts and jailed by the thousands with substantial public approval. Although restricted activities carried on underground, the Egyptian campaigns represented the convergence of Victorian morality, wartime anxiety about the health of fighting forces, and codes of conduct rooted in Islamic principles.[36]

The interplay of local and imperial interests also influenced approaches to syphilis in southern Africa, including the British protectorate of Uganda. As discussed in chapter 7, Ugandan societies were profoundly disrupted by the arrival of Europeans and diseases that had sweeping effects upon livestock as well as humans. When the colonial relationship was formalized in 1894, colonial officials believed—as they did elsewhere—that syphilis was rampant in the region. Attention focused on the disruption of "traditional" social patterns under colonial rule and the consequences for the behavior of ethnic Baganda women. In 1908, the British medical journal *The Lancet* even suggested that when these women were freed from previous social constraints, "[t]hey were, in effect, merely female animals with strong passions, to whom unrestricted opportunities for gratifying these passions were suddenly afforded."[37] To British officials, it seemed that the authority of Bagandan chiefs should be reinforced to counter the disruptive effects of Christianity and "civilization." The message was well received by the chiefs, who in 1913 promulgated laws that would compel treatment for infected individuals. The chiefs also provided laborers to construct the Mulago Hospital, in Uganda's capital city of Kampala, which included isolation wards for people believed to have "contagious venereal diseases." Faced with profound social disruption, Bagandan elites used concerns over sexually transmitted diseases to exert some control over gender relations. By 1930, the initiative ebbed somewhat, in part because it became increasingly clear that the most widespread disease was yaws rather than venereal syphilis.

During the world wars, the global movement of millions of young soldiers enabled the spread of venereal syphilis and gonorrhea on a large scale. The cost of sick soldiers was substantial: in the year 1918 alone, 60,000 members of the British Expeditionary Force in France were admitted to a hospital for venereal disease, and the actual number of infected men was likely much higher.[38] The continuing difference between Anglophone and Continental approaches to prostitution was also apparent. While Germany and France sponsored military brothels, soldiers from the United States and Britain were sometimes discouraged from resorting to prostitutes. Although British troops patronized French brothels (*maisons de tolérance*) through most of the war, in spring 1918 the British Cabinet bowed to public pressure and decreed that such establishments were now off limits. Rubber condoms that were available to other combatants were not provided by the British until 1917 or to US troops at all. For soldiers from these countries, the approved prophylaxis (i.e., prevention) was a small kit with washcloths and calomel, a mercury-based ointment used to wash the genitals after sex.

Attitudes did not shift greatly prior to the start of World War II, although latex condoms, which could be stored longer and provided more cheaply, were now available. Public opinion in the United States remained ambivalent toward condoms—in part because they provided contraception as well as protection from disease—and military leaders continued to emphasize abstinence. In 1942, the US army enlisted the growing movie industry to spread the message. Movies, posters, and pamphlets warned of the dangers of casual sex and urged restraint out of patriotism as well as for personal safety. But these campaigns were ineffective for tired soldiers far from home. In 1945, sexually transmitted diseases were diagnosed in more than 7 per cent of the soldiers in the US army and the actual rate may have been substantially higher.[39]

After 1943, the widespread use of penicillin decisively blunted the impact of syphilis and gonorrhea. Penicillin's ability to cure these ailments and many others had a profound effect on health worldwide. No statistics fully account for penicillin's impact on global syphilis prevalence, but its swift cure of both syphilis and gonorrhea accelerated a steep drop in STIs that was already underway in some affluent countries. Between 1946 and 1956, rates of infection in the United States plunged more than 90 per cent, from 66 cases per 100,000 people to 4 cases per 100,000.[40] By 1959, a year when drug companies produced more than 600 tons of penicillin, in most populations around the world the prevalence of syphilis dropped below 1 per cent and deaths attributed to the disease almost disappeared. For a brief time, public health officials glimpsed the prospect of eliminating syphilis from some countries. But the achievements were neither universal nor permanent: during the 1960s, broad changes in sexual behavior and drug use touched off increases in STIs across the Western world.

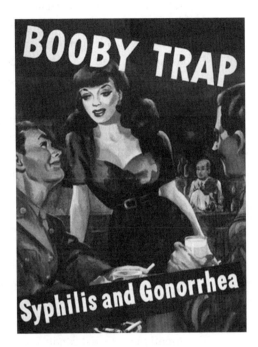

IMAGE 2.5 "Booby Trap"—Public health poster for US military forces (ca 1942–1944). The US Army attempted to prevent casualties from syphilis and gonorrhea by warning recruits about prostitutes and casual encounters. Young men on leave were expected to consume alcohol liberally and behave in ways that might expose them to disease.

In North America during the last few decades, cases of syphilis and other STIs have concentrated in underserved populations and disadvantaged minorities, including residents of Canada's northern territories, African Americans in the US, intravenous drug users, and men who have sex with men (MSM).[41] As of 2017, rates of infection were well below the pre-penicillin era but they have risen steadily since 2000 and are now over ten times the level of the 1950s. This may partly reflect growing social awareness and testing for infection among at-risk populations. However, some public health experts link the increase in syphilis to the reduced impact of AIDS. During the 1980s and 1990s, high AIDS mortality encouraged safer-sex practices. As improved therapies are transforming AIDS into a chronic, manageable disease, some research suggests that sexual networks are returning to higher-risk patterns and individuals are foregoing protective measures such as condoms.[42] In developed countries, MSM are at highest risk for syphilis, and the stigma that often surrounds same-sex relationships influences their ability or willingness to seek medical care. The fact that infection rates have increased in rural areas as well as cities further indicates a need for comprehensive efforts to prevent and treat sexually transmitted diseases. The recent history of syphilis confirms an observation made by epidemiologist William Brown more than fifty years ago: "as a disease program approaches the end point of eradication, it is the program, not the disease, which is more likely to be eradicated."[43]

Conclusion

The emergence of AIDS in the 1980s prompted historians and public health officials to reconsider the historical impact of syphilis and other sexually transmitted diseases. Like AIDS today, over the centuries these maladies have focused attention on sexual conduct, created hostility toward certain stigmatized groups, and engendered debates concerning the role of government in public health. The analogies between the emergence of the pox and AIDS have deepened as the imprint of AIDS has changed, especially in Western societies. Just as the pox became a chronic, persistent presence in European cities during the sixteenth century, in the last two decades AIDS-related mortality has declined but the disease remains a fixture in many communities.

Aspects of Europe's experience with the pox presaged challenges now faced by public health advocates. While MSM are at greatest risk for STIs in developed countries, around the world social inequality between men and women and high levels of poverty foster the spread of disease today just as they did in the sixteenth century. In South Africa, for example, STIs remain especially prevalent among young women, particularly those who are unmarried and have little or no education.[44] In other societies as well, poverty and social vulnerability prompt some women to engage in sex work or to enter relationships involving transactional sex in which they cannot insist on safer-sex practices. Patterns of migrant labor disperse infected individuals between urban centers and rural communities. As we will also see in the chapter exploring AIDS, the reduction of poverty is a key element in efforts to reduce the spread of STIs.

Right from the 1490s, European physicians and other authorities considered the pox a treatable disease, and this belief spurred innovation in both medical theory and treatment. The desire to prevent disease motivated governments to control individuals, such as prostitutes, who were blamed for spreading physical and moral corruption. Although syphilis may now be cured with antibiotics, access to treatment varies across countries and among social groups within countries. Debates continue over the most appropriate strategies to reduce infection among populations. Some programs emphasize education and sexual abstinence, while others promote tools to reduce infection (such as condoms) and encourage widespread diagnosis and treatment. Vaccine research programs have also made recent strides and may soon provide an important preventive tool. But, for now, history suggests that a combination of preventive, educative, and therapeutic measures holds the most promise for reducing the disease's global burden.[45]

Many researchers have pondered the pox's origins and consequences for Europe. This should not obscure the fact that, after 1500, Europeans spread the disease around the world through direct contact and indirectly through trading networks. Nor were the material causes of infection the only exports: in contrast to other parts of the world, Christianity and Western science fostered an association of disease and immorality that persisted even after germ theories transformed the scientific understanding of syphilis's causes and cure. The pathogen that initially gave rise to the pox may have come from outside Europe, but thereafter Europeans exported the concept of a sexually transmitted disease that has profoundly influenced public health throughout the modern era.

While the pox was an important social force, its main impact did not stem from the mortality it caused. Quite different were the epidemics of smallpox and other diseases that crossed the Atlantic from Europe and Africa beginning around 1500. In the centuries that followed, the Americas and isolated island peoples experienced depopulation that transformed many cultures, destroyed some forever, and enabled the spread of Europeans into vast reaches of a continent they considered new.

WORKSHOP: SEX AND DISEASE IN SEVENTEENTH-CENTURY LONDON

By the late sixteenth century, Europeans recognized the pox as a contagious disease that inflicted lasting damage on bodies and relationships. Although other explanations (such as divine displeasure) were not abandoned entirely, the spread of the pox and its long-term effects concentrated attention on human actions. This did not escape the attention of Elizabethan dramatists, whose success depended on their ability to link topical concerns to enduring themes of human experience. Many authors believed that the pox, which was particularly rampant in London and other cities, provided fertile ground to reflect on relationships between men and women, the corrupting influences in society, and the danger of deceit in human affairs.

Likewise, recent historians have suggested that Elizabethan literature illuminates how people explained and learned to live with a disease that was often chronic and sometimes devastating. Indeed, numerous sources of the period present a seemingly coherent picture of how the pox evoked horror and encouraged suspicion in a world full of rapid social change. However, the picture from such literary works is not complete: plays and poetry may illuminate widespread attitudes, but they do so to serve dramatic or didactic purposes for an author and the perceived audience. While drawing from them, it is also necessary to consider what may have been exaggerated—or what has been ignored and left out.

Plays and poems from the distant past pose a challenge to modern readers because of their unfamiliar spellings, vocabulary, and syntax. Working slowly, or reading aloud—with reference to the notes that are provided—will enable appreciation of the wordplay that Elizabethan audiences savored in dramatic performances.

> **Lues Venerea [Venereal Disease]—William Clowes (1579)**
>
> These passages are from the opening of a lengthy treatise on the symptoms and treatment of the pox. Clowes was a well-regarded surgeon who served at London's St Bartholomew Hospital, which was founded in the Middle Ages and re-established by Henry VIII in 1548. Clowes claims that both government action and moral reform are necessary to combat the pox. While the text begins with conventional criticism of "lewd" behavior, Clowes also suggests that the disease spreads by routes other than sexual transmission. To medical practitioners, it was far harder to assign blame—or, for that matter, to avoid catching the pox oneself—than it was to offer moral commentary.

CAP. I: THE CAUSES OF THIS DISEASE IN ENGLAND

First I say, the disease itself was never in my opinion more rife among the Indians, Neapolitans, yea in Italy, France or Spain, than is at this day in the realm of England. I pray

God quickly deliver us from it, and to remove from us that filthy sin that breedeth, nurseth, and disperseth it.

It is wonderful [*i.e., astonishing*] to consider the huge multitudes of those infected with it, that daily increase, to the great danger of the commonwealth & the stain of the whole nation. The causes whereof: I see none so great as the licentious and beastly disorder of a great number of rogues, and vagabonds, the filthy life of many lewd and idle persons, both men and women, about the city of London, and the great number of lewd ale houses, which are the very nests and harbors of such filthy creatures....

I may speak boldly, because I speak truly, and yet I do speak with great grief of heart, that in the Hospital of St. Bartholomew in London, there have been cured of this disease, by me and three others, within five years, to the number of one thousand and more. I speak nothing of Saint Thomas Hospital and other houses about the city, wherein an infinite multitude are daily in cure. So unless the Lord [*God*] is merciful to us, and the magistrates do with great care seek correction & punishment of that filthy vice, as also for the reformation of those places above mentioned; and unless the people of this land do speedily repent their most ungodly life, & leave this odious sin, it cannot be but that the whole land will shortly be poisoned with this most noisome [*i.e., disgusting*] sickness....

CAP. II. THE MANNER OF TAKING THIS SICKNESS, ITS CAUSES AND SIGNS

This sickness is said first to be engendered by the accompanying with unclean women, which although it be most commonly true, yet it is not always so, nor in all persons. For I myself have known both men and women grievously infected with this sickness, who have had those parts that bring the most suspicion thereof and are most speedily infected [*i.e., the genitals*] free and clear from all kind of malady or show of any such disease. Whereas, if the infection had happened by that means, those parts should in reasonable likelihood have been first touched, as being most apt to putrefy, by reason of the looseness and moistness of the part....

What should I say of young children, whereof diverse have been grievously vexed with this disease, and some of them three or four months old, some of them a year old, some four or five years old.... And I may not here in conscience overpass to forewarn of lewd and filthy nurses, for that in the year 1583 it chanced that three young children all born in this city of London, and all of one parish, or very near together, were put to nurse, the one in the country, and the other two were nursed in the city, but within less than half a year, they were all three brought home to their parents, grievously infected with the pox, by their wicked and filthy nurses....

Moreover, this sickness is many times bred in the mouth by eating and drinking with infected persons, sometimes in other parts of the body, sometimes by lying in the bed with them, or by lying in the sheets after them. Sometimes also it is said to come by sitting on the same stool of easement, where some infected person frequenteth. Sometimes those who have been cured of this disease fall into it again by wearing their infected clothes. All which causes of this disease I wish to set down, for that I would thereby admonish as many as shall read this treatise to be careful of themselves in this behalf, and to shun, as much as may be, all such occasions.

Pleasant Quippes for the Upstarte Newfangled Gentlewoman—Stephen Gosson (1595)
A former actor, Gosson wrote several tracts that mingled wit and pointed social commentary. This poem depicts several forces at work in London—fashion, prostitutes, disease—as emblems of moral decay. Fears of foreign influence merge with warnings about female deceit; those ensnared by the Devil's wiles run the risk of contracting disease.
The poem's text is in the left-hand column and commentary on the right.

These fashions fond of country strange
which English heads* so much delight,   *heads=people (or their tastes)
through town and country which do range
and are embraced of every wight*   *wight=country bumpkin
So much I wonder still to see,
That nought so much amazeth me ...

And when old beldames, withered hags,*   *beldames ... hags=old women past
whom hungry dogs cannot require,   childbearing age
Will whinny still, like wanton nags,*   *wanton nags=horses in heat who try
and saddled be with such attire,   to attract attention
A patient heart cannot but rage
To see the shame of this our age.

These Holland smocks* so white as snow,   *Holland smocks=linen brought from
and gorgets* brave with drawn-work wrought,   Holland
A tempting ware they are, you know,   *gorgets=decorated collars or
wherewith (as nets) vain youths are caught;   neckbands
But many times they rue* the match,   *rue=regret
When pox and piles* by whores they catch.   *piles=inflamed hemorrhoids

These flaming heads with staring hair,
these wires turned like horns of ram,

These painted faces which they wear,*
can any tell from when they cam?
Don* Sathan, lord of feign-ed lies,
All these new-fangles did devise ...

*wires ... wear=headgear
and makeup (see reference
to wigs and other ornaments)
* Don=Master

These periwigs, ruffs armed with pins,
these spangles, chains and laces all;
These naked paps,* the Devil's gins,**
to work vain gazers painful thrall,*
He fowler* is, they are his nets,
Wherewith of fools great store he gets ...

*paps=bosoms revealed by low-cut
dresses
**gins=wiles, traps
*thrall=entrapment
*fowler=one who catches birds

These hoops, that hips and haunch do hide,
and heave aloft the gay hoist train,*
As they are now in use for pride,
so did they first begin of pain;
When whore in stews had gotten pox,
This French device kept coats from smocks ...*

*hoops ... train=the supports that hold
a dress up off the ground.

* When ... smocks=dress hoops, it is
claimed, are designed for whores with
undergarments soiled by disease. A
"French device" to hide the "French
disease."

The better sort that modest are,
whom garish pomp doth not infect,*
Of them Dame Honour hath a care,
with glorious fame that they bedeckt:

*garish ... infect=the wish to impress is
like a disease that one should avoid

Their praises will for aye remain,
When bodies rot shall virtue gain*

*praises ... gain=the renown of true
virtue grows after mortal lives are over

Let fearful poets pardon crave ...
that seek for praise at every lips;
Do thou not favor, nor yet rave:
the golden mean is free from trips.*
This lesson old was taught in schools,
It's praise to be dispraised of fools.*

*golden ... trips=modest people will
avoid life's pitfalls
* praise ... fools=criticism by a fool
brings honor

Timon of Athens—William Shakespeare (1607)

This play is set in the Athens of Greek antiquity. The title character, Timon, is a popular nobleman who enjoys acclaim as long as he spends lavishly. His reputation is dashed after his true financial circumstances are revealed. When his former friends refuse to help, he leaves Athens for bitter exile. In the following excerpt, Timon, scratching the ground like a beggar, is visited by a friend (Alcibiades) and two prostitutes (Phrynia and Timandra). He rages against humanity and urges his surprised visitors to return and destroy the city by spreading riot and the pox.

Like Stephen Gosson's poem, the play draws on the familiar web of imagery surrounding prostitutes, deceit, and disease. But whereas Gosson concentrates on women and the dangers of a superficial focus on current fashions, the Timon text indicts all of society for hypocrisy. No one escapes his diatribe, but he reserves special scorn for lecherous priests and mercenary lawyers. The passage is notable for its detailed references to the pox and its treatment. The closing speech is a concise catalogue of visible pox symptoms that Shakespeare and his associates routinely observed and experienced.

The text of the play is in the left-hand column; commentary is supplied on the right.

*Enter Alcibiades with Drumme
and Fife in warlike manner,
and Phrynia and Timandra.*

Alc: What art thou there? Speak.

Timon: A beast, as thou art*. Cankers* gnaw thy heart/
For showing me again the eyes of man ...

* beast ... art=Timon is a beast, like Alcibiades.
* canker=cancer, ulcer, corruption

Alc: I've heard in some sort* of thy miseries.

* sort=way, manner

Timon: Thou sawest them when *I* had prosperity.

Alc: I see them now, then was a blessed time.

Timon: As thine is now, held with a brace* of harlots.

* brace=a pair (Alcibiades' harlot companions)

Timandra: Is this th'Athenian minion,* whom the world
Voic'd so regardfully?*

* minion=chosen one, favourite
* Voic'd regardfully=acclaimed with praise

Timon: Art thou *Timandra?*
Timandra: Yes.
Timon: Be a whore still,* they love thee not that use thee. Give them diseases, leaving with thee their lust. Make use of thy salt* hours. Season* the slaves/ For tubs* and baths, bring down rose-cheeked youth*

* still=constantly
* salt=lustful
* Season=prepare, make fit
* tubs=sweating tubs for curing the pox
*youth=young lovers should not escape
*tubfast=fasting tub

To the tubfast* and the diet.**
Timandra: Hang thee,* monster.
Alc: Pardon him, sweet *Timandra*, for his wits
Are drowned and lost in his calamities.
I have but little gold of late, brave* *Timon*,
The want* whereof doth daily make revolt**
In my penurious band*....

** diet=cure regime
* Hang thee=Curse you!

* brave=noble, excellent
* want=need, necessity
** revolt=rebellion
* penurious band=poor and needy group (the harlots want money)

(Alcibiades reveals his plan to return to Athens with soldiers and cause an uproar. Timon offers gold and dismisses him.
Alcibiades and the harlots ask for more gold; Timon insults them but encourages them to spread disease among their corrupt clients. He concludes with a catalogue of familiar pox complaints and sends them off with a curse.)

Timon: ... There's gold to pay thy soldiers.
Make large confusion;* and thy fury spent,
Confounded be thy self!* Speak not, be gone.
Alc: Hast thou gold yet? I'll take the gold thou givest
me, not all thy counsel.
Tim: Dost thou, or dost thou not, Heaven's curse
upon thee.
Both Timandra and Phrynia: Give us some gold,
good Timon: hast thou more?

* large confusion=widespread destruction or ruin
* Confounded ... self=may you be ruined as well

Timon: Enough to make a whore forswear* her trade,
And to make whores, a bawd.* Hold up, you sluts,
Your aprons mountant*; you're not oathable**,
Although, I know, you'll swear; terribly swear,

*forswear=abandon, renounce
*bawd=madam or pimp (they will earn enough money to have other women work under them)
*mountant=lifted skirts signify sexual availability
**oathable=fit to take an oath

Into strong shudders, and to heavenly agues*...
Paint till a horse may mire upon your face;*
A pox of wrinkles!
Timandra & Phrynia: Well, more gold—what then?
Believe, that we'll do anything for gold.

* agues=fever, feverish shaking
* Paint ... face=apply concealing makeup so thickly a horse could get stuck in it

Timon: Consumptions sow*
In hollow bones of man, strike their sharp shins,
And mar men's spurring.* Crack the lawyer's voice,

* Consumptions sow=spread wasting disease
* shins ... spurring=damage to the tibia and ankle bones were signs of long-term pox infection

That he may never more false title* plead,
Nor sound his quillets* shrilly. Hoar the flamen,**
That scolds against the quality of flesh,

* false title=weak, illegitimate claim
*quillets=hair-splitting distinctions
**Hoar the flamen=whiten (hoar) the skin of a hypocrite priest (flamen) who catches the pox

And not believes himself. Down with the nose,
Down with it flat; take the bridge quite away* Of him,
that his particular to foresee
Smells from the general weal.* Make curled-pate**
ruffians bald
And let the unscarred braggarts of the war
Derive some pain from you.* Plague all;
That your activity may defeat* and quell
The source of all erection.* There's more gold.
Do you damn others, and let this damn you,
And ditches grave* you all.

*Down ... away=a flattened nose (the pox damaged nasal cartilage)
* him ... weal=a man who tends selfishly to his own affairs (general weal=common good)
** curled-pate=curly-haired (the pox caused hair loss)
*unscarred ... you=the whores should infect bragging, uninjured soldiers
*defeat=ruin
*quell ... erection=destroy men's ability to perform sexually
*grave=entomb, bury

INTERPRETING THE DOCUMENTS

1. The two paragraphs by surgeon William Clowes express very different sentiments about the kinds of individuals who contract the pox. How do you account for the contrast? What conclusion do you draw concerning how Clowes might have dealt with his actual patients?

2. Gosson's poem and the passage from *Timon of Athens* are both critical of society but in different ways. What are the targets of each? How does each passage use the fact that catching the pox was a genuine fear for Londoners of their day?

3. Plague remained a very real threat to the inhabitants of Elizabethan England. Why do you suppose the pox, rather than plague, seemed to present a better dramatic opportunity?

MAKING CONNECTIONS

1. Compare the discourse concerning the spread of the pox with the discourse concerning plague that you explored in the last chapter. How did each disease seem to pose the problem of human accountability?

2. Consider how the spread of the pox and plague were understood in earlier centuries. How does the means by which the disease was seen to spread influence the kind of social criticisms that are made in connection with it?

3. In a comment on *Timon of Athens*, two authors recently suggested that "Shakespeare and his contemporaries imagined, and hence made imaginable for future generations, the possibility of bioterrorism." How do you evaluate this claim? What are the differences between the modern concept of bioterrorism and the assault on Athens that Timon proposes?

For further reading: Louis F. Qualtiere and William W.E. Slights, "Contagion and Blame in Early Modern England: The Case of the French Pox," *Literature and Medicine*, vol. 22, no. 1 (Spring 2003): 1–24.

Notes

1. Ulrich von Hütten, *Of the Wood Called Guaiacum That Healeth the Frenche Pockes...*, trans. Thomas Paynel (London, 1536), 5r–5v.

2. Alfred Crosby, *The Columbian Exchange: Biological and Cultural Consequences of 1492* (Santa Barbara: Greenwood Publishing, 1972).

3. Rebecca E. LaFond and Sheila A. Lukehart, "Biological Basis for Syphilis," *Clinical Microbiology Reviews* 19, no. 1 (2006): 30–33.

4. Fernando Lucas de Melo et al., "Syphilis at the Crossroads of Phylogenetics and Paleopathology," *PLOS-Neglected Tropical Diseases* 4, no. 1 (2010): 7–9.

5. Lorenzo Giacani and Sheila A. Lukehart, "The Endemic Treponematoses," *Clinical Microbiology Reviews* 27, no. 1 (2014): 89–115.

6. John Arrizabalaga, John Henderson, and Roger French, *The Great Pox: The French Disease in Renaissance Europe* (New Haven: Yale University Press, 1997), 145–70.

7. Claudia Stein, *Negotiating the French Pox in Early Modern Germany* (London: Palgrave Macmillan, 2003), 125–50.

8. Robert S. Munger, "Guaiacum, the Holy Wood from the New World," *Journal of the History of Medicine and Allied Sciences* 4, no. 2 (1949): 202–203.

9. Vivian Nutton, "The Reception of Fracastoro's Theory of Contagion: The Seed That Fell among Thorns?" *Osiris* 6 (1990): 196–234.

10. Mitchell Hammond, "'Ora Deum et Tribuas Medicum': Medicine in the Theology of Martin Luther and Philipp Melanchthon," in *Religion und Naturwissenschaft im 16. und 17. Jahrhundert*, ed. Kaspar von Greyerz (Gütersloh: Schriften des Vereins für Reformationsgeschichte, 2010), 33–50.

11. Anna E. Winterbottom, "Of the China Root: A Case Study of the Early Modern Circulation of *Materia Medica*," *Social History of Medicine* 28, no. 4 (2014): 22–44.

12. Desiderius Erasmus, "The Unequal Match," in *Collected Works of Erasmus: Colloquies*, ed. and trans. Craig R. Thompson (Toronto: University of Toronto Press, 1997), 846.

13. Sharmaine van Blommestein, "Aquinas, Thomas," in *Encyclopedia of Prostitution and Sex Work: Vol. 1, A–N*, ed. Melissa Hope Ditmore (Santa Barbara: Greenwood Publishing Group, 2006), 39–40.

14. Johannes Fabricius, *Syphilis in Shakespeare's England* (London: Jessica Kingley, 1994), 98.

15. Simon Szreter, "Treatment Rates for the Pox in Early Modern England: A Comparative Estimate of the Prevalence of Syphilis in the City of Chester and Its Rural Vicinity in the 1770s," *Continuity and Change* 32, no. 2 (2017): 197–203.

16. Barnabe Rich, *My Ladies Looking Glass* (London, 1616), 36.

17. Amy Stanley, *Selling Women: Prostitution, Markets and Household in Early Modern Japan* (Berkeley: University of California Press, 2012), 194–95.

18. Joan Sherwood, *Infection of the Innocents: Wetnurses, Infants and Syphilis in France, 1780–1900* (Montreal: McGill-Queen's University Press, 2010).

19. Alfred Fournier, *Syphilis and Marriage*, trans. P. Albert Morrow (New York, 1882), 5.

20. John E. Lesch, *The First Miracle Drugs: How the Sulfa Drugs Transformed Medicine* (Oxford: Oxford University Press, 2007), 3.

21. Paul Brack, "Norman Heatley: The Forgotten Man of Penicillin," *The Biochemist* 37, no. 5 (2015): 36–37.

22. Andreas-Holger Maehle, "'God's Ethicist': Albert Moll and His Medical Ethics in Theory and Practice," *Medical History* 56, no. 2 (2012): 227.

23. Cynthia J. Tsay, "Julius Wagner-Jauregg and the Legacy of Malarial Therapy for the Treatment of General Paresis of the Insane," *Yale Journal of Biology and Medicine* 86, no. 2 (2013): 245–54.

24. Allan M. Brandt, "Sexually Transmitted Disease: Shadow on the Land, Revisited," *Annals of Internal Medicine* 112, no. 7 (1990): 481.

25. James H. Jones, *Bad Blood: The Tuskegee Syphilis Experiment*, rev. ed. (New York: The Free Press, 1993); Presidential Commission for the Study of Bioethical Issues, *"Ethically Impossible."*

26. R.M. White, "Misrepresentations of the Tuskegee Study of Untreated Syphilis," *Journal of the National Medical Association* 97, no. 11 (2005): 564–81.

27. Henrik L. Blum and Charles W. Barnett, "Prognosis in Late Latent Syphilis," *Archives of Internal Medicine* 82, no. 4 (1948): 393–409.

28. United States Public Health Service (USPHS), *VD Fact Sheet. No.* 10 (1953), 20.

29. Presidential Commission for the Study of Bioethical Issues, *'Ethically Impossible': STD Research in Guatemala from 1946 to 1948* (Washington, DC: www.bioethics.gov, 2011).

30. S. Smith, "Wellesley Professor Unearths a Horror: Syphilis Experiments in Guatemala," *The Boston Globe*, 2 October 2010.

31. Presidential Commission for the Study of Bioethical Issues, *"Ethically Impossible,"* 74.

32. Philippa Levine, *Prostitution, Race and Politics: Policing Venereal Disease in the British Empire* (New York: Routledge 2003), 72.

33. J.E. de Becker, *Nightless City of the Geisha*, rev. ed. (London: Kegan Paul, 2002), 163.

34. Milton J. Lewis, "Public Health in Australia from the Nineteenth to the Twenty-First Century," in *Public Health in Asia and the Pacific: Comparative Perspectives*, ed. Milton J. Lewis and Kerrie L. MacPherson (New York: Routledge, 2008): 222–49.

35. Karen Jochelson, *The Color of Disease: Syphilis and Racism in South Africa, 1880–1950* (New York: Palgrave, 2001).

36. Mark Harrison, "The British Army and the Problem of Venereal Disease in France and Egypt during the First World War," *Medical History* 39 (1995): 133–58.

37. Quoted in Megan Vaughan, *Curing Their Ills* (Cambridge: Polity Press, 1991), 133.

38. Harrison, "British Army," 145.

39. US Army Medical Department, Office of Medical History, *Preventive Medicine in World War II*, vol. 5, Appendix 4, http://history.amedd.army.mil/booksdocs/wwii /communicablediseasesV5/appendixd.htm.

40. Judith N. Wasserheit and Sevgi O. Aral, "The Dynamic Topology of Sexually Transmitted Disease Epidemics: Implications for Future Strategies," *Journal of Infectious Diseases* 174, suppl. 2 (1996): S206.

41. Public Health Agency of Canada, *Canada Communicable Disease Report*, 44, no. 2 (2018): 37–54; CDC, "Sexually Transmitted Disease Surveillance" (July 2018), https://www.cdc.gov /std/stats17/minorities.htm; Winston E. Abara et al., "Syphilis Trends among Men Who Have Sex with Men in the United States and Western Europe: A Systematic Review of Trend Studies Published between 2014 and 2015," *PLOS One* 11, no. 7 (2015), https://doi.org/10.1371 /journal.pone.0159309.

42. Chris Richard Kenyon et al., "The Changing Relationship between Bacterial STIs and HIV Prevalence in South Africa: An Ecological Study," *International Journal of STD & AIDS* 26, no. 8 (2015): 556–64.

43. William J. Brown, "The First Step toward Eradication," *Proceedings of the World Forum on Syphilis and Other Treponematoses* (Washington: US Government Printing Office, 1964), 23.

44. Sarita Naidoo et al., "High Prevalence and Incidence of Sexually Transmitted Infections among Women Living in Kwazulu-Natal, South Africa," *AIDS Research and Therapy* 11, no. 31 (2014), http://www.aidsrestherapy.com/content/11/1/31.

45. Allan M. Brandt, "The Syphilis Epidemic and Its Relation to AIDS," *Science* 239, no. 4838 (1988): 380.

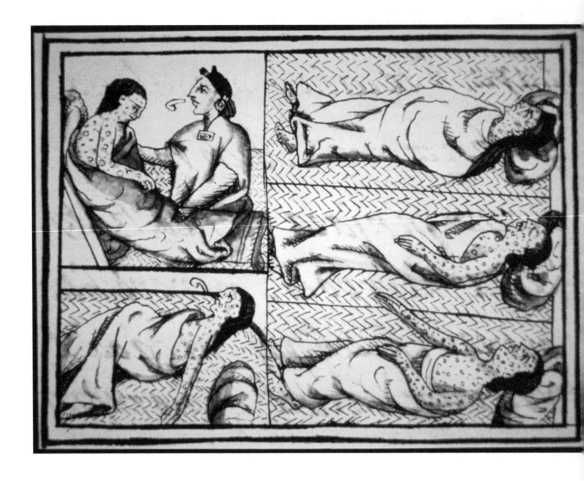

IMAGE 3.1 Smallpox in the Valley of Mexico. Indigenous Caribbean and American peoples confronted various devastating diseases, especially smallpox, after the arrival of Europeans beginning in the late fifteenth century. In this drawing that is preserved in the Florentine Codex manuscript (ca 1575), a scribe recalled the suffering of the years 1520–21 in the city of Tenochtitlán.

SMALLPOX AND AMERICAN CATASTROPHE

On a mid-November day in 1620, the English ship *Mayflower* finished its Atlantic voyage and dropped anchor at the coast of a North American territory controlled by the Wampanoag people. The few inhabitants avoided the newcomers who came ashore. Instead, the English found vacant houses, buried food, and graves covered with mats and boards. It was several months before a man boldly approached the settlers and surprised them by speaking in halting English and naming several ship captains. The settlers called him Samoset—one of their chroniclers wrote that the man "told us the place where we now live, is called Patuxet, and that about foure yeares agoe all the Inhabitants dyed of an extraordinary plague, and there is neither man, woman, nor childe remaining, as indeed we have found none, so as there is none to hinder our possession, or to lay claime unto it."[1] As if by miracle, stretches of fertile land had suddenly been vacated just before the English arrived and established the community later known as Plymouth, Massachusetts.

Not for the first time, or the last, Europeans believed that their prayers were answered by what they saw and heard on American shores. A century before, in 1519, Spaniards led by Hernán Cortés (1485–1547) were lured by hints of gold to the densely populated Valley of Mexico. In the mid-seventeenth century, French Jesuits proclaimed a harvest of converts to the Catholic church. Indigenous Americans were peripheral to the grand drama that one prominent historian described, in 1956, as "the movement of European culture into the vast wilderness of America."[2] Until the later twentieth century Indigenous Americans mostly appeared in history as foils to European conquerors, missionaries, and freedom seekers.

They also appeared as victims of European diseases that struck with unbeliev-able ferocity. Early in the twentieth century, scholars such as S. Lyle Cummins used the concept of "virgin soil" to explain why Indigenous Americans apparently had such little resistance to European diseases. In 1976, Alfred Crosby applied the term "virgin soil epidemic" to the sixteenth-century outbreaks of smallpox, influenza, and measles that exploded among Indigenous populations throughout North and South America.[3] Other authors also linked the impact of disease to a momentous accident of global geography. Over millennia, the argument went, peoples of Eurasia and Africa had exchanged microbial agents with their domesti-cated animals. Their abilities to resist diseases evolved as they lived side by side with pigs, goats, horses, and chickens. Indigenous Americans, on the other hand, remained "immunologically naïve," even "born to die," because their environ-ments offered less opportunity for this development.[4] Scholars suggested that the arrival of Europeans began an irresistible microbial onslaught that combined with other stressors to overwhelm resistance to colonizing forces.

Recent researchers have challenged this explanation, arguing that it mini-mizes the active role that Europeans played in the destruction of Indigenous American societies. Archaeologists and anthropologists have attempted to dispel the aura of inevitability around European dominance and to draw attention to social inequities that still affect Indigenous communities. The challenge for historical analysis, therefore, is not to highlight the destructive force of epidemics but rather to assess their impact in relation to other factors.

In this regard, smallpox provides a particularly apt focus. Many diseases accompanied Europeans on their global travels after 1500, but none seemingly fostered their dominance in the modern world more than the disease known as "the speckled monster." Its disfiguring and lethal effects were obvious throughout the Americas and island communities, all the more so because most adult Europeans were affected far less severely than Indigenous peoples. In early modern Europe it was children who usually contracted smallpox, but this threat, too, was eventually overcome by the preventive power of vaccination. Europeans began to export this technique in the early nineteenth century. In the late 1970s, a global campaign successfully eradicated smallpox from the natural world. As countless lives were saved, this "conquest of smallpox" also demonstrated the ability of Western experts to intervene in public health throughout the world.

Etiology and Early History

Alone among the great human pathogens, smallpox has been eradicated from nature by human efforts. Unlike plague and syphilis, smallpox was caused by a **virus**—a strand of DNA surrounded by a protein sheath that enters a host cell in order to reproduce. The smallpox *Variola* virus is now classified in a genus that also includes the microbes that cause horsepox, monkeypox, cowpox, and tater-apox (the latter is a disease of small rodents). Two strains of smallpox circulated at least since the later nineteenth century: *Variola major*, which resulted in case fatality rates of up to 30 per cent, and *Variola minor*, a milder variant that resulted in mortality closer to 1 per cent. The welcome disappearance of smallpox has led to historical amnesia about its impact. Smallpox killed roughly 300 million people in the twentieth century alone, far more than the number who died as a result of armed conflict. Even in the late 1960s, it is estimated that between 10 and 15 million people contracted smallpox annually and of these roughly 2 million died.

Twentieth-century observations yielded extensive evidence concerning smallpox's symptoms. The disease transmitted easily from dried scabs or through infective droplets spread by coughs and sneezes. After an **incubation period** (the interval between infection and the appearance of symptoms) that averaged roughly twelve days, sufferers experienced high fever, muscle pain, and headaches as the virus multiplied in the bloodstream and proceeded to the spleen, bone marrow, and lymph nodes. Two weeks after infection, reddish spots appeared in the mouth, throat, and mucous membranes, followed by skin eruptions that swiftly covered the face and the body. The lesions became hard pustules that resembled small beads buried in the skin with a characteristic dimple. These usually dried and formed scabs after about two weeks but less commonly, in confluent smallpox, the pustules merged to form a painful layer of infection across large expanses of skin. Perhaps one in ten sufferers developed either malignant smallpox with flattened lesions or hemorrhagic smallpox with internal bleeding, both of which usually caused death. The lasting effects of smallpox often included blindness and pitted scars, the latter a result of damage to the skin's **sebaceous** glands.

Until recently, researchers believed that smallpox, measles, and influenza emerged about 10,000 years ago as some societies became sedentary and created dense settlements that encouraged the exchange of microbial material with domesticated animals. Humans are the sole host of the *Variola* virus—the disease passed only from one person to another—and the pathogen required a substantial population of susceptible individuals for an epidemic to take place. The evolution of human diseases seemed to fit neatly with other key developments in the evolution of human societies.

However, analysis in the last decade has revised our understanding of smallpox viruses and the limit of what scientists can infer from the current evidence. The study of the ancient DNA of bacteria such as *Y. pestis* (see the chapter 1 Science Focus) has progressed further than the harvesting and analysis of ancient viral DNA. For viral mutations, it is not yet possible to conduct phylogenetic analysis with physical evidence that is more than a few centuries old. Instead, scientists mostly extrapolate backwards from more recent samples of smallpox that were collected from the 1940s to the 1970s. This procedure relies on a **molecular clock hypothesis**: the assumption that genetic sequences of DNA or other proteins will evolve in an organism (such as a virus) at a relatively constant rate.[5] Such conjecture faces difficult questions. How much does the rate of evolution vary among organisms? What does the rate of evolution in one organism—such as a virus—tell us about the rate for another similar organism? And how might the rate of evolution for an organism change over time in response to various environmental factors? The way that scientists answer such questions influences how they "calibrate" the molecular clock, or estimate rates of evolutionary change over thousands or millions of years.

The estimate of when the smallpox virus evolved, therefore, is a time range rather than a date. One projection points to smallpox's separation from taterapox in Africa roughly 3,000–4,000 years ago, but origins as early as 50,000 years ago have not been ruled out. The earliest extant genetic sample—from a mid-seventeenth-century mummy found in Lithuania—has characteristics that are ancestral to all the other more recent samples that have been analyzed.[6] Thus, some mutations that were critical to the evolution of modern smallpox probably took place in the last few centuries, not thousands of years ago. Accounts from the eighteenth century describe cases of smallpox that varied in severity. This offers more evidence that viral strains other than *V. major* and *V. minor* circulated in earlier times. These considerations introduce notes of caution: our knowledge of how smallpox behaved in recent history is, at best, a rough guide to its impact in the more distant past.

Likewise, researchers have cast doubt on the claim that Indigenous populations were especially susceptible to frequent or more lethal cases of smallpox. Earlier scholars had proposed that genetic diversity among Eurasia's peoples blunted smallpox's impact, particularly after many centuries of exposure. In the smaller, homogeneous populations of the Americas, the argument went, the smallpox virus rapidly gained virulence as it moved among genetically similar human hosts.[7] However, no genetic basis for immunity to smallpox has been identified, and the "gene pools" in various populations do not account for smallpox-related mortality or for the ultimate fate of various social groups struck by the disease.[8]

Researchers have pointed instead to the important—but not exclusive—role played by **adaptive** (or **acquired**) **immunities** that create differential susceptibility to infection. In parts of Eurasia where smallpox was common, survivors of smallpox infection developed antibodies that enabled them to resist contracting the disease again. Mothers who had survived cases of smallpox passed on antibodies to protect their children in the first months of life. Owing to the influence of acquired immunity, the timing of more severe outbreaks tended to be cyclical as the disease preyed upon children born since the previous episode. While smallpox might still flare up and cause substantial mortality, the pathogen and its host peoples developed an equilibrium as smallpox became endemic in many regions. European adults who survived mild childhood cases were substantially more equipped to face the virus than American communities without any prior exposure. But this was an outcome of prior exposure to smallpox among (some) Europeans, rather than evidence of an inherent genetic difference.

Substantial evidence suggests that smallpox exerted considerable influence in antiquity, although the lack of early DNA evidence introduces an element of doubt into retrospective diagnoses. Populations in regions of India, China, and the Nile River valley were all sufficiently large to support smallpox in ancient times. Pockmarks visible on an Egyptian mummy from the twelfth century BCE, and written evidence from China ca 250 BCE attest to its probable influence. In 165 CE, Roman soldiers returned from Mesopotamia with a pestilence that may have been smallpox that caused high mortality in Rome and elsewhere in the Mediterranean. This epidemic, which possibly originated in China, weakened the Roman army's ability to defend against Germanic peoples who eventually occupied Roman territory. Smallpox may also have accompanied the tide of Arabic peoples that moved into North Africa and brought Islam to the Iberian Peninsula in the early eighth century. In addition to the DNA evidence noted above, textual evidence from earlier times suggests that smallpox's virulence varied and that observers in some times and places did not consider it a lethal disease. Thus, one of the earliest clear descriptions of smallpox, from the Arabic author Rhazes (ca 865–925) in the tenth century, describes it as a common childhood ailment that was less severe than measles.

Defending
against Disease:
Innate and
Adaptive
Immunity

When we consider transmissible infections, no aspect of human physiology receives more attention than the immune system. Military metaphors are often employed to describe it—we refer to pathogens that "penetrate" the body, cells that "mount a defense," and health that returns when the invaders are "destroyed." However, the immune system does more than fight; it balances or regulates the activity of trillions of microbes and human cells (figure 3.1).

Many immune functions help humans resist infection and respond to **antigens** (material that is foreign to the body). Scientists distinguish between **innate immunity** that develops independently of any environmental stimulation and **adaptive immunity** that changes over a lifetime in response to many forces. Innate immune responses include many of the body's first responses to injury or the entrance of microbes: mucus, fever, inflammation, and swelling. At the cellular level, certain white blood cells move freely through the blood stream and swallow up, dissolve, or burst foreign microbes and cells that are dead or compromised. Parts of the innate immune system also target certain viruses and bacteria, including the microbes that cause colds, flu, and tuberculosis. **Cytokines**, or signaling proteins, are released and trigger further immune responses.

The adaptive immune system develops more specific responses to various antigens that a body encounters. Two types of white blood cells, B and T lymphocytes, perform complementary functions. **B lymphocytes**, which work outside of cells, produce vast quantities of antibody proteins. These neutralize pathogens by latching onto them or otherwise blocking entry into cells. **T lymphocytes**, in contrast, react to signals emitted by infected or damaged cells and release chemicals that destroy them. Other T cells coordinate immune response by secreting cytokines that attract other cells to the site of an infection. Importantly, some B cells and T cells survive as "memory cells" that prompt a swifter immune response if a similar pathogen enters the body later.

Adaptive immunities are produced by both natural and artificial means. Children receive protective maternal antibodies before birth

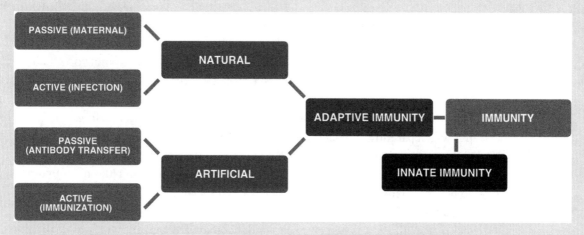

FIGURE 3.1 Outline of the human immune system.

and in infancy through breastmilk. When mothers have no prior exposure to a lethal disease—as in the case of smallpox's arrival in the Americas—childhood mortality can reach very high levels. Beginning in infancy, children also develop their own antibodies as their bodies respond to infections. The impact of those first infections may be far reaching—some evidence suggests that they deeply influence how the immune system responds to different strains or types of a virus (such as different subtypes of influenza virus) throughout life.

The most common artificial method of inducing adaptive immunity is vaccination. In this procedure, a small amount of a dead or weakened pathogen is introduced into the body. The intended effect is to mobilize antibodies and induce cellular memory of the pathogen without causing a full-blown case of symptomatic disease. Another tactic is to introduce antibodies taken from another person or animal. For

example, doctors first treated diphtheria in the 1890s with blood serum taken from infected sheep and horses. The animals had produced antibodies that neutralized a causal toxin emitted by the bacteria.

The eradication of smallpox from nature testifies to the potential for vaccines to transform human health. However, many diseases pose greater challenges to public health campaigns than smallpox did. Microbes have tricks of their own. Some, such as influenza viruses, mutate swiftly; others, including the bacteria that cause tuberculosis, can hide in a dormant state for years; and human immunodeficiency virus (HIV) inserts itself into strands of DNA in its host's cells. Some adaptive immunities, such as resistance to malaria, disappear unless a person is routinely exposed to the patho-gen. And many other human factors, such as fatigue or nutrition, influence immunity in ways that often remain mysterious.

Useful comparative evidence for the impact of smallpox in the Middle Ages comes from the Japanese islands, where population densities were higher than Europe and systematic descriptions of important events began around 700 CE. It is not clear when it first arrived, but an especially severe epidemic of *mogasa*, or "bean-pod pox," swept through the islands in 735–37.[9] Thereafter, outbreaks recurred with increasing regularity; by the twelfth century, if not before, smallpox was apparently an endemic disease that infected the vast majority of Japanese children in periodic waves until the mid-nineteenth century. Smallpox was a ritual of childhood that may have caused aggregate mortality in cities of around 10 per cent. This was enough to have a marked social impact but not sufficient to halt an overall growth in population. Moreover, as Akihito Suzuki suggests, the fact that smallpox was perceived as a childhood malady meant that it was dealt with primarily within family units, rather than through sweeping public health interventions of the sort inspired in Europe by bubonic plague.[10] In Europe, there is little evidence of severe smallpox until the later sixteenth century, but by the mid-seventeenth century its experience seems to have been similar to Japan's. After 1630, records from London suggest that the "background" annual mortality from smallpox crept upward to about 5 per cent of the population.[11] More severe outbreaks every few years killed slightly more than 10 per cent on average, with mortality concentrated in young children.

In eighteenth-century Europe, smallpox remained a feared killer that eventually inspired important therapeutic innovations. But it did not cause the level of suffering and upheaval experienced in the Americas. Accounting for the role of smallpox, inevitably, raises one of the most charged questions that recent historians have faced: the causes of Indigenous American decline in the face of European imperialism.

Smallpox and Social Upheaval in the Americas

A comparison with Europe's experience after 1348 may illuminate the stakes in this debate. As explained in chapter 1, during the Black Death and its aftermath Europe faced profound social disruption and its population declined by an estimated 50 per cent, mostly (but not exclusively) because of disease-related mortality. Within a century, however, Europe's population began to recover and some regions, notably city-states in Italy, entered an era of great vitality. Beginning in the sixteenth century, American societies also began to experience very high disease-related mortality whenever they first encountered Europeans.

Over decades, however, population fell even more in the Americas than it did in Europe during the Black Death era. The decrease was over 50 per cent overall and in some regions substantially greater. Many communities did not recover until the twentieth century or died out altogether.

What caused this terrible decline, and why did American populations not recover as Europe's had? Earlier scholars such as Alfred Crosby suggested that the cumulative impact of various diseases was even more devastating in the Americas than in Europe—so devastating that almost all of America's Indigenous inhabitants died and the remnants that were left could not resist the incursion of Europeans. From this perspective, the demise of Indigenous peoples is not best explained by European aggression; rather, as Francis Jennings noted in a book titled *The Invasion of America* (1975), "the Europeans' capacity to resist certain diseases made them superior, in the pure Darwinian sense, to the Indians who succumbed."[12]

As noted previously, however, no persuasive evidence suggests that susceptibility to smallpox among Indigenous Americans differed markedly from that of Europeans, or that genetic homogeneity in Indigenous populations helped the virus move more easily from host to host. Some recent scholars have, instead, emphasized the "structural violence" of regimes that mounted sustained attacks on Indigenous societies and also initiated ecological changes with consequences that ranged far beyond direct human action.[13] Although the introduction of novel pathogens played a role, they suggest that warfare, famine, and forced migration accounted for high mortality more than the susceptibility of Indigenous bodies to disease. It has also become increasingly clear that the experience of Indigenous communities varied widely and that regional case studies are preferable to broad generalizations.

One such case study of great importance is the Valley of Mexico during and after the capture of Tenochtitlán, capital of the Mexica (or Aztec) people, in 1521. At the time, the Valley of Mexico was the most densely inhabited region of the Americas; with a population that may have approached 200,000, Tenochtitlán was an imperial metropolis comparable in scale to European cities such as Paris or Florence. The attack of fewer than 1,000 Spaniards under the leadership of Hernán Cortés triggered an extraordinary sequence of events that upended a powerful empire. For centuries, few episodes apparently illustrated the superiority of European culture more dramatically than the exploits of the resourceful Spanish conquistador. It is now clear, however, that the invasion could not have succeeded without assistance from Indigenous allies and deaths caused by disease.

Following the first voyages of Christopher Columbus (1451–1506) to the Caribbean in the 1490s, the Spanish had established outposts on the islands of

Isabella (now Cuba) and Hispaniola (now Haiti and the Dominican Republic). In two decades, diseases and Spanish aggression decimated the Indigenous population. The need for more "Indian" laborers was one of Cortés's stated reasons for a renegade expedition to the mainland. His force departed from Isabella in April 1519 against the orders of the island's governor. Smallpox was probably conveyed to Mexico in May 1520 by men led by Pánfilo de Narváez, who were dispatched to restrain Cortés but eventually joined him instead. As Europeans and Americans negotiated and fought, smallpox apparently reached the Mexica capital in fall 1520. Among its many victims was the leader Cuitláhuac (ca 1476–1520), whose brother Moctezuma II (ca 1466–1520) had first received Cortés after the Spanish arrived. As disease continued to spread, Cortés forged alliances with other chiefs and laid siege to Tenochtitlán in May 1521. Within a few months, the city was destroyed. As Europeans arrived in greater numbers, the Indigenous population declined over the next century to a fraction of the level it had been in 1520.

A Franciscan monk, Bernardino de Sahagún (ca 1500–1590), collected some of the most moving testimony about the first years of conquest from native informants in the 1540s. Sahagún eventually oversaw the production of a large manuscript—the Florentine Codex, completed around 1575—that contained a wealth of information about traditional Mexica society and history. Book XII of this work describes the suffering from disease that the Mexica experienced after Europeans arrived:

> It was in Tepeilhuitl [*during October*] that there spread over the people a great destruction of men. Some of it indeed covered; they were spread everywhere, on one's face, on one's head, on one's breast. There was indeed perishing; many indeed died of it.... And when they bestirred themselves, much did they cry out. There was much perishing. Like a covering, covering-like, were the pustules. Indeed many people died of them, and many just died of hunger. There was death from hunger; there was no one to take care of another; there was no one to attend to another.[14]

This testimony and other accounts strongly suggest that smallpox caused great suffering soon after Europeans arrived and probably during the siege of Tenochtitlán. But how large was the overall population loss in the Valley of Mexico, and what role did smallpox and others diseases play in it? In part, answers to these questions reflect estimates of the population in the valley before Europeans arrived. On one extreme, Woodrow Borah and Sherburne Cook claimed that up to 25 million inhabitants lived in the Valley of Mexico in 1520, and that just over 1 million Indigenous people remained in 1600. Most scholars have shied away from the high initial figure and offered estimates in the range of 4 million initial inhabitants. From this starting point, the combined effect of disease, ecological disruption, and warfare reduced the population by roughly 75 per cent in less than a century.[15]

To what extent could smallpox account for this high mortality? In most European populations at this time, overall mortality rates during smallpox epidemics were lower because of high levels of immunity among individuals who previously had been exposed. However, as James Riley has pointed out, mortality among nonimmune people in isolated regions such as Iceland could still approach 40 per cent in the early eighteenth century.[16] Among the Mexica, initially no one was immune and children who did not benefit from maternal antibodies were especially vulnerable. Behavior may also have increased the Mexica's susceptibility. If they ate and slept in tight quarters, almost everyone would be infected in a single outbreak. In sum, smallpox probably caused very high mortality in American Indigenous communities, but it behaved no differently than among Europeans with a similar lack of exposure.

As more Europeans arrived and the impact of violent conquest rippled through the Valley of Mexico, other diseases caused mortality in ways that varied among peoples and regions. Measles was an especially serious threat. Prior to the era of vaccinations, the disease was extremely common among children. Recent studies have confirmed that measles causes significant immune suppression and may reduce resistance to other infectious diseases for years.[17] Once measles was introduced to the Americas, Indigenous communities may have been more vulnerable to outbreaks of pneumonia, diarrheal diseases, and other conditions that caused both adult and childhood mortality. In any case, sufficient evidence exists to indicate that diseases other than smallpox caused lethal epidemics. For example, recent genetic investigation suggests that an epidemic of an enteric (intestinal) disease caused by a *Salmonella* bacteria contributed to high mortality between 1545 and 1550 among Mixtec-speaking peoples who lived south of Tenochtitlán.[18] The expanded use of genetic analysis may enable future historians of this era to describe the full extent of disease-related events in greater detail.

In the sixteenth century, the greatest upheavals took place in the Caribbean, Central America, and South America as Spanish influence emanated outward from Mexico and the Portuguese established a colony in Brazil. In the Andes Mountains during the late 1520s, smallpox apparently preceded Europeans and aggravated social disruption and civil war among the Incas. The turmoil prevented effective resistance against a small force led by Francisco Pizarro that captured an Incan prince, Atahualpa, and toppled the Inca regime in the early 1530s. On the Atlantic coast of South America, smallpox arrived in Brazil from Lisbon in the 1560s. While the region's low population did not permit the disease to establish a stable foothold, thereafter smallpox frequently crossed the Atlantic with slaves that were imported from Africa to replace dwindling Indigenous populations.

To the north, expeditions around the Gulf of Mexico and as far as the Great Plains did little to add to Spanish wealth but introduced European diseases to the local inhabitants. Epidemics became more frequent as religious missions spread from Mexico and fostered more frequent contact between Europeans and Indigenous peoples. Beginning in 1593, Spanish Jesuit priests recorded that waves of disease swept northern New Spain every five to eight years.[19] Smallpox was the greatest killer, but not the only one: measles, influenza, and tuberculosis claimed many lives, and some episodes of high mortality were probably caused by a combination of diseases that struck at once. Sexually transmitted diseases such as gonorrhea (brought by Europeans) may have contributed to lower birth rates. As discussed in chapter 4, the introduction of yellow fever also had important consequences for the Caribbean, Latin America, and the southern United States.

Smallpox in North America

Beginning in the early seventeenth century, Indigenous peoples in North America faced many stressors as they encountered French, English, and Dutch arrivals. Up and down the Atlantic coast—at Jamestown in 1607, Quebec in 1608, Plymouth in 1620, and New Amsterdam (later New York) in 1624—Europeans established tentative footholds while Indigenous communities made guarded overtures and regarded the newcomers with a mixture of curiosity, pity, and suspicion. Coastal ship traffic and substantial contact preceded the settlers, and in some areas diseases preceded them as well. Reports of the epidemic that Samoset described— its cause remains unclear—suggest that it devastated numerous coastal communities but did not progress far inland. Quite different was a wave of pestilence in 1633, most likely smallpox, which originated in the Connecticut River valley and progressed north into New France. This epidemic had wide-ranging repercussions. High mortality among Mohegan and Pequot peoples encouraged English settlers to move into the Connecticut valley, and a successful war against the Pequots (1636–37) supported the founding of a new colony.

Throughout North America, epidemic diseases accompanied war, social upheaval, and ecological change that ensued from colonization. The dynamics varied from place to place. North and east of the Great Lakes, French traders and settlers entered relationships with Huron-Wendats, members of the Iroquois Confederacy, and other communities. Population losses fed an escalating cycle of warfare as Indigenous groups protected trade networks and replaced lost community members with captives. In 1648–49, a series of Iroquois attacks destroyed the villages of 2,000 Huron-Wendats. They abandoned their homeland and sought refuge with other groups. In the American southeast, beginning in the late 1690s, smallpox from the English colonies caused a major epidemic in the Indigenous territories east of the Mississippi River.[20] By the late 1730s, a series of disease outbreaks had weakened Cherokee communities who lived in the southern Appalachian Mountains, undermining their position against the colonies and their main Indigenous rivals, the Creek Confederation. Further west, where written evidence for this period is scant, oral histories suggest that, by the early eighteenth century, smallpox accompanied the expansion of Spanish Catholic missions and the arrival of horses from Mexico. Equestrianism transformed life for peoples of the Great Plains as they oriented to buffalo herds for their livelihood. However, rapid horse travel also facilitated the spread of smallpox across a vast territory from the Rio Grande River valley to the Saskatchewan River valley. In sum, by 1750 distinct patterns of disease and conflict caused upheaval for Indigenous communities throughout North America.

Initially, European settlers often resorted to providential explanations of events. Thus, in the aftermath of the 1633 epidemic, the Puritan John Winthrop (1587–1649) discerned a divine blessing behind his colony's good fortune: "if God were not pleased with our inheriting these parts," Winthrop asked, "why did he drive out the natives before us? and why dothe he still make roome for us, by deminishinge them as we increace?"[21] But not all European perceptions were self-justifying. At times, colonists and missionaries acknowledged responsibility for the disruption of Indigenous traditional customs and, when pressed, they considered their role in spreading disease. For example, in 1639, a group of Hurons accused the Jesuit missionary Jerome Lalemant (1593–1673) of bringing smallpox to their villages. "These poor people are in some sense excusable," Lalemant wrote ruefully, "for it has happened very often, and has been remarked more than a hundred times, that where we were most welcome, where we baptized the most people, there it was in fact where they died the most."[22] As David Jones suggests, during the early years of encounter settlers did not consider

Indigenous Americans to be intrinsically different from them on a physical level. Suffering and death brought by starvation, frostbite, and disease reminded the colonists that divine favor did not promise safety from natural dangers. Notions of divine providence, although powerful, coexisted with a belief that European and Indigenous bodies were subject to the same natural forces.[23]

However, attitudes hardened in the eighteenth century as competition for American territory intensified among the French, British, and various Indigenous communities. Armies contemplated how to use smallpox infections for tactical advantage. In 1763, after smallpox broke out among British troops at Fort Pitt (later Pittsburgh), some commanding officers concocted a plan to infect Delaware tribe warriors with infected blankets. A militia captain who ran the local trading post, William Trent, acted on the idea. British officers later approved reimbursement for a "gift" of two blankets and a handkerchief from the smallpox hospital. (The Delawares did suffer an outbreak of smallpox, but the part played by the contaminated cloth is unclear.) Veterans of the British army warned colonists about the tactic, and during the Revolutionary War (1775–82) the British were periodically accused of sending infected individuals into the American camps.[24]

The colonists' fears seemed justified, not only in view of British actions at Fort Pitt but also because the British army inoculated its troops against smallpox. As discussed later in this chapter, Britons were the first Europeans to expose individuals to smallpox material in order to provoke a mild case of the disease and thereby induce lasting resistance. The increasing prevalence of **inoculation** among Europeans and their descendants widened the gap between many Indigenous Americans and colonists in the region. In Central and South America, some Indigenous communities practiced inoculation extensively beginning in the 1760s, but there is little evidence that Indigenous peoples in North America employed the practice. British authorities, such as those who managed Hudson Bay Company outposts, were reluctant to attempt inoculations among their Indigenous associates, even when smallpox outbreaks threatened lucrative trade.[25]

The Revolutionary War coincided with a series of smallpox epidemics that eventually spanned much of North and South America. New England experienced outbreaks during the war's first battles in 1775, and smallpox hampered the American army when it unsuccessfully besieged Quebec City early in 1776. The following year, General George Washington (1732–1799) ordered his troops to undergo the inoculation procedure. Nonetheless, smallpox continued to spread south and west—precise routes of transmission have not been reconstructed—and also apparently came north from the Gulf of Mexico after an outbreak in the port of Pensacola. At Yorktown and elsewhere, the disease even hampered the efforts of British forces—although the troops were inoculated, smallpox took a heavy toll upon former slaves who assisted the British against their rebelling masters.[26]

In the summer of 1779, smallpox broke out in Mexico City, and tens of thousands of people died. This outbreak was probably not connected directly to the outbreaks further north, as the disease had struck Mexico City every fifteen years or so throughout the eighteenth century. In this case, however, smallpox coursed throughout the American West, spreading to New Mexican pueblos, into the Great Plains, and even north of the Great Lakes region. Written and oral accounts offer substantial evidence that smallpox came to the Pacific Northwest via the Columbia River with Indigenous groups that had crossed the Rocky Mountains.[27] Contemporary reports have not survived for the northwest coast but, in 1792, the English mariner George Vancouver (1757–1798) found numerous abandoned villages as he sailed the Juan de Fuca Strait between the mainland and the island now named for him. By this time, even remote northern communities were drawn into the orbit of epidemic diseases. One trader with the Hudson's Bay Company described bodies eaten by dogs and survivors in such a state of despair that they could barely speak. Another explorer and fur trader, Samuel Hearne, recounted in 1782 that disease had devastated "Northern Indians" at Churchill after they contracted smallpox from trading partners to the south. Outbreaks of other diseases followed in the region during the early nineteenth century.[28]

Elizabeth Fenn has suggested that smallpox "forged a horrific common experience that spanned the continent."[29] However, events of this era and subsequent decades also pushed European and Indigenous societies further apart. For groups such as the Cherokee, who had their villages burned to the ground after they sided with the English against American revolutionaries, the violence of war inflicted even greater harm than disease. In the 1830s, in several episodes later known collectively as the "Trail of Tears," more than 40,000 Indigenous Americans were forcibly marched from southern US states to territories west of the Mississippi River. An especially severe wave of smallpox killed many thousands of people in 1837–38. In the prairies and western regions of the United States and Canada, Indigenous communities later experienced outbreaks of various diseases as settlers moved westward and white militias sought to crush Indigenous groups.

In the late nineteenth century, the lives of Indigenous Americans increasingly were remote from the experience of the white majority. The understanding of earlier times that Indigenous and non-Indigenous bodies shared the same

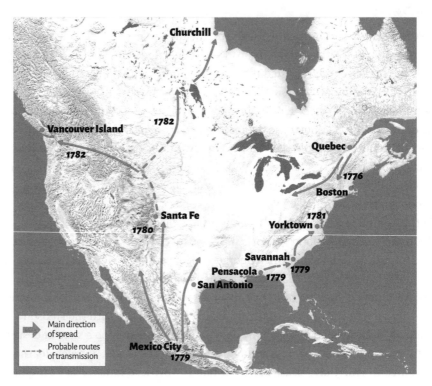

MAP 3.1 Smallpox in North America, 1775–1782.

vulnerabilities began to disappear. After the publication of Charles Darwin's epochal work on evolution, *On the Origin of Species* (1859), many whites applied the concept of "natural selection" among animals to envision human societies on an evolutionary scale. The experience of previously isolated Pacific peoples, such as Australian Aborigines and Hawaiian islanders, seemed to offer further confirmation that European dominance was inevitable. In the century after 1778, when a British expedition led by James Cook (1728–1779) reached the Hawaiian archipelago, missionaries documented a population decline that even by conservative estimates was over 80 per cent.[30] Westerners found various reasons for Indigenous decline: in addition to lethal epidemics, it might be explained by apparent flaws in traditional society—the communal ownership of land, for example—or as the result of exposure to trappings of "civilization" such as alcohol or venereal disease. Indigenous peoples appeared unequipped to thrive in a world dominated by Europeans and their (white) descendants in former colonies. As we have seen, recent research has modified this picture. However, as the quote above from

Francis Jennings illustrates, Darwinist assumptions remained influential among historians long after they dispensed with notions of inherent European cultural superiority.

By 1900, warfare, disease, and poverty had reduced the Indigenous population of North America to 400,000 or less. In the twentieth century other diseases took a heavier toll, as some Indigenous Americans adapted to life on designated reserves that usually had poor living conditions. As explored in chapter 6, the impact of tuberculosis provides additional evidence that social inequities and persecution heightened Indigenous susceptibility to infectious diseases. The impact of smallpox ebbed, in part because of the benefit of a new technology—vaccination—that eventually lifted the burden of smallpox from all peoples.

From Inoculation to Vaccination

Through the eighteenth century, smallpox was a routine cause of death, especially for children, throughout Eurasia and Africa. In Europe, where its severity had actually worsened, it accounted for between 5 per cent and 10 per cent of all mortality. And it struck people from all walks of life, including rulers and, more often, their young heirs. Then, in the late 1790s, an ancient folk practice was refined and recast as a signal achievement of modern science. The vaccination technique, proposed by the English physician Edward Jenner (1749–1823), won rapid acceptance from many, but it also inspired controversial questions that have echoes today: should governments be empowered to enforce an invasive procedure in the name of public health? And how will the safety of any such procedure be guaranteed?

A doctor in the rural county of Gloucestershire, England, Jenner lived in a milieu in which many elites felt increased confidence in the human ability to understand and control the natural world. It was fashionable for gentlemen to contribute to natural knowledge with observations and experiments. Scientific information spread through personal circles of communication and learned associations such as the Royal Society of London, which had been founded in 1662. The Latin language enabled research findings to disseminate across national boundaries. Jenner had tapped into learned circles during his medical training in London with a leading surgeon, John Hunter (1728–1793). Like his teacher, Jenner was an avid naturalist; his research interests ranged from hibernating hedgehogs to migrating birds, and he earned membership in the Royal Society with a well-regarded essay on the nesting habits of cuckoos.

In England at the time, the inoculation technique—also known as **variolation**—had begun to make inroads against smallpox. The idea was simple: individuals received material from a smallpox sufferer to cause a (hopefully) mild bout of the disease. Those who recovered would never have smallpox again. Peoples in many parts of Eurasia and Africa had acted on this premise for centuries, mostly by exposing children to infected clothing or blankets. In China, practitioners collected material from smallpox scabs, stored it for a period to reduce its potency, and then used a silver tube to blow ground scabs into a child's nostrils. In Turkey, fluid (**lymph**) was collected from a pustule and then inserted into scratches or shallow cuts. These practices had substantial risk—on occasion, the inoculated contracted full-blown smallpox—but they allowed the inoculators to adjust the strength of the infective dose and to safely isolate the subjects for several weeks.

While much remains obscure concerning the global spread of inoculation techniques, in the British Isles some practitioners reported that Welsh commoners knew of the practice from at least the early seventeenth century.[31] Interest grew among elite observers after the Royal Society published a detailed account of "Turkish inoculation" in 1714. Thereafter, the wife of Britain's ambassador in Constantinople, Mary Wortley Montagu (1689–1762), had both her children inoculated and she promoted the practice when she returned to England. After one successful trial with orphans, and another with convicts, within a year the British king set an example by having his own children inoculated. Additional support also came from Boston, the largest port in colonial New England. A fervent proponent of the procedure, the Puritan minister Cotton Mather (1663–1728), was prodded into action after he learned of it from his slave Onesimus (late 1600s–1700s) and other West Africans. Although most Bostonians were skeptical, physician Zabdiel Boylston (ca 1680–1766) reported in 1726 that he had inoculated 282 people and only 6 had died.[32] A mortality rate of roughly 2 per cent would not be counted a success today, but it was deemed vastly preferable to Boston's experience overall: in a town of 10,500 residents nearly 6,000 people had contracted smallpox and roughly 800 died.

In the next half century, inoculation spread to other European countries and their colonies. The practice was especially popular among the middle classes in Britain, and charities and orphanages began to provide it to poor children as well. After the 1760s, many Britons were inoculated by the "Sutton method," popularized by apothecary Robert Sutton and his sons, in which a pronged instrument called a **lancet** was used to introduce smallpox lymph into a shallow puncture. Jenner learned of inoculation through John Hunter's surgical practice and later performed the procedure himself. Although mild cases of smallpox were expected after the procedure, along the way Jenner learned of individuals who apparently were not affected at all. They had previously contracted cowpox, a disease of cattle that caused lesions and mild, flu-like symptoms in humans. In farm country, the malady was well known among dairy workers, who recognized that a "case of cowpox" could provide resistance to smallpox. Several practitioners in England and elsewhere had inoculated individuals with cowpox material in the belief that this would provide similar protection. Jenner attempted to prove it, and he described his observations and experiments in *An Inquiry into the Causes and Effects of the Variolae Vaccinae* (1798).

Jenner's treatise reflected his observation of the entire farm environment. He believed that cowpox actually originated with horses that suffered from "grease," an inflammation that caused their heels to ooze a dark fluid discharge. Jenner named this infected material with a Latin word, *virus*, which was usually translated in English as "poison." He suggested that farm workers spread the material from horses to cows, and dairy maids were infected when they milked cows that had lesions on their udders. The main question was whether inoculation with this milder material would induce resistance to smallpox. On 14 May 1796 Jenner inoculated an eight-year-old boy, James Phipps (1788–1843), with cowpox material taken from a dairy maid named Sarah Nelmes (or Lucy, as Jenner's notes once refer to her).[33] When Phipps was inoculated with smallpox he displayed no signs of disease. In subsequent tests with more children, Jenner further demonstrated that cowpox could be "passaged" by physical contact from one person to another and still confer protection to smallpox. Inoculation with cowpox was called **vaccination** because the Latin word for cow is *vacca*. The new procedure was much less risky than traditional inoculation. No smallpox was needed and, as long as cowpox material was preserved or passed arm to arm, no infected cows were required, either. This eventually proved important since cowpox was not widespread around the world.

It is not clear what horse disease Jenner called "grease"—it may have been a now-extinct variety of horsepox or (more likely) the symptoms of another bacterial or fungal infection. In his later years, as he encountered criticism, Jenner retreated from claims about a horse disease, and historical accounts often ignore his interest in it. However, Jenner's initial theory reveals a great deal about his mindset. Jenner used the term *virus* much as his predecessors had: he referred to a poison that, he believed, originated with horses and then spread to cows and humans. Although Jenner did not claim that this poison was a living entity, he thought it changed as it moved through the bodies of various animals. Jenner thought this accounted for the different symptoms of grease and cowpox, and that it might also explain why some cases of human smallpox were more severe than others. His conception of a changing poison differed from later germ theorists who attributed diseases to distinct, living pathogens. This is not surprising when we consider that Jenner did not use a microscope or consider a role for microbes in the spread of disease.

It is also not surprising that Jenner encountered controversy in 1798 when he sought supporters in London. The city had its share of sharp-elbowed opportunists, and inoculation was a profitable business that inspired competition. Many practitioners resisted a change to the untested vaccination procedure, while others, such as physician George Pearson (1751–1828), attempted to take credit for vaccination and push Jenner aside. Questions also arose as hundreds of vaccinations were performed at a smallpox hospital directed by physician William Woodville (1752–1805). After the procedure many people experienced severe skin eruptions that were considered little better than smallpox itself. To Jenner, this suggested that some batches of Woodville's vaccine had been contaminated by smallpox material. Jenner cautioned that vaccinators must use lymph taken from cases of "true" cowpox, not material taken from old lesions or from skin outbreaks that were not caused by cowpox at all.[34]

Jenner's claim about Woodville was never proven, but questions about the makeup of the earliest vaccines have persisted ever since. Amid various allegations about contamination, one of Jenner's opponents, Dr Benjamin Moseley (1742–1819), even asserted that cowpox was actually a form of syphilis that had no protective value against smallpox. More recent scientists have approached the issue from a different perspective. In the 1930s, after techniques were developed to distinguish various viral agents, it was shown that the vaccine agent that was in use by then differed from the cowpox that was found in animals. The virus that served as the basis for the global eradication campaign has never been observed outside a laboratory. Was it the result of contamination, a mutation created during countless vaccinations, or a naturally occurring virus that died out? We may never know.

Vaccination, Adaptation, and Resistance

Despite the questions raised about vaccination in London, after 1798 enthusiasm for the practice spread through international networks of diplomats and bureaucrats with astonishing speed. Within five years, translations of Jenner's treatise circulated throughout Europe. Cowpox material was soon sent to Switzerland, Austria, and further afield on threads that contained dried lymph or between small glass plates encased in wax. Although France and England were combatants during the Napoleonic wars, high-level diplomatic exchanges won over officials in Paris to the new procedure. French and Dutch doctors also orchestrated vaccinations on islands in the Indian Ocean that were under colonial control. Knowledge of vaccination spread quickly in the United States, especially after it received vigorous support from the influential statesman Thomas Jefferson (1743–1826), who served as the third president from 1801 to 1809. Some Indigenous communities in the United States also received vaccinations, notably the Cherokees in the 1820s, although the procedure did not supplant other antidisease strategies that had developed in these societies over time.

Remarkable campaigns enlisted children to deliver cowpox material by the arm-to-arm technique to regions where cowpox did not occur in nature. The first was organized by officials in imperial Spain for the benefit of American colonial territories. In November 1803, with the blessing of King Carlos IV, twenty-two orphan boys set sail for New Spain under the direction of Dr Francisco Xavier de Balmis (1753–1819). After arriving in Caracas (now in Venezuela), de Balmis sent one team south and went north himself to work in Mexico. De Balmis taught the arm-to-arm technique to Mexicans and then set off across the Pacific with more boys to visit outposts in Malaysia, the Philippine Islands, and China's coast.[35]

In 1849, Japanese doctors performed a similar feat after they made a special request for cowpox scabs from the island colony Batavia that was controlled by the Netherlands. (The island is now part of Indonesia.) Japan's ruling Tokugawa shogunate restricted European trade, and previous attempts to deliver cowpox lymph had failed because the material lost its potency during the long voyage. A vaccine derived from the scabs did the trick. Beginning with a single boy in the port city of Nagasaki, visiting children were vaccinated arm-to-arm and sent home to distribute cowpox material to other children. The procedure reached clinics throughout the Japanese islands in only six months. This effort was also remarkable because initially it was not encouraged by a colonial power or actively sponsored by Japan's rulers. Vaccination was promoted by a medical elite outside of government circles, and during the first decade it was sponsored and supervised by local officials. Thereafter, however, vaccination became a cornerstone of a modernizing national public health scheme, particularly after the Tokugawa family relinquished power in 1868 and regional leaders reinstated a Japanese emperor.[36]

Through the nineteenth century, governments in Europe considered vaccination both an opportunity and a challenge. It offered the potential to eliminate a disease rather than stop it at a border, but successful campaigns depended on individual compliance. The question was how to encourage everyone to undergo the procedure. Some early requirements for vaccination targeted people who participated in government institutions. For example, in 1805 Bavaria required vaccination for all schoolchildren who had not had smallpox, and in 1807 it mandated the same for its army conscripts. Other European jurisdictions followed suit with vaccination requirements for orphans or families that received public support. The tactics and timing varied among countries. Russia, Sweden, and Denmark all had national vaccination laws by 1816. France, in contrast, relied on a patchwork of requirements for groups such as the military, university students, and government workers until 1902. England was initially hesitant as well, but in 1853 Parliament passed a measure requiring the vaccination of all infants. Laws enacted in 1867 and 1871 provided for enforcement by vaccination officers and penalties for noncompliance.[37] Less overt forms of persuasion were often more effective than the threat of punishment. Encouragement by doctors or clergy, instructions by an employer, the refusal of an insurance company to provide benefits to the unvaccinated—all became powerful incentives for individuals to accept a vaccine.

Although the number of vaccinated people steadily increased, large cities continued to experience periodic outbreaks, including Paris in 1825 and London between 1837 and 1840. In Canada, when smallpox threatened Quebec City in the 1870s and 1880s, conflict erupted between an English-speaking government that pressed for vaccination and a French majority that angrily resisted the practice. The most significant European pandemic in the later nineteenth century broke out in 1870 among French troops in the Franco-Prussian War. The death rate among those who contracted the disease was exceptionally high, often exceeding 15 per cent. As smallpox spread to France's general population and to other countries, the total deaths numbered in the hundreds of thousands. Especially after this episode, various countries tightened their vaccination requirements but this also had a reverse effect: as rules and their enforcement increased, the opponents of vaccination were also energized.

The Opponents of Vaccination

As explained in chapter 1, over the long term there was no inherent conflict between religious and medical practices for most Europeans. But the invasive vaccination procedure struck a nerve. Critics had already suggested that inoculation was an attempt to interfere in God's sovereign control over life and death. Vaccination raised the same objection; moreover, some people claimed that it was an abomination to mix material from cows with human bodies. Cartoonists played upon this anxiety with memorable satires of vaccinators and their opponents. As early as 1802, for example, British illustrator Charles Williams vividly depicted a monstrous cow that consumed baskets of infants in one end and excreted them with horns out the other (image 3.2). Opponents of vaccination also argued that the exchange of bodily material could spread corruption between persons. In a sermon preached in August 1882, the British archdeacon Thomas Colley claimed that the procedure "mingles, in a hideous communion of blood, all the disease and taints of the community. Every hereditary sewer is made to open up in the nursery, through the unsanitary process of vaccination." Much like the anxieties that concerned syphilis, such statements did not distinguish between physical and spiritual defilement. Colley simply argued that vaccination would soil "the life-blood of our little ones."[38]

Not all criticisms of vaccination reflected a knee-jerk moralism or wholesale rejection of science. The idea that vulnerability to one disease (smallpox) could be removed by causing another (cowpox) simply struck many laypeople as implausible. In an era when both the content of vaccines and inoculation procedures were almost completely unregulated, there were legitimate fears of infection from puncture wounds or the transfer of other diseases from the cowpox donor. Attention centered most often upon syphilis, a disease that spread by intimate contact and which, as Benjamin Moseley had noted, caused ulcers that somewhat resembled cowpox lesions.

Although doctors often protested that vaccinations were safe, fear sometimes was fed by more than mere appearances. Several widely publicized cases revealed that cowpox lymph could be tainted by even a tiny amount of blood. In 1861, at the Italian town of Rivalta, lymph that had been taken from an eleven-month-old boy infected fifty other children with syphilis. It later emerged that the wet nurse of the first boy had syphilitic ulcers around her nipples.[39] Cities in the United States faced a similar panic in 1901 during a national smallpox epidemic. In the rush to meet surging demand for vaccines, some doses were apparently contaminated with tetanus that caused fatalities in New Jersey, Pennsylvania, and Ohio. Partly because of this crisis, President Theodore Roosevelt signed the 1902 Biologics Control Act, which restricted the sale of vaccines and related products to establishments that were licensed annually by the national Public Health

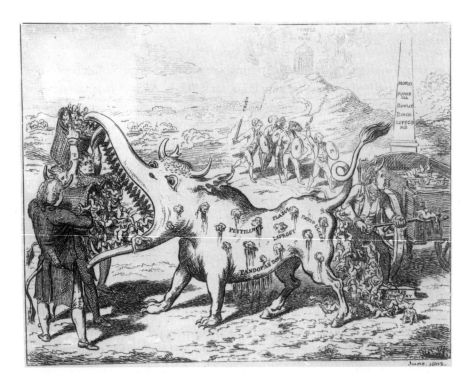

IMAGE 3.2 "Vaccination." Critics of vaccination decried what they considered a bestial intermixing of animal and human. This cartoon by Charles Williams (1802) depicts vaccination as a monster that Edward Jenner feeds with a basket of infants. (Jenner is demonized, literally—note his tail and horns.) The infants poured into the beast's maw emerge from its rear with horns on their heads; weeping sores on the hide bear labels that include "leprosy," "plague," and "fetid ulcers." Jenner's henchman tramples a book labeled "Lecture in Botany"—a symbol of learned science—as he shovels an infant into a cart. Vaccination's opponents, bearing swords of "truth," descend the hill from a "temple of fame." The monument behind the wagon bears the names of vaccination's foremost opponents, including Benjamin Moseley.

Service.[40] Long into the twentieth century, however, such episodes continued to provide ammunition for both learned and popular rejection of vaccination.

The opponents of vaccination had their most tangible success in Britain after an Anti-Compulsory Vaccination League was founded in 1867 in response to laws that required the procedure. Many people who did not oppose vaccination on medical grounds nonetheless believed that citizens should have the liberty to refuse it. The British system of vaccinations for the poor, which was begun in 1840, created particular grounds for concern. To obtain a free vaccination,

families were required to bring their children to workhouse clinics twice, once
to undergo the procedure and eight days later to confirm that it had "taken."
Those children with fully developed pustules were required to provide lymph to
vaccinate others, but there was no means of ensuring that the lymph was free of
other diseases. Reformers railed against a system that many considered degrad-
ing and dangerous for the lower classes. The businessman William Tebb
(1830–1917) used mortality statistics to argue that vaccination was responsible
for rising death rates from syphilis, bronchitis, and cancer.[41] The height of
Britain's vaccination controversy coincided, in the 1870s and 1880s, with the
debate over the Contagious Disease Acts, which were also accused of targeting
poor and marginal women (see chapter 2). In 1898, Parliament amended the
vaccination law so that children could undergo the procedure in their homes and
receive vaccine from a regulated supply of calf lymph. Significantly, the new law
also allowed for "conscientious objection" by parents who refused vaccination
altogether, and the statute was modified in 1907 to require a mere declaration
instead of a written certificate. A principle of conscientious objection is still
invoked in some contexts by individuals who refuse invasive medical interventions, including blood transfusions and transplants as well as vaccinations.

To nineteenth-century Europeans, vaccination could be considered either a
lifesaving social practice or an unnecessary imposition by scientific and social elites.
A further example illustrates how it also was perceived as a tool of empire. In colonial
India, where vaccine material first reached British doctors in 1802, smallpox killed
many thousands of people annually during the nineteenth century. Inoculation
practices were already widespread in the subcontinent's diverse Hindu and Muslim
communities. Especially among Hindus, the *tikadar*—or inoculator—was a familiar
figure who often traveled from village to village in the months after the harvest.
Inoculation had ritual connotations because it was understood to invoke the protective power of the goddess **Sitala**, who was closely identified with smallpox.

British officials hoped that vaccination would illustrate their benevolent
intentions and the benefits of European science. However, owing to various
logistical and cultural factors, attempts to replace inoculation with vaccination
made only halting progress. Cowpox lymph lost its effectiveness in warm weather,
so it was difficult to keep a steady supply. In the absence of fully standardized
procedures, a great deal depended on the vaccinator's ability to introduce the
cowpox material properly, either with a lancet or arm to arm. Because of the
difficulties involved in transporting and storing lymph, the arm-to-arm method
was more practical but it was resisted by Hindus who considered the transfer of

bodily fluids between people unclean. Some Hindu parents were appalled when vaccinators took young children with "ripe" cowpox lesions door to door to provide material to others. Efforts to create a local Indian supply of calf lymph were no better since Hindus viewed this as mistreatment of a sacred animal.

As David Arnold has suggested, vaccination was held in suspicion as a colonial import, although some middle-class Indians supported the practice by the 1880s.[42] By 1900, millions of children were vaccinated annually but, among India's population of over 300 million people, a substantial cohort of rural villages paid no attention. Moreover, beginning in the 1910s, India's influential leader Mohandas Gandhi criticized vaccination as a "savage custom," although he did support sanitary measures that were informed by Western science.[43] Gandhi's view of vaccination apparently softened over time and did not cause an end to anti-smallpox campaigns. However, soon after his death in 1948, opponents of the practice cited Gandhi's criticism in an effort to stymie government-led tuberculosis vaccination campaigns (see chapter 6).

Vast and culturally diverse, through the 1970s India remained one of the last outposts of smallpox in nature. But the challenges in India were not entirely unique. After World War II, public health officials faced a broad range of geographic, cultural, and political challenges as they considered the prospects of global eradication. Scientific innovations were necessary but not sufficient—the ultimate success of vaccination technology depended on adaptation to local conditions and collaboration across cultures.

From Vaccination to Eradication

Some observers glimpsed the prospect of a world without smallpox within a few years of the beginning of vaccination. **Eradication** (the complete removal of a disease from nature) became a topic of earnest discussion after World War II with the founding of the World Health Organization (WHO) in 1948. By this time, smallpox **elimination** (removal from a given region) had been accomplished in many nations of Eurasia and North America. Vaccination had played an important role in this development, but elimination was also abetted by the increased circulation of *V. minor*, the milder smallpox variant that rarely caused life-threatening disease but conferred lasting immunity. In wealthier countries, smallpox was no longer a domestic challenge but, owing to its virulence and the swift spread enabled by commercial air travel, the disease remained a threat that could not be ignored. The postwar diplomatic milieu encouraged large-scale international collaboration. In a quarter century that Randall

Packard has called an "era of eradication," frontal assaults were mounted on malaria, tuberculosis, smallpox, and other infectious diseases.[44]

We will see in later chapters that efforts to combat malaria and tuberculosis foundered by the late 1960s, but hope remained that smallpox eradication was feasible. Smallpox caused highly visible symptoms that enabled cases to be identified swiftly. It had no reservoir in other animals, and the virus was transmitted solely from one human case to another. The disease thus posed fewer challenges than vector-borne diseases—such as malaria or plague—or widespread, often dormant infections such as tuberculosis. Moreover, the Soviet Union had demonstrated success with a smallpox elimination campaign in the 1930s. The Soviet deputy health minister, Victor Zhdanov (1914–1987), was instrumental in persuading WHO delegates to approve a global campaign in 1959. At first, efforts against smallpox competed with other public health priorities in individual countries. Then, in 1966, the WHO secured funding for an intensified eradication program in regions where smallpox had the most stubborn presence. These included sub-Saharan Africa, where large distances, a lack of infrastructure, and tropical temperatures had long made vaccination efforts impractical.

Shifts in technology increased the capacity to store and more easily administer vaccines in remote areas. **Lyophilization** (freeze-drying), a procedure refined during World War II for transporting blood plasma, enabled public health workers to carry vaccine material into mountainous or jungle areas that were isolated from transportation networks. In large communities, workers initially used compressed-air guns to rapidly inject vaccine into hundreds of people per hour. While this reduced the need for sterilized needles and syringes, experience showed that the guns required skill to operate and sometimes malfunctioned. Vaccinators turned to a far simpler technique: the **bifurcated needle**, created by clipping the eye of an industrial sewing needle to produce two prongs that would hold an ideal liquid dose of vaccine. Volunteers could learn the procedure in an hour; they were instructed to give fifteen jabs in a circle and watch for a drop of blood to indicate that they had reached the right depth. Simple and reliable, the bifurcated needle enabled broad community participation that contributed to the success of vaccination campaigns.[45]

Of equal importance was a shift in the strategy for whom to vaccinate in order to break chains of person-to-person transmission. Until the late 1960s, the preferred strategy was mass vaccination in a given geographic area. A sufficiently vaccinated population would attain **herd immunity**, meaning that the probability of one person infecting another would fall so low that the disease would fail to spread. Many observers considered this impractical for countries such as India

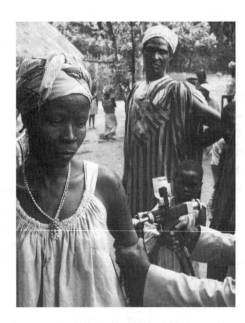

IMAGE 3.3a Smallpox vaccination with an injector gun. This photograph from 1969 depicts a villager in Niger receiving vaccines for smallpox and measles in front of concerned onlookers. Jet injector guns used compressed air instead of needles to administer vaccine doses.

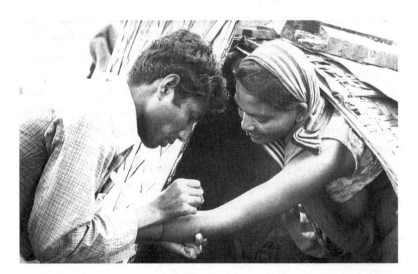

IMAGE 3.3b Smallpox vaccination with a bifurcated needle. This photograph from 1975 depicts a volunteer vaccinator and vaccine recipient in Bangladesh during the global smallpox eradication campaign. The woman lived in an unofficial settlement where occupants otherwise had little access to health care. Success of the eradication campaign required action among the world's most remote and impoverished communities.

where inhabitants were numerous and dispersed. Then, in December 1966, a fortuitous test took place when a team in eastern Nigeria confronted a smallpox outbreak with an insufficient supply of vaccine. Using radios and motorcycles, the team isolated new cases, traced the people who had been in contact with the infected, and created perimeters of vaccinated individuals. Within five months, the chain of transmission was broken, although less than 10 per cent of the population had been vaccinated. This strategy of "surveillance and containment" was soon used in the Indonesian province of West Java and in India's state of Tamil Nadu. Success in India was especially important because of the continued prevalence of smallpox and the need for willing engagement at local, regional, and national levels in other parts of that country. These results were in contrast to British attempts to stamp out bubonic plague decades earlier, when heavy-handed coercion had inspired protests and encouraged individuals to conceal their infections.

As WHO's director-general at the time, Dr Halfdan Mahler (1923–2016), later observed, the smallpox program was "a triumph of management, not of medicine." In October 1977, a man named Ali Maow Maalin (1954–2013) was identified in Somalia with the last known natural case of smallpox. A hospital cook in Mogadishu, Maalin contracted smallpox (fortunately, *V. minor*) as he drove an infected family to a clinic. He knew about the eradication program but was, as he later acknowledged, also afraid of needles. Two years later, the WHO declared smallpox eradicated from nature on 9 December 1979. Maalin recovered, and decades later he led vaccination campaigns for polio in war-torn parts of southern Somalia. He carried out this work until shortly before his death from malaria in July 2013.[46]

Conclusion

In the summer of 2016, near the Arctic Circle in northern Siberia, melting permafrost uncovered animal graves contaminated with anthrax bacteria that spread among local animals. Researchers called to the area also found something else: fragments of smallpox DNA in a corpse that bore marks of infection from the disease. In an era of swift climate change in the far north, could smallpox rise from a frozen grave? Scientists consider it highly unlikely that a complete virus could survive the region's cycles of freezing and thawing intact. Another remote but unwelcome prospect is the use of smallpox for an intentional biological attack. Although there are only two known stocks of smallpox samples—in the United States and Russia—the possibility of another source has never been ruled out completely. In the event of a smallpox outbreak, the strategy of surveillance and containment would be the measure of first resort, particularly since vaccine material does not exist in sufficient quantities for a mass campaign. Not every disease is easily controlled by surveillance and containment, but smallpox's highly visible symptoms and relatively short incubation period enabled health workers to track its transmission and forestall a wider disaster.

Smallpox and other diseases contributed to a drastic depopulation of the Americas, Australia, and many islands. What Indigenous peoples experienced as catastrophe, Europeans and their descendants considered an astonishing windfall that enabled a far-reaching exploitation of the world's natural and human resources. Moreover, to many Europeans and their descendants, the lesson of smallpox was that their triumph against other peoples was fore-ordained. Over the centuries, the explanations for Western success varied: they included divinely appointed victory in conflict, Darwinist notions of an evolutionary hierarchy, and the biological advantages conferred by life in more complex societies. Regardless, as European states created colonial empires, and as American and Canadian colonists moved westward, they carried with them a belief in their ability to spread "civilization" into the wilderness and among more primitive peoples.

However, diseases were not isolated forces, nor did they reveal fundamental biological differences between Indigenous Americans and European invaders. The impact of novel diseases was magnified, either indirectly by forced labor, resettlement, and other conditions imposed by settler colonialism or, in a few cases, directly through the intentional spread of infected materials. The infamous episode at Fort Pitt has played an outsized role in the history of smallpox. But the intentional spread of disease has had far less profound consequences for Indigenous Americans than the health-related effects of marginalization and deprivation that persist today. Alongside disease and warfare, Indigenous health has been deeply influenced by environmental change, the disruption of livelihood, and relatively poor access to housing, health care, and other necessities. These contemporary challenges require exploration as much as the history of highly visible atrocities.

One of the greatest repercussions of depopulation in the Americas was the vast expansion in trans-Atlantic migration, and especially the forced migration of Africans. In an effort to extract profits from the Americas and the Caribbean, over several centuries colonists imported roughly 10 million slaves and created new landscapes to produce sugar and other tropical goods. The resulting ecological changes had important consequences for the plants, animals, and peoples that populated the region. Within the new societies that took shape, yellow fever and malaria influenced the geopolitics of an entire hemisphere.

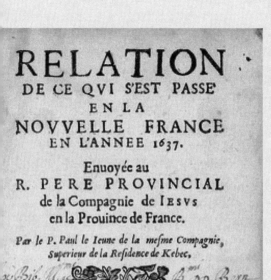

RELATION
DE CE QVI S'EST PASSE'
EN LA
NOVVELLE FRANCE
EN L'ANNEE 1637.

Enuoyée au
R. PERE PROVINCIAL
de la Compagnie de IESVS
en la Prouince de France.

Par le P. Paul le Ieune de la mefme Compagnie,
Superieur de la Refidence de Kebec,

T
IHS.

A ROVEN,
Chez IEAN LE BOVLLENGER, prés le
College des PP. Iefuites.

M. DC. XXXVIII.
AVEC PRIVILEGE DV ROY.

[IMA]GE 3.4 *Jesuit Relations* title page (1638).

WORKSHOP: INDIGENOUS AMERICANS, JESUIT MISSIONARIES, AND DISEASE IN NEW FRANCE

Scholars of early North American history encounter a challenging problem. Undoubtedly, the arrival of Europeans and their diseases transformed many Native American communities. However, in most cases the surviving written sources reflect the perspective of European explorers and religious missionaries. Even when these writers attempted to represent people and events faithfully, they wrote with specific objectives and certain convictions that shaped their accounts. We therefore face a conundrum that often arises with European depictions of other peoples around the world: the challenge is to "read behind" the sources, taking into account the authors' perspectives without disregarding them as "biased" because they represent views about Indigenous people, religion, or medicine that reflect their era and not ours.

This is very much the case with the remarkable narratives of the *Jesuit Relations*, descriptions of life in New France that were written by Catholic Jesuit missionaries and published in Europe (at first in Latin and French) between 1632 and 1672. In these decades, small numbers of missionaries went to great lengths to travel to remote Indigenous villages, acquaint themselves with the way of life, and convert Huron and Algonquin peoples to Christian beliefs. They provided accounts of their work and observations to the head of the Jesuit order in Quebec. Selections were then delivered to Paris where they were edited and published.

For their intended European audience, the *Jesuit Relations* served multiple purposes: as adventure literature for an interested public, advertisements for the missionaries' activities, and narratives of the successful spread of Catholicism for a Europe bitterly divided between

Catholics and Protestants. While the Jesuits are at the center of the accounts, a careful reading of the *Relations* also suggests that Indigenous communities and individuals acted with a complex range of motives. Amusement and genuine curiosity are mixed with suspicion and, certainly by the mid-seventeenth century, an awareness that Europeans were a significant trading partner and military force whose wishes could not be ignored. Indigenous people also wrestled with the inescapable fact that they were more vulnerable to many serious illnesses than Europeans.

It might seem logical to reject the *Relations* as accounts that are unreliable or biased. Despite the missionaries' efforts, they clearly understood Indigenous languages imperfectly, and sometimes scarcely at all. The Jesuits often expressed a low opinion of "savages" who differed fundamentally from them in beliefs and social practices. Most of all, the Jesuits perceived the hand of God behind every event and even interpreted their own failures as part of a divine master plan that ultimately advanced the cause of Catholicism. But there are reasons to make the most of these historical sources rather than dismiss them. The Jesuits were astute observers who did their best to understand Indigenous ideas and practices. It is possible to analyze and interpret their descriptions of events, not only to learn about European attitudes and experiences but also to better understand Indigenous peoples whose own words are lost. Although the testimony is indirect, these documents illuminate the great suffering and resourcefulness of the Hurons and other Indigenous peoples across North America as they faced terrifying challenges that changed their communities forever.

"Jesuit Efforts to Heal Sick Hurons"—François le Mercier (1636)

Le Mercier arrived at a Huron settlement called Ihonatiria in August 1636. A disease that may have been influenza struck the missionaries and was often lethal among the native inhabitants. Le Mercier's account reflects the importance of the European Galenic medicine to which Jesuits were accustomed and suggests that his Huron acquaintances were receptive to it.

From about the 15th of October, when our patients [*Le Mercier refers here to some of his fellow Jesuits who had fallen ill*] were entirely out of danger and began again to take the ordinary food of the country, our principal occupation up to the 17th of November was to assist the sick of our village.... We visited them twice a day, morning and evening, and carried them soup and meat, according to the condition and disposition of the patients, always taking occasion to exhort them to have recourse to God, and to gently influence them to baptism. We ate during our own sickness a few of the raisins and prunes, and some little remedies that your Reverence [*the head of the Jesuit order in Quebec*] had sent us, using them only in cases of necessity, so that we still had a good part of them, which we have made last up to the present. Everything was given by count, two or three prunes, or five or six raisins to one patient; this was restoring life to him. Our medicines produced effects which dazzled the whole country, and yet I leave you to imagine what sort of medicines they were! A little bag of senna served over fifty persons; they asked us for it on every side; and sometimes the joke of it was that if the patient found himself troubled by a retention of urine, our medicine acted only as a specific for that ailment. [*Senna is an herb; its seeds and pods were used in Galenic medicine as a laxative and sometimes as a diuretic.*] Simon Baron [*a Jesuit*] rendered us good service at this time; for, having learned before at Chibou, during a period of like necessity, to handle the lancet [*i.e., to perform bloodletting*], he did not fail to exercise it here throughout the winter; and lancets were more deficient with us than was good will with him, and [*the same was true*] for the desire to be bled on the part of our savages. They had seen the good effects of it in the recovery of several persons who had been almost given up....

"Smallpox Strikes the Hurons"—Jerome Lalemant (1639)

The following two passages were written by a prolific contributor to TheJesuit Relations. Lalemant first describes how images of Jesus and the Virgin Mary, portrayed in European artistic styles, evoked wonder and then suspicion as people fell ill. Lalemant hints at the hostility that he and his associates encountered, and he also refers to divisions among the Hurons between those who chose to help the Jesuits and those who did not.

Our Fathers [*other Jesuits*] had erected a sort of altar where they had placed some little pictures, in order thus to secure opportunity to explain to them [*the Hurons*] what was the principal motive that brought us here and had attracted us to their village. The whole cabin resounded with expressions of admiration at the sight of these extraordinary objects; above all, they could not weary of gazing at two pictures—one of Our Lord [*Jesus Christ*], and the other of Our Lady [*the Virgin Mary*]. We had some difficulty in making them believe that these were only flat paintings, especially as these pictures were of life size, for the small figures make but little impression upon their minds. We had to leave them exposed all day in order to satisfy all the people.

This first view cost us very dear; for, without speaking of the annoyance that inquisitive persons have since caused us—that is to say, all the people who arrive from other villages—if we derived thence some advantage for speaking to them of our Holy mysteries and disposing them to the knowledge of the true God, some of them took occasion to spread new reports and to authorize the previous calumnies, namely, that we were causing the death of these peoples by our images.

In a few days the country was completely imbued with this opinion, that we were, without any doubt, the authors of this so universal contagion. It is very probable that those who invented these slanders did not believe them at all; yet they spoke in so positive terms that the majority no longer doubted them. The women and children looked upon us as persons who brought them misfortune. God be forever blessed, who willed that for the space of three or four months, while these persecutions were at their height, we should be deprived of nearly all human consolation. The people of our village seemed to spare us more than the others, yet these evil reports were so persistent, and were such a common subject of conversation in their assemblies, that suspicion began to take hold upon them; and the most prominent ones, who had loved us and had been accustomed to speak in our favor, became entirely mute, and when they were constrained to speak, they had recourse to excuses, and justified themselves as well as they could for having built us a cabin.... [*Lalemant's account continues in 1640, when a renewed outbreak of disease arouses fresh suspicions about the influence of the missionaries. It is not clear how this epidemic spread. Lalemant attributes its origin among the Hurons to contact with Algonquins, and he also suggests that the Hurons' living practices are at least partly to blame. But Lalemant also acknowledges the coincidence of timing between disease outbreaks and missionary presence. Although Europeans were not directly responsible for introducing diseases in all cases, the overall dynamic could not be ignored.*]

It was upon the return from the journey which the Hurons had made to Kebec [*Quebec*], that it started in the country, our Hurons, while again on their way up here, having thoughtlessly mingled with the Algonquins, whom they met on the route, most of whom were infected with smallpox. [*Algonquins spoke a different language than Hurons but at the time were allied with them. Algonquin communities were often mobile and disseminated ideas, products, and sometimes diseases.*] The first Huron who introduced it came ashore at the foot of our house, newly built on the bank of a lake—whence being carried to his own village, about a league distant from us, he died straightway after. Without being a great prophet, one could assure one's self that the evil would soon be spread abroad through all these regions: for the Hurons, no matter what plague or contagion they may have, live in the midst of their sick, in the same indifference, and community of all things, as if they were in perfect health. In fact, in a few days, almost all those in the cabin of the deceased found themselves infected; then the evil spread from house to house, from village to village, and finally became scattered throughout the country....

The villages nearer to our new house having been the first ones attacked, and most afflicted, the devil did not fail to seize his opportunity for reawakening all the old imaginations, and causing the former complaints of us, and of our sojourn in these quarters, to be renewed; as if it were the sole cause of all their misfortunes, and especially of the sick. They no longer speak of aught else, they cry aloud that the French must be massacred.... They observed, with some sort of reason, that, since our arrival in these lands, those who had been the nearest to us, had happened to be the most ruined by the diseases, and that the whole villages of those who had received us now appeared utterly exterminated; and certainly, they said, the same would be the fate of all the others if the course of this misfortune were not stopped by the massacre of those who were the cause of it....

Wherein truly it must be acknowledged that these poor people are in some sense excusable. For it has happened very often, and has been remarked more than a hundred times, that where we were most welcome, where we baptized most people, there it was in fact where they died the most; and, on the contrary, in the cabins to which we were denied entrance, although they were sometimes sick to extremity, at the end of a few days one saw every person prosperously cured. We shall see in heaven the secret, but ever adorable, judgments of God therein.

"Huron Healing Beliefs"—François du Peron (1639)

Du Peron worked in a village called Ossassoné, a center of Jesuit activity that was struck by a severe smallpox outbreak in 1639. As his account indicates, Huron healing practices often focused on the mental state of the sufferer. The Jesuits viewed Indigenous healing practices, and especially shamans (or "sorcerors") who commanded respect in their community, as potential competition with the new Catholic teachings.

To cure a sick person, they summon the sorcerer, who, without acquainting himself with the disease of the patient, sings, and shakes his tortoise shell; he gazes into the water and sometimes into the fire, to discover the nature of the disease. Having learned it, he says that the soul of the patient desires, for his recovery, to be given a present of such or such a thing—of a canoe, for example, of a new robe, a porcelain collar, a fire-feast, a dance, etc., and the whole village straightway sets to work to carry out to the letter all the sorcerer may have ordered.

At other times, to cure the sick, the old men of the village go to see the sick man, and ask him what his soul desires. He answers according to his dream, which will sometimes be extravagant and abominable. He will ask as many as twenty-five important presents, which are immediately furnished him by the village; if they failed in a single one, they would consider this the cause of the patient's death. Hence, since we cry out against these deviltries and refuse to contribute anything of ours to them, the devil, because he would like either to exact from us some homage, or to direct upon us all their envy, is sure to make the patient dream for something that we alone possess, or to make the sorcerer specify it.

As I was writing this, on the 13th of April, about noon, a savage, greatly excited, came from a neighboring village, and begged us to give him a piece of red stuff [*perhaps a piece of dyed cloth*], because the sorcerer had said that one of his sons, who was sick, desired for his recovery this bit of stuff. It was not given to him; but one of our Fathers immediately repaired [*i.e., went*] to the place "quasi aliud agenda" [*Latin for 'on the pretext of another errand'*] and baptized the little patient. These continual refusals cause them often to threaten to split our heads, attributing to us the cause of their diseases, saying that, since they believe, they have sickness among them. Each family has certain maladies, and consequently certain abominable remedies.

> **"Jesuit Attempts at Baptism"—Pierre Chastelain (1639)**
>
> *The following anecdotes recount the experience of Pierre Chastelain, a missionary at work in villages the Jesuits called St Joseph, St Michel, and St Ignace. The accounts apparently are based on real events but they are constructed to emphasize Jesuit success and the miraculous ability of the Christian Holy Spirit. They illustrate the Jesuits' persistent attempts to baptize the sick. The missionaries believed baptism would enable eternal salvation, but some Hurons questioned the intrusion upon the dying. As with other passages in the* Jesuit Relations, *boundaries are drawn between individuals who apparently believe and support the Jesuits and those who do not.*

Another time, wishing to enter a cabin to visit a very sick woman, they tell me at first that it was all over with her, and that she had expired two hours before. As they do not willingly see us where there are any dead, I enter a neighboring cabin, but I cannot be at rest there; I feel myself inwardly impelled to return, and enter the house of the woman reported dead. Her husband keeps her as a corpse, with much sadness: nevertheless I perceive her still breathing. I commend myself to God, and—fearing nothing but my sins in such matters, and having asked his pardon—I draw near to instruct her, with confidence in his goodness. They make sport of me, saying that she had long ago lost hearing and speech; I insist, saying that I had already found several others who, having lost their faculties for ordinary things, had by an incomparable mercy of God understood the matter of their salvation, and spoken sufficiently for that. At the same time, I draw near and instruct her with a confidence extraordinary for a heart faithless to its God, like mine. I ask her consent; whereupon, motionless as she was, she begins to move her head, arms, and all her body, and speaks enough to show me her desire; her husband insists that what she signifies is an aversion for what I say to her—he does not wish me to baptize her. I maintain what I had asserted: he questions her himself, urges her to say 'teouastato,' 'I am not willing;' whereto she says not a word. I ask her again, at the same time, whether it be not true that she desires to be baptized: she distinctly answers 'Yes.' The husband, surprised, says to her: 'What, then? Do you wish to leave your relatives, your fathers, mothers, and children who are dead, in order to go with strangers?' God knows whether I redoubled my prayers: she answers with an effort and a fervor that I would not have dared to hope for—'Yes.' I baptize her; she dies immediately after....

There, also, I secretly baptized two little innocents, who straightway took flight for heaven. I know not whether these losses did not irritate the demons: be this as it may, a young man of this cabin stands up, and begins to blaspheme in my presence. I rebuke him, and say to him that he was taking the way to Hell; 'I am quite resolved on that,' he answered me; 'You will see what it is like,' I say to him, and then I leave. Evening sets in, the night comes on; the devil appears to him, and tells him that he wants a head, that otherwise he may work mischief for him. The devil possesses this man; he becomes furious, he runs through the village, hatchet in hand, looking for a Frenchman. Some captains came to beg us not to go out; the chief of the cabin came to tell me in private that this madman was expressly seeking me, as having cursed him and having caused him this misfortune. They tie him, they put a double piece of leather over his eyes; he looks through it like a demon, this man told me; in short, to hear him speak, they had never seen anything like it. Finally they bethink themselves to offer him the head of an enemy, lately seized, and thus he was immediately cured—the devil, by his duplicity, having turned his thought upon the head of a Frenchman.

INTERPRETING THE DOCUMENTS

1. The Jesuits' narratives sometimes refer to disagreements among the Hurons concerning how the Jesuits should be received. What factors influenced the Hurons' perception of the Jesuits? How do you assess the Jesuits' own interpretation of the motivations that are at work?
2. The Hurons' approach to healing emphasized spiritual or psychological therapy as much as physical treatment. Review the Science Focus in chapter 2. How would you compare the description of Huron healing methods to the European Galenic medicine that the Jesuits practiced?
3. Consider Chastelain's account of the dying woman that he baptizes. What is the conflict he describes and how do you assess his narrative of what took place? How does this passage contribute to our understanding of the Jesuit mission and Huron responses to it?

MAKING CONNECTIONS

1. How would you compare the experience of the Hurons with the inhabitants of Mexico a century earlier?

2. The level of mortality from smallpox in the Americas was comparable to the Black Death in Europe. Do you think that perceptions of these catastrophes were also similar?

3. As with the "great pox" (syphilis), European accounts of disease reflected their attempts to explain the susceptibility of Indigenous peoples to an apparently contagious disease. What do European explanations of these two diseases have in common? How are they different?

For further reading: Bruce G. Trigger, *Children of Aataentsic: A History of the Huron People to 1660* (Montreal: McGill-Queen's University Press, 1988), 572–602.

Notes

1. This passage of the anonymous chronicle, now attributed to William Bradford and Edward Winslow, was initially credited to George Mourt and published under his name beginning in 1622. The quote is from a later edition, *Mourt's Relation, Or Journal of the Plantation at Plymouth* (Boston, 1745), 84–85.

2. Perry Miller, *Errand in the Wilderness* (Cambridge, MA: Belknap Press, 1956), vii.

3. Alfred Crosby, "Virgin Soil Epidemics as a Factor in the Aboriginal Depopulation in America," *William and Mary Quarterly* 33, no. 2 (1976): 289–99.

4. David S. Jones, "The Dynamics of Mortality," in *The Oxford Handbook of Native American History*, ed. Frederick E. Hoxie (Oxford: Oxford University Press, 2016), 420; Noble David Cook, *Born to Die: Disease and the New World Conquest, 1492–1650* (Cambridge: Cambridge University Press, 1998).

5. Simon Ho, "The Molecular Clock and Estimating Species Divergence," *Nature Education* 1, no. 1 (2008): 168.

6. Ana T. Duggan et al., "17th Century Variola Virus Reveals the Recent History of Smallpox," *Current Biology* 26, no. 24 (2016): 3407–12.

7. Francis L. Black, "Why Did They Die?" *Science* 258 (1992): 1739.

8. James Riley, "Smallpox and American Indians Revisited," *Journal of the History of Medicine and Allied Sciences* 65, no. 4 (2010): 466–68 and 475–77.

9. Ann Bowman Jannetta, *Epidemics and Mortality in Early Modern Japan* (Princeton: Princeton University Press, 1987), 65–70.

10. Akihito Suzuki, "Smallpox and the Epidemiological Heritage of Modern Japan: Towards a Total History," *Medical History* 55, no. 3 (2011): 313–18.

11. Anne G. Carmichael and Arthur M. Silverstein, "Smallpox in Europe before the Seventeenth Century: Virulent Killer or Benign Disease?" *Journal of the History of Medicine and Allied Sciences* 42, no. 2 (1987): 147–68.

12. Quoted in David S. Jones, "Death, Uncertainty and Rhetoric," in *Beyond Germs. Native Depopulation in North America*, ed. Catherine M. Cameron, Paul Kelton, and Alan C. Swedlund (Tucson: University of Arizona Press, 2015), 22.

13. Clark Spencer-Larsen, "Colonialism and Decline in the American Southeast: The Remarkable Record of La Florida," in *Beyond Germs*, 87–90.

14. Bernardino de Sahagún, *The Florentine Codex: General History of the Things of New Spain*, trans. Arthur J. O. Anderson and Charles E. Dibble (Santa Fe: School of American Research, 1982), Book 12, p. 83.

15. Robert McCaa, "Spanish and Nahuatl Views on Smallpox and Demographic Catastrophe in Mexico," *Journal of Interdisciplinary History* 25, no. 3 (1995): 428–31.

16. Riley, "American Indians Revisited," 474–75.

17. Kartini Gadroen et al., "Impact and Longevity of Measles-Associated Immune Suppression: A Matched Cohort Study Using Data from the THIN General Practice Database in the UK," *BMJ Open* (2018), https://doi.org/10.1136/bmjopen-2017-021465.

18. Åshild J. Vågene et al., "*Salmonella enterica* Genomes from Victims of a Major Sixteenth-Century Epidemic in Mexico," *Nature Ecology & Evolution* 2, no. 3 (2018): 520–28.

19. Daniel T. Reff, "The Introduction of Smallpox in the Greater Southwest," *American Anthropologist* 89, no. 3 (1987): 704.

20. Paul Kelton, *Cherokee Medicine, Colonial Germs* (Norman: University of Oklahoma Press, 2015), 47.

21. Quoted in David S. Jones, *Rationalizing Epidemics: Meanings and Uses of American Mortality since 1600* (Cambridge, MA: Harvard University Press, 2004), 37.

22. Jerome Lalemant, "Relation of 1640," in *The Jesuit Relations and Allied Documents*, vol. 19, ed. Reuben Gold Thwaites (Cleveland: Burrows Bros, 1898), 96.

23. Jones, *Rationalizing Epidemics*, 32–36.

24. Elizabeth A. Fenn, *Pox Americana: The Great Smallpox Epidemic of 1775–82* (New York: Hill and Wang, 2001), 90–91.

25. F.J. Hackett, "Averting Disaster: The Hudson's Bay Company and Smallpox in Western Canada during the Late Eighteenth and Early Nineteenth Centuries," *Bulletin of the History of Medicine* 78, no. 3 (2004): 576–89.

26. Philip Ranlet, "The British, Slaves, and Smallpox in Revolutionary Virginia," *Journal of Negro History* 84, no. 3 (1999): 221–24.

27. Cole Harris, "Voices of Disaster: Smallpox around the Strait of Georgia in 1782," *Ethnohistory* 41, no. 4 (1994): 601–607; Fenn, *Pox Americana*, 250–58.

28. Liza Piper and John Sandlos, "A Broken Frontier: Ecological Imperialism in the Canadian North," *Environmental History* 12, no. 4 (2007): 764–65.

29. Elizabeth A. Fenn, "The Great Smallpox Epidemic of 1775–82," *History Today* 53, no. 8 (2003): 17.

30. A.W. Crosby, "Hawaiian Depopulation as a Model for the Amerindian Experience," in *Epidemics and Ideas: Essays on the Historical Perception of Pestilence*, ed. Terence Ranger and Paul Slack (Cambridge: Cambridge University Press, 1992), 175–202.

31. Arthur Boylston, "The Origins of Inoculation," *Journal of the Royal Society of Medicine* 105, no. 7 (2012): 309–13.

32. Zabdiel Boylston, *An Historical Account of the Smallpox Inoculated in New England upon All Sorts of Persons, Whites, Blacks, and of All Ages and Constitutions* (London, 1726), 39–40.

33. Derrick Baxby, "The Genesis of Edward Jenner's *Inquiry* of 1798: A Comparison of the Two Unpublished Manuscripts and the Published Version," *Medical History* 29 (1985): 194.

34. Derrick Baxby, "Edward Jenner, William Woodville, and the Origins of the Vaccinia Virus," *Journal of the History of Medicine and Allied Sciences* 34, no. 2 (1979): 141–51.

35. Ann Jannetta Bowman, *The Vaccinators: Smallpox, Medicine and the "Opening" of Japan* (Stanford: Stanford University Press, 2007), 41–52.

36. Ann Jannetta, "Jennerian Vaccination and the Creation of a National Public Health Agenda in Japan, 1850–1900," *Bulletin of the History of Medicine* 83, no. 1 (2009): 129–34.

37. Peter Baldwin, *Contagion and the State in Europe, 1830–1930* (Cambridge: Cambridge University Press, 1999), 254–66.

38. Thomas Colley, "Vaccination: A Moral Evil; a Physical Curse; and a Psychological Wrong," *The Medium and Daybreak* 13, no. 651 (1882): 602.

39. Gareth Williams, *Angel of Death: The Story of Smallpox* (New York: Palgrave Macmillan, 2010), 265.

40. Terry S. Coleman, "Early Development in the Regulation of Biologics," *Food & Drug Law Journal* 71 (2016): 548–51.

41. Williams, *Angel of Death*, 262.

42. David Arnold, *Colonizing the Body: State Medicine and Epidemic Disease in Nineteenth-Century India* (Berkeley: University of California Press, 1993), 157.

43. Christian W. McMillen and Niels Brimnes, "Medical Modernization and Medical Nationalism: Resistance to Mass Tuberculosis Vaccination in Postcolonial India, 1948–55," *Comparative Studies in Society and History* 52, no. 1 (2010): 193.

44. Randall M. Packard, *A History of Global Health: Interventions in the Lives of Other Peoples* (Baltimore: Johns Hopkins University Press, 2016), 133–80.

45. WHO, *Bugs, Drugs and Smoke: Stories from Public Health* (San Francisco: Center for Tobacco Control Research and Education, 2012), 10–12.

46. Michaeleen Doucleff, "Last Person to Get Smallpox Dedicated His Life to Ending Polio," National Public Radio, 31 July 2013, https://www.npr.org/sections/health-shots/2013/07/31/206947581/last-person-to-get-smallpox-dedicated-his-life-to-ending-polio.

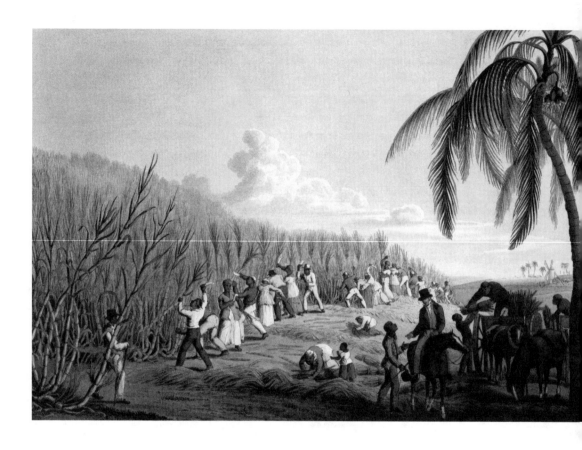

IMAGE 4.1 *Cutting the Sugar Cane*. This lithograph by William Clark (1823) appeared in a series that depicted plantation life on the Caribbean island of Antigua. Clark's rather idealized depiction suggests that slavery in the region differed little from farmwork in Europe. In reality, alongside the hardships of forced labor, plantations created a distinct ecosystem where mosquito-borne pathogens exacted a heavy toll for more than three centuries. Differences in immunity to disease among the region's inhabitants shaped the revolutionary history of Hispaniola and the mainland of the Americas.

YELLOW FEVER, RACE, AND THE ERA OF REVOLUTION

4

I n April 1802, heavy rains drenched the large Caribbean island of Hispaniola, including the French colony of Saint-Domingue that occupied its western third. In coastal towns and plains, a French-led expeditionary force of roughly 65,000 men sought to subdue a rebellion of ex-slaves led by the freedman Toussaint L'Ouverture (1743–1803). The rebels camped in the forested mountains and raided their larger, better-armed adversary. And they awaited the arrival of their most powerful ally: yellow fever. As the rains went on through the spring and summer, troops died from a disease that discolored their skin and caused profuse vomiting. The outbreak gained momentum, and the French lost over 100 men per day. By mid-September, the French command reported 28,000 dead, the vast majority from disease. The rebels soon counterattacked, and in the following summer thousands of European reinforcements met the same fate as their predecessors. A disappointed Napoleon relinquished his dream of an American empire and ceded a large mainland territory claimed by France—Louisiana—to the United States. Within months, in January 1804, the new nation of Haiti proclaimed its independence. Victory belonged to former slaves and to what the prologue of Haiti's independence act called "our avenging climate."

The Haitian Revolution was sparked by the intellectual ferment of the French Revolution. It was sustained by epidemics of yellow fever that ravaged European troops. After 1791, amid shifting conflicts and alliances in the Caribbean, first British and then French forces failed to quell the uprising. Contaminated ships also brought the disease north to Philadelphia, the capital of the new United

States of America. Epidemics stoked tensions among political factions in the nascent republic. While the influence of yellow fever was exceptional in this decade, similar dynamics played out elsewhere in the early nineteenth century as colonial peoples in the Americas wrested autonomy from European regimes.

The events of this revolutionary era are part of a remarkable history that intertwines politics, race, disease, and the consequences (both intended and unintended) of human impact upon landscapes. In the Caribbean, Latin America, and the eastern United States, two mosquito-borne diseases—malaria and yellow fever—played especially prominent roles and often caused destruction together. Before 1900, it was yellow fever that was more feared among soldiers and mariners for its gruesome symptoms and high mortality. As steamship traffic increased, no Atlantic port city was safe. Yellow fever outbreaks were recorded from Quebec City in the north to Rio de Janeiro in the south. In the early twentieth century, as the United States expanded its Caribbean influence, encounters with yellow fever and other diseases fueled a racial ideology that legitimized imperialist actions to provide sanitation and security from disease.

For several decades, mosquito control measures and the development of vaccines dramatically reduced the risk of yellow fever infection in many nations. However, tens of thousands of people still die annually from yellow fever in Africa and central and South America. Its resurgence in the twenty-first century is indicative of a disparity among nations in public health capacity and the mixed legacy of recent efforts to reduce infection.

Etiology and Early History

"There is always something new coming out of Africa," wrote the ancient Greek authority Aristotle.[1] The renowned philosopher himself viewed novelty with suspicion. He described Africa as the home of wild hybrid animals that were outside the normal order of things. Twenty-three centuries later, the phrase "out of Africa" similarly attaches to notions of the continent as a primeval spawning ground of exotic, threatening diseases such as yellow fever, malaria, AIDS, and Ebola. But ancient stereotypes can be misleading. Although researchers have traced yellow fever's origins to Africa, the disease's beginnings do not explain very much about its impact on the modern world. Far more important is the way that yellow fever left Africa and the features of the Caribbean and American societies in which it has caused the greatest devastation.

Yellow fever virus (YFV) has lent its name to the genus *Flavivirus*—"flavus" is Latin for yellow—in which it is now classified with about seventy other viruses. Along with **dengue** virus, West Nile virus, and tick-borne encephalitis virus, YFV is an **arthropod**-borne virus, or **arbovirus**, that inhabits a variety of *Aedes*, *Haemagogus*, and *Sabethes* species of mosquitoes. While mosquito-borne diseases have infected animals for millions of years, the ingredients for large-scale yellow fever outbreaks apparently did not converge until relatively recently. A major outbreak requires a large and densely populated settlement, in part because the virus has an incubation period in mosquitoes of about twelve days before it can be passed on. Yellow fever outbreaks are associated historically with cities, while malaria traditionally was known as a swamp disease.

Yellow fever's most common urban vector, the mosquito species *Aedes aegypti*, has received the unflattering label "most dangerous animal in the world."[2] True or not, the species stands out among the 3,500 known species of mosquitoes as a cause of human suffering. In addition to yellow fever, *A. aegypti* is a major vector of pandemics caused by three other viral diseases: dengue, chikungunya, and Zika virus disease. It is considered a "house-haunting mosquito" that thrives in close proximity to humans in cities or military camps.[3] The species has a flight range of only a few hundred meters. The females are choosy about their food and surroundings—they strongly prefer human blood, and their favored egg-laying perch is just above small pools, exactly the conditions offered by an uncovered rain barrel, a gutter, a broken pot, or an empty tire. A shift in the environmental conditions that affect mosquitoes can also influence the spread of the virus and the severity of epidemics.

To Westerners before the twentieth century, yellow fever's disturbing symptoms reinforced its association with the wild and primitive. During an initial phase, the virus multiplies in the human host and enters the bloodstream. (The presence of viruses in the blood is called **viremia**.) Individuals are asymptomatic and noninfectious for several days but then develop high fever, intense headache, abdominal pain, and vomiting. This is followed by a remission of symptoms that lasts 12–24 hours, and many patients recover at this stage. In 15–25 per cent of cases, severe symptoms ensue during an intoxication phase: the kidneys fail, severe liver damage causes the characteristic yellowed skin (jaundice), and vomit assumes the consistency of coffee grounds as the result of internal bleeding. The final stages of infection are marked by delirium, sometimes accompanied by seizures or muscle spasms that horrified observers. Although vaccines were first developed in the 1930s and are highly effective, there remains no treatment for full-blown yellow fever and the mortality rate in severe cases varies from 20 to 50

Vector
Connections:
Mosquitoes,
Fleas, Lice,
and Disease

The facts of microbe transmission change according to one's point of view. This is especially true when there are several actors involved: a human, a microbe, and an organism that links the two. An understanding of vector-borne diseases benefits from an ability to shift from one vantage point to another.

Mosquitoes mostly seek to feed and breed, but they play two additional roles in the spread of diseases such as yellow fever or malaria. From the microbes' standpoint, mosquitoes are a host in which they live and reproduce unless they are deposited into a human or other mammal when the mosquito feeds. Where mammals are concerned, the mosquitoes are vectors that both transmit and receive harmful pathogens in blood meals. Cycles of transmission vary with the environment and the organisms involved.

Yellow fever provides an example. As shown in figure 4.1, different species participate in distinct cycles. In the sylvatic (forest) cycle, most transmission occurs between monkeys and various *Aedes* mosquito species in the tree canopies. In the urban cycle, *A. aegypti* mosquitoes cause transmission between infected humans, which can result in explosive outbreaks. In the zone of emergence, mosquitoes feed on both humans and monkeys, resulting in small-scale outbreaks.

With every vector species or subspecies, the epidemiologist's puzzle grows: various types of mosquitoes inhabit different parts of the jungle, feed at different times of day, and prefer a different range of hosts. Temperature shifts caused by seasonal change or broader climate trends also affect mosquito behavior and may alter the prevalence of disease.

Other microbes, arthropods, and mammals create transmission cycles of comparable complexity. The action is not all in the air. For example, various burrowing mammals host flea species that carry the plague bacterium, *Yersinia pestis*. Prairie dogs and marmots are susceptible to environmental forces just as mosquitoes are, and environmental disruptions have probably played a role in plague outbreaks through the centuries. Some researchers have even raised the possibility that another type of arthropod, lice, contributed to the spread of plague during the Black Death. Lice also host the bacteria that cause the most severe form of typhus. Humans contract typhus from louse excretions that contain the microbes.

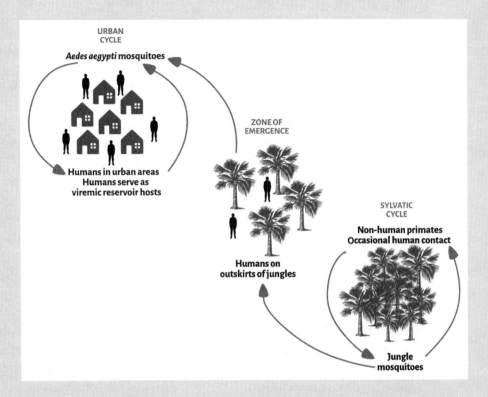

FIGURE 4.1 Yellow fever transmission cycles in Africa.

Vector-borne infections such as malaria have posed a disease-control conundrum: should health measures target the microbes, insect hosts, or humans? For malaria, the answer has varied according to the strategies that are available. Prior to the 1940s, authorities in southern Europe relied on a combination of a parasite-killing drug—**quinine**—and instructions to inhabitants to avoid mosquitoes. As discussed in chapter 9, the introduction of a powerful pesticide, DDT, refocused efforts toward an attack on mosquito vectors. However, both malaria parasites and mosquitoes have developed resistances to the measures used against them.

Will rising global temperatures increase the impact of vector-borne diseases? There is no single answer, since climate change will have variable effects on local weather conditions such as the amount or intensity of rainfall. Because arthropods cannot regulate body temperature physiologically, a persistent change in temperature may alter their population levels or their geographic range of activity in unexpected ways. However, the occurrence of serious disease will also depend on the characteristics of human settlements, especially the level of sanitation and the development of health infrastructure.

per cent. Recent analysis suggests that the yellow fever virus evolves relatively slowly, and manifestations of the disease have apparently not changed dramatically over the centuries.[4] However, different strains of the virus currently circulate, and historical sources reported outbreaks that varied widely in the severity of symptoms. Mariners and medical officers feared outbreaks of the disease they called "black vomit" (*vomito negro*); historians rely on such references to identify probable episodes, but it remains difficult to separate epidemics of yellow fever from the possible effects of other diseases.

Analysis of twentieth- and twenty-first-century viral samples suggests that the strains of yellow fever that circulate today originated no more than roughly 1,500 years ago. The evidence points to an origin in either central or East Africa, where older variants of the virus may have circulated for several thousand years among small populations of humans and other primates. At some point, the virus's *A. aegypti* carrier adapted to human settlements. One attractive scenario to explain this is that North African *A. aegypti* mosquitoes evolved to survive near human-made watering holes as the Sahara Desert expanded during a continental dry spell 4,000–6,000 years ago. However, recent genetic analysis of the *A. aegypti* mosquitoes (as opposed to the virus) suggests that some mosquitoes oriented to human settlements in West Africa 400–550 years ago.[5] Either way, domesticated *Aedes aegypti* mosquitoes had arrived in West Africa by 1500 or soon after, and they accompanied ships bound for the Caribbean and Brazil.

A related question concerns the perception that ethnic groups vary in their susceptibility to the disease. Since YFV originated in Africa, the claim has persisted that many West and central Africans and their descendants are either innately immune to yellow fever or resistant to its most severe effects. As with smallpox, no genes that confer inherited resistance have been identified, and recent researchers have suggested that the idea should be abandoned.[6] However, earlier observers had a basis for the belief—widespread among Europeans, at least—that individuals from tropical environments were less vulnerable to yellow fever. For reasons that are still unclear, children usually experience milder symptoms than adults, and antibodies convey lifelong immunity after even a mild case. Accordingly, individuals who grew up in regions where yellow fever was endemic often enjoyed immunity after childhood, while adult immigrants from elsewhere bore the full brunt of infection. In the Caribbean, the resulting differential immunity between populations had far-reaching biological and political consequences. And it provided a rationale for Western ideologies concerning disease, climate, and race that persisted well into the twentieth century.

Paradise Found: Mosquitoes on the Tropical Plantation

Although yellow fever's first arrival in the western hemisphere cannot be dated with confidence, by 1650 A. *aegypti* mosquitoes had gained a foothold in the Caribbean and in Central America. By this time, Portuguese nobles had been refining both sugar and techniques of human exploitation for two centuries. Sugar cane, a succulent grass that is native to Southeast Asia, had been grown in India and China for centuries and was brought west to North Africa and the Mediterranean. Beginning in the 1450s, the nobles who controlled the island of Madeira, about 600 miles southwest of the Portuguese coast, shifted from logging tropical woods and farming wheat to planting sugar crops with cane root transplanted from Sicily. The whole operation required large amounts of financial capital and labor: workers cut down trees and rooted out stumps, planted roots once the soil was tilled, and carried bundles of mature cane to mills where they were crushed to yield sap. Fields had to be watered with irrigation ditches, and the mills were often powered by waterwheels constructed by skilled carpenters. Additional wood was cut for fuel to heat and filter the sap, which yielded several grades of sugar and liquid for rum. One observer of this emerging economy was the Genoese sailor Christopher Columbus, who lived for several years in Madeira before striking out further across the Atlantic in 1492.[7] Similar agricultural techniques and social arrangements, which scholars have labeled the **plantation complex**, eventually dominated the Caribbean islands, coastal regions of South America, and the southeastern region of North America.

Madeira's slave labor, obtained from raids along the Sahara Coast or the Canary Islands, was expensive and furnished a small proportion of the workforce. It was different on the island of São Tomé, 155 miles off the west coast of Africa, which the Portuguese first settled in the 1480s. Here, where growing conditions favored sugar cane but few immigrants came voluntarily, plantations relied on slaves obtained in West Africa. Portuguese traders established especially close ties with the Kingdom of Kongo, which became an important supplier of slaves for São Tomé and later colonies. Although São Tomé's sugar economy grew gradually, by the end of the sixteenth century its output was around 2,000 tons annually, comparable to that of Madeira. Island plantations and a few coastal outposts were all that Europeans could manage on Africa's west coast. Yellow fever, malaria, and other diseases closed the door on the continent's interior: for centuries, European expeditions on the Congo, Zambezi, and Niger rivers ended in disaster. As Philip Curtin demonstrated in a trailblazing analysis of British military records, into the

nineteenth century roughly half the Europeans who sailed to West Africa succumbed to disease.[8] Recognition of this fact has far-reaching implications for the
history of the Atlantic slave trade. As John Thornton has pointed out, Europeans
did not have the military means to raid West African communities for slaves or
compel African leaders to sell them. Europeans were forced to rely upon cooperation from African elites and their intermediaries. Whereas much scholarship casts
Africans as passive victims of European aggression, Thornton's more complex
picture suggests that Africans shaped the slave trade and the important transfer of
African cultures across the Atlantic.[9]

At the same time, the reputation of the West African coast as "the white man's
grave" reinforced European perceptions that African bodies were suited to withstand yellow fever and other diseases of tropical climes. As Europeans expanded
slave-trading networks across the Atlantic, they carried with them the notion that
darker-skinned peoples were naturally conditioned for plantation labor.

Slavery and Disease in the Caribbean

As importation of slaves continued at São Tomé, its labor model spread to islands
ruled by Spain (Cuba and Hispaniola) and to Portuguese territory on the South
American mainland (Brazil). Cotton, coffee, and tobacco joined sugar as commercial crops. The plantation model was also adopted in the seventeenth century by
English colonists in Virginia, the Carolinas, and the island of Barbados (first
occupied by the English in 1625). Similarities in climate fostered close linkages
among English landholders and merchants throughout the region. After 1663, the
region that became the colonies of North and South Carolina was often overseen
by governors who hailed from Barbados.

The Caribbean economy created new havens for African mosquitoes, which
frequently arrived after hatching from eggs laid in the bilge tanks and moist
crevices of slaving vessels. From a mosquito's vantage point, sugar plantations
had very attractive features: abundant sources of fresh water in canals and
shallow containers, a supply of humans who worked in the open air for female
mosquitoes that took blood meals, supplies of sweet liquid for both male and
female mosquitoes, and a climate that offered warm temperatures year-round
but avoided extremes of heat and cold. Seasonal variations in rainfall did not
pose an intractable problem. *A. aegypti* eggs may survive for several months in a
suspended state, known as diapause, until they are immersed in water and their
larval development continues. Accordingly, mosquito populations exploded

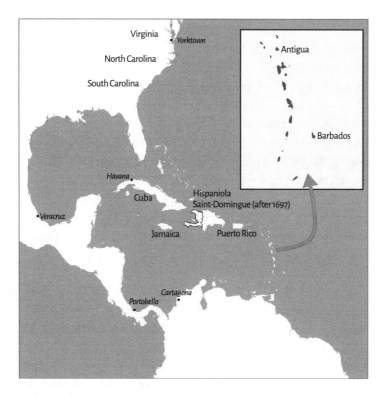

MAP 4.1 The greater Caribbean

when the Caribbean rainy seasons commenced in April or May. Humans could scarcely have devised a more perfect ecology for *A. aegypti* and the large yellow fever outbreaks that ensued when large populations of nonimmune adults arrived.

Between 1550 and 1850, roughly 10 million Africans reached Caribbean and American destinations after harrowing voyages that, in the sixteenth century, sometimes lasted months. Traffic reached its peak in the later eighteenth century, the era of large wooden galleons with creaking masts and billowing sails. Some of the largest ships were modified to warehouse hundreds of slaves in crowded cargo holds. A freed slave named Olaudah Equiano (ca 1745–1797) vividly described this "Middle Passage" in a memoir, published in 1789, that became one of the first widely read narratives of freed and escaped slaves. Equiano related that he was captured with his sister as a young child in the 1750s. After brief service in West Africa, he was taken aboard an English slave ship bound for Barbados. At first,

Equiano was allowed to remain on deck, but as the ship filled the boy was taken below:

> The closeness of the place, and the heat of the climate, added to the number in the ship, which was so crowded that each had scarcely room to turn himself, almost suffocated us. This produced copious perspirations, so that the air soon became unfit for respiration, from a variety of loathsome smells, and brought on a sickness among the slaves, of which many died, thus falling victims to the improvident avarice, as I may call it, of their purchasers. This wretched situation was again aggravated by the galling of the chains, now become insupportable; and the filth of the necessary tubs, into which the children often fell, and were almost suffocated. The shrieks of the women, and the groans of the dying, rendered the whole a scene of horror almost inconceivable.[10]

Slaving ships harbored a host of lethal or debilitating diseases. These included epidemic typhus, a lice-borne bacterial infection; malaria, caused by parasites that were spread by mosquitoes (see chapter 9); and **dysentery**, which is a condition of severe intestinal inflammation and diarrhea that may be caused by various pathogens. Although yellow fever caused mortality as well, many West Africans were immune because they had faced mild bouts of the disease as children in regions where it was endemic. This was one reason why the level of mortality among the crew of slaving ships departing from West Africa often exceeded death rates among the prisoners. In some cases, slaves had also survived previous exposure to malaria, and this conveyed some resistance to the disease. When travelers from Europe arrived in the Caribbean, their bodies were less prepared to withstand various diseases than the slaves who had endured capture and the long Atlantic voyage. The winnowing of the Middle Passage thus contributed to the European belief that Africans were immune to tropical maladies and, therefore, naturally suited to the environment of plantation labor.

Yellow Fever and the Caribbean "Wilderness"

Africans transplanted to the Caribbean offered food for blood-sucking mosquitoes and a few hosts for the yellow fever virus. They did not provide a large population of nonimmunes that could generate a large-scale outbreak of disease. Europeans, on the other hand, considered tropical voyages as dangerous journeys from temperate civility into a wilderness of heat and moisture. Observers described a vaguely defined process called **seasoning** through which European bodies became acclimated and better able to withstand the onslaught of novel ailments. In practice, this probably meant survival of one or more bouts of malaria, perhaps a mild case of yellow fever, or experience with other maladies not limited to warmer climes, such as the waterborne disease **typhoid fever**. "Unseasoned" sailors sometimes refused to join voyages or mutinied after a Caribbean destination was disclosed. Particularly after the arrival of yellow fever, their fear was entirely justified.

The disastrous attempt of Scottish settlers to colonize the isthmus of Panama in 1698–1700 illustrates how yellow fever influenced almost any undertaking involving newcomers from temperate regions.[11] Control of the isthmus and access to both Atlantic and Pacific coasts was (and is) a prize of great strategic value. Since the early sixteenth century, the Spanish had fortified one port named Portobello on the isthmus and another several hundred kilometers northeast named Cartagena. About 1,200 Scottish colonists—religious Protestants, and hence rivals of the Catholic Spaniards—arrived on the isthmus in November 1698 with intentions to found a colony named Caledonia. The initial signs were encouraging. The native inhabitants were neither numerous nor hostile, and the forests were full of edible plants and game. However, as the cooler season ended and diseases began to flare up, supply ships that were anticipated failed to arrive. After hundreds of deaths, probably caused by yellow fever in combination with other maladies, the colonists gave up and set sail in June 1699. A second contingent, unaware that the first group had departed, arrived in November to find an abandoned settlement with no usable supplies. The Scots persevered but, as the toll of disease mounted again, the Spanish sent a detachment of soldiers from Cartagena to lay siege. By April 1700 they had driven the Scots off the isthmus.

A Scottish minister, Francis Borland, blamed the failure to repel the Spanish on "a sore, contagious, raging and wasting sickness, which was now become epidemical." He thought the expedition's leaders had no choice but to surrender. "Otherwise," Borland added bitterly, "they had been foolishly fond of filling this place with their dead bodies, and of coveting graves in this wilderness."[12] Disease followed the retreating Scots onto their ships and killed off eight or nine men each day as the expedition limped to safety in British-held Jamaica. Out of nearly 2,500 participants in the venture only about 500 returned to Scotland.

We may note in passing that Europeans generally drew a very different lesson from such terrible episodes than from their observations of smallpox. To them, a relative immunity to smallpox demonstrated an innate or divinely sanctioned superiority to Indigenous peoples. Deaths from "tropical fevers," on the other hand, signified European susceptibility to a hostile environment. The tropics were out to get them.

The obvious risks did not deter European navies from Caribbean ventures, particularly as the West Indies trade increased in importance. As the galleons and expeditions grew larger, Spanish defenders placed their trust in fortifications and the superior resistance to disease among their seasoned troops and local militias. In March 1741, an enormous British force of 29,000 attacked Cartagena on the mainland and Guantánamo Bay on the island of Cuba. The assaults failed utterly and cost more than 20,000 lives. Two decades later, Britain occupied Cuba and then, after losing about 10,000 troops, returned the island to Spain in a treaty signed in 1763. In both campaigns, disease killed well over ten times the number of troops who fell in combat. A French attempt to colonize Guiana on the mainland in 1764–65 fared just as poorly. Out of perhaps 14,000 participants 11,000 died, a mortality rate approaching 79 per cent.[13]

In the eighteenth century, because of disease, no foreign military force could hold its own in the Caribbean for more than a few months, especially in the spring or summer. Until the 1770s, this ecological reality undergirded the Spanish empire even as its economic and military vitality ebbed. However, European immigrants to the Caribbean and the mainland increasingly were outnumbered by native sons and daughters who felt little loyalty to distant mother countries across the Atlantic. Beginning in 1775, the revolution of English colonists offered a model of resistance. The far larger French Revolution provided a revolutionary ideology and caused a quarter century of turmoil that occupied Europe's colonial powers. Homegrown patriots seized the opportunity to rebel; differential resistance to malaria and immunity to yellow fever gave them a significant advantage against colonial overlords.

Disease in the Era of Revolution, 1775–1825

As we have seen, in the Caribbean and South America yellow fever and malaria often acted in tandem, with yellow fever causing high mortality in explosive outbreaks. While this remained the case through the early nineteenth century, malaria played the more prominent role further north in the revolution of British colonists that began in 1775. The plantation colonies, which included Virginia, North Carolina, and South Carolina, cultivated rice more frequently than sugar or cotton. This pattern of land use, combined with warmer summer temperatures than the Caribbean and abundant swamps with brackish water, provided a congenial habitat for *Anopheles*-species mosquitoes that carry the malarial parasite. A bout with malaria does not convey full immunity, but American colonists—the Southerners, at least—were less susceptible overall than newly arrived British troops. For years, this differential resistance hobbled British efforts as they played a cat-and-mouse game with small forces that avoided pitched battles. Malaria apparently affected the readiness of British forces in the Carolinas and motivated their commander, the Earl Cornwallis, to move the troops north to Virginia. In October 1781 the British surrendered after they were pinned at the port of Yorktown between opposing ground troops and a French naval force.[14] Yellow fever's role in the conflict, although indirect, was also significant. Thousands of British troops died or were incapacitated in the Caribbean during the American Revolution, mostly from yellow fever. By 1781, the supply of recruits available to fight the colonists had run dry.

Between 1788 and 1804, events around the world related to the French Revolution were influenced by dramatic shifts in climate as well as geopolitical factors. Recent studies of climate data indicate that the years 1788–96 were one of the most pronounced **El Niño** events of the last millennium, meaning that typical temperature and rainfall patterns were severely disrupted worldwide. In Europe, the result was prolonged drought and exceedingly poor crop yields. Richard Grove has suggested that food shortages contributed to the popular unrest that preceded the storming of the Paris Bastille in July 1789. In the Caribbean for some years thereafter, extremes of rain and drought fostered *A. aegypti* breeding and multiplication of yellow fever virus.[15]

This had important consequences for the political twists and turns that followed a great slave uprising in the French colony of Saint-Domingue. After 1697, when France acquired the western third of Hispaniola from a treaty with Spain, the colony became one of the world's largest producers of sugar and coffee. It was home for roughly half a million slaves, 40,000 whites, and 30,000 people of mixed ancestry (*gens de couleur*), many of whom owned slaves themselves. In 1789, France's revolution raised fundamental questions concerning the legitimacy of slavery and the extent of political equality that would ensue for the various factions in Saint-Domingue. As France's policy toward its prize colony vacillated, an unsuccessful rebellion by some *gens de couleur* in 1790 was followed by the revolt of tens of thousands of slaves that began on 22 August 1791. After months of violence and shifting alliances, the political landscape changed again in February 1793 when France declared war on Britain. A key part of Britain's military strategy was to deprive France of its profits from Saint-Domingue. Much as it had done against Spain in the previous century, between the fall of 1793 and the summer of 1796 Britain dispatched about 30,000 soldiers to capture the island and otherwise interfere with French interests.

Soon the rebels found their champion: a literate former slave, Toussaint L'Ouverture, who used extraordinary tactical skill to manipulate foreign adversaries and defeat rivals in his ranks. L'Ouverture proclaimed loyalty to revolutionary France. In practice, he fought against Saint-Domingue's former plantation owners and the European armies that supported them. As he noted in correspondence, L'Ouverture placed his trust in the rainy season, which he believed would do more to destroy his foreign enemies than any weapon. Events proved him right. The rebels conducted guerrilla warfare and forced British troops to stay near port cities where they died in droves. When the British withdrew in the summer of 1798, about 15,000 troops had lost their lives on Saint-Domingue, the vast majority from disease.

Yellow fever also struck the United States capital, Philadelphia, beginning with an outbreak in the summer of 1793 that killed an estimated 5,000 people. Eighteenth-century Philadelphia had grown rapidly to a population of roughly 50,000. It was one of the few North American cities large enough to support outbreaks of diseases such as measles, smallpox, and yellow fever. Since Philadelphia was also a center of sugar refining, it had close Caribbean ties and received about 2,000 refugees who fled the violence of the Saint-Domingue rebellion. As the death toll from disease mounted, a heated debate about the epidemic's causes was fueled by broader disagreement concerning policy toward France, the former colonies' ally against Britain.[16] Politicians who were suspicious of France and foreign influence in general (the Federalists) blamed contaminated ships for the epidemic and supported strong quarantine measures. Advocates of close ties with France and trade with Saint-Domingue (the Republicans) opposed quarantine and attributed disease to the city's corrupt physical and moral environment. The apparent immunity to yellow fever among people of African descent also took on political significance after Philadelphia's leaders asked them to assist with burials and treating the sick. Supported by white antislavery advocates, some Africans used Philadelphia's crisis to assert a higher standing in US colonial society.

On Hispaniola, yellow fever continued to benefit the rebels of Saint-Domingue. In 1802, France duplicated Britain's failure when Napoleon sent 65,000 soldiers and sailors to the island. Napoleon had hoped to use Saint-Domingue to promote his ambitions for the vast Louisiana territory that lay to the west of the United States. However, the French were powerless against Saint-Domingue's diseases. Although L'Ouverture was captured in June 1802, the French withdrew seventeen months later after tens of thousands of troops died, mostly from yellow fever. This setback, combined with changing political realities in Europe, persuaded Napoleon to abandon his American plans. In short order, title to the Louisiana territory was sold to the United States, speeding the young nation's expansion across the continent. Saint-Domingue proclaimed its independence as Haiti in January 1804.[17]

To a degree that is exceptional in the history of disease, yellow fever served as a *virus ex machina* that enabled the Haitian Revolution. A decade later, it was one of many challenges that loosened Spain's grip on the territory of New Granada, which included much of modern-day Venezuela, Ecuador, Colombia, and Panama. Independence movements in this region began when Napoleon's forces disrupted Spain's ruling regime and occupied the Iberian Peninsula between 1808 and 1814. After Spain's monarchy was restored, King Ferdinand VII sent about 12,000 soldiers to reassert colonial rule across the Atlantic. As in Saint-Domingue, resistance coalesced around a charismatic leader, a young aristocrat named Simón Bolívar (1783–1830). And as in Saint-Domingue, yellow fever and other diseases whittled away a European force sent to subdue the rebels. The Spanish commander, Pablo Murillo, fretted about the impact of "black vomit," and complained in 1817 that "the mere bite of a mosquito often deprives a man of his life."[18] Murillo had no specific knowledge of how mosquitoes spread yellow fever and malaria, but he viewed insects as a cause of suffering that worsened his chances of success. As Spanish prospects dwindled, the king attempted to send another force in January 1820. Some of Murillo's veterans who had returned to Spain warned the recruits about the dangers that lay in wait. The army mutinied and never left port.

For almost three centuries, a Spanish empire had straddled the Atlantic. By 1826, its claim to vast territories had nearly evaporated: only Cuba and Puerto Rico remained under its control in the Atlantic and the Philippine Islands in the South Pacific. Henceforth, in the Americas at least, powerful nations would pursue their interests through trade policy as well as colonial occupation. The increasing scale and speed of commerce added urgency to the measures that countered yellow fever.

Trade, Imperialism, and Yellow Fever

In the mid-eighteenth century, yellow fever replaced plague as the disease that most endangered Atlantic maritime trade. Particularly after the outbreaks of the 1790s, authorities debated whether or not yellow fever was contagious and how (or whether) to quarantine incoming ships. An answer to the first question was elusive, since the prevailing theories of disease transmission did not consider a role for tiny insects or invisible microbes. For experts of the time to consider a disease contagious, it had to be shown that some kind of physical or chemical influence passed from a sick person to a susceptible one through direct contact, fomites, or the air. Many observers associated the arrival of ships from the Caribbean with outbreaks of disease, but no one could demonstrate a causal connection. Outbreaks seemed to begin as soon as ships reached port, not when they were unloaded; people who fled from epidemics did not seem to cause outbreaks elsewhere; and most people who attended the sick did not fall ill themselves. Moreover, yellow fever outbreaks always occurred in warm weather, which suggested a seasonal or atmospheric cause rather than contagion. Accordingly, yellow fever was often considered alongside other vaguely defined "fevers" that were thought to have local environmental causes (such as filth) and to vary with climate conditions.

As Philadelphians had learned, uncertainty concerning the spread of yellow fever opened room for debate over the second question, the usefulness of quarantine. Even to many people who were concerned about the spread of disease, the isolation of passengers and goods for thirty or forty days was a costly burden that seemed of little use. Beginning with England and the Dutch Republic in 1825, many European nations and individual ports relaxed their quarantine measures for several decades. Historians have considered various factors that tipped the scale as governments reconsidered these policies. In a classic essay, Erwin Ackerknecht suggested that many nineteenth-century physicians held liberal political views that influenced their approach to contagion and quarantine. Liberals wished to promote individual liberty and curb state interference; a support of contagion theory, which would justify quarantine measures and government controls, was incompatible with these goals.[19]

While political commitments may have influenced perceptions of quarantine and other disease control measures, other factors were important, too. As Peter Baldwin has pointed out, economic considerations and the simple realities of geography influenced quarantine policies as much as political ideology did. British merchants, who lived far from the tropics, had less incentive to guard against yellow fever than those in ports further south. Those British merchants also had large financial interests in colonial India, which dampened their interest in protective measures against cholera as well as yellow fever. Conversely, in cities such as Marseille, merchants remembered the horrific plague outbreaks of the past, and they often supported quarantine measures to secure their community's reputation as a safe place of business. In sum, everyone could agree that disease prevention was an important issue, but the lines of debate shifted according to local circumstances as well as national trade strategies.[20]

The room for discussion was ample because there were many ways to account for yellow fever's transmission. For example, in 1821 the French military physician Mathieu Audouard (1776–1856) suggested that slave ships carried the disease. In these filthy vessels, the wood tar became contaminated and dung was trapped between planks in the hulls. Audouard claimed that heat from summer months would then release "deadly emanations" that would spread even if port cities were not contaminated beforehand.[21] Other investigators found evidence that local causes, such as miasmas caused by sewers, provided an adequate explanation. The most influential European authority, another French doctor named Nicolas Chervin (1783–1843), toured the American coastline from Guiana to Maine and found that the vast majority of his colleagues had anti-contagionist views. Overall, the debate over yellow fever lent support to so-called **sanitarian** measures designed to rid streets of filth or reduce the stench of garbage, animal droppings, and noxious trades such as tanning or butchering.

But European and American perceptions of yellow fever and quarantine shifted in the 1850s and 1860s. As chapter 5 will discuss, from the 1830s forward successive pandemic waves of cholera alongside yellow fever motivated careful attention to quarantine. However, the most important catalyst was improvement in shipping technology. In the nineteenth century, the great wooden galleons were replaced by iron-hulled steamships. After 1850, the scale of maritime traffic increased dramatically, and many vessels were equipped with screw propellers that cut the trans-Atlantic sailing time by more than half.[22] Yellow fever could now travel in a few days from the Caribbean to almost any Atlantic port, often before sufficient time had elapsed for infected passengers to develop symptoms. In 1853, an outbreak in New Orleans killed almost 8,000 people, and several more outbreaks in the 1850s forced officials all along the Mississippi River to reconsider quarantine measures.[23] The growth of railway networks in the United States provided another avenue for yellow fever's rapid movement inland. As the threat to European shores also increased, several minor outbreaks provided opportunities for physicians to meticulously track cases of disease back to their first local source. During outbreaks at St Nazaire on France's northwest coast (1861) and at the Welsh industrial seaport Swansea (1865), French and British officials reached similar conclusions: a precise source of infection could not be found, and person-to-person transmission could not be shown, but yellow fever was a specific imported disease, not a heightened version of a local fever.

The information yielded from these outbreaks encouraged European nations, reluctantly, to reinstitute routine quarantines. The case tracing performed at Swansea and St Nazaire eventually became an important component of epidemiological practice (now more commonly called **contact tracing**).[24] Although the movement of yellow fever from port to port was now beyond question, the means of transmission remained opaque and many American ports continued to resist quarantine measures. Outbreaks of yellow fever in Buenos Aires and Rio de Janeiro ended thousands of lives. In 1878, about 20,000 people died in the United States when a wave of disease traveled upriver and via railway arteries from the Gulf of Mexico. This catastrophe and many smaller episodes encouraged some southern US states to institute boards of health to manage quarantine measures. In April 1878, the United States Congress enacted legislation that created a Division of Quarantine within the United States Marine Hospital Service (MHS), a branch of government that formerly had focused upon the care of sick sailors. Thereafter, the MHS's authority expanded to include supervision of quarantine, inspection of immigrants, disease control measures among the US states, and the weekly reporting of disease outbreaks.

Although many people opposed vigorous quarantines for economic reasons, few US observers could deny the coincidence of shipping traffic from Cuba and yellow fever outbreaks. As the nation grew in economic and military power, public health concerns underscored the usefulness of a Caribbean beachhead. In January 1898, a fiery explosion destroyed an American ship, the USS Maine, in the harbor at Havana, Cuba's capital city, and 266 servicemen died in the catastrophe. Although it was later shown that a coal bunker fire onboard caused the explosion, an initial outcry inflamed hostility in the United States against a Spanish regime on its southern doorstep. On a pretext of self-defense, the United States exploited the weakness of Spanish rule in both the Caribbean and Pacific outposts in the Philippine Islands. The invasion of Cuba marked a turning point in US foreign policy; it was also an important chapter in the development of a new discipline, "tropical medicine," that supported imperial ventures in the Americas and around the world.

The Roots of Tropical Medicine

As discussed more fully in the next chapter, during the late nineteenth century researchers used new methods of microbiology to link specific bacteria to specific diseases. The first scientist to accomplish this was the physician Robert Koch, who, in 1876, clarified the life cycle of the pathogen that causes anthrax.

Scientists soon applied similar techniques to "diseases in the tropics" that had thwarted Europeans for centuries. Tropical medicine coalesced as a discipline that embraced disparate inquiries connected in some way to European endeavors, including naval medicine and ship hygiene.[25] The category of "tropical" diseases did not necessarily reflect the characteristics of the diseases themselves or the geographic range where they appeared. Some maladies, such as malaria or hookworm (a parasitic infection that can cause anemia), were prevalent in parts of Europe and the United States but were deemed "tropical" when they interfered with colonial interests. Other diseases were mostly unknown in temperate climes but caused great suffering in warmer regions—and, in some cases, still do.

One example is lymphatic **filariasis**, a disease that still affects more than 100 million people worldwide in tropical and subtropical regions of Africa, Asia, and the Caribbean. Filariasis is caused by tiny parasitic worms that begin their larval development in the gut of mosquitoes. When the infected mosquitoes feed, the larvae enter the human body and proceed to inhabit lymphatic vessels. Mature worms produce millions of larvae that migrate to lymph and blood vessels near the skin. When they are ingested by more mosquitoes the cycle begins again. In the disease's most severe manifestation, elephantiasis, blockage of lymph vessels creates roughened skin and painful, disfiguring swelling in limbs and the lower body.

In the 1870s, filariasis attracted the interest of Patrick Manson (1844–1922), a Scottish doctor who worked with British customs officials in Chinese ports. From blood samples and numerous dissected mosquitoes, Manson established that the worms caused human disease and that mosquitoes served as their intermediate host. These insights, which Manson first published in 1878, provided a model for understanding malaria, a disease in which parasites divide their life cycle between humans and mosquitoes. Manson eventually moved to London where he advised colonial officials and founded a research institute that was based in the Albert Dock Seamen's Hospital.

After its opening in October 1899, the London School of Hygiene & Tropical Medicine and a similar institute founded the previous year in Liverpool were recognized as leading centers for knowledge about the diseases of tropical regions. Within a few years, researchers from these institutes or from the University of Edinburgh in Scotland identified the cause of sleeping sickness (parasites called **trypanosomes**), established the life cycle of the worm that caused **Guinea worm disease**, and staged a dramatic demonstration in London to prove that mosquitoes transmitted malaria to humans. The London School's first class of twenty-eight students included three women, which was notable since no university in London admitted women at the time. Manson also supported the work of Ronald Ross (1857–1932), a medical officer in India who conducted groundbreaking research on the transmission of malaria from mosquitoes to birds (see chapter 9). In August 1897, Ross claimed that mosquitoes were also the vector for human malaria, a hypothesis that was independently confirmed a few months later by Italian researchers led by Giovanni Battista Grassi (1854–1925).[26]

Tropical diseases had long been feared, but scientists had generally assumed that they resembled infections found in Europe and could be explained by conventional medical theory. Instead, the investigation of filariasis, malaria, and other diseases revealed that the ecology of vectors, hosts, and pathogens involved many organisms and was far more complex than researchers had realized. Tropical diseases now appeared fundamentally different from the maladies of temperate regions, and combat against them seemed to require a new, comprehensive approach to hygiene. Researchers further argued that a mastery of tropical medicine required training at dedicated institutes such as the ones in London or Liverpool that were founded at the end of the 1890s. In consequence, the discipline evolved independently from other branches of medicine, and it was closely aligned with the colonial enterprises that would benefit from its findings. The supporters of tropical medicine often claimed that new cures and hygiene standards would benefit less civilized colonial peoples. For many individuals in India or Africa this was undoubtedly true, but the discipline's first allegiances were to the physical health, business interests, and political objectives of European colonizers.

While chapters 7 and 9 will consider tropical medicine in relation to rinderpest, sleeping sickness, and malaria, aspects of this new discipline naturally influenced the scientific approach to yellow fever in the Caribbean and the Americas. Among scientists in the United States, the most significant initiatives in tropical medicine were linked to military enterprises. Hostilities in Cuba provided the first occasion for US medical officers to make their mark in the field. The so-called Spanish-American War, which lasted four months between April and August 1898, was a late stage in a broader conflict that was far more destructive for Spaniards and Cubans than for Americans. After decades of unrest, Cubans revolted against Spanish rule in 1895. In a scenario that resembled events in Saint-Domingue a century earlier, Spanish expeditionary forces concentrated in port cities and attempted to subdue guerrillas in the countryside. Mortality from smallpox was extremely high among Cubans since Spanish troops forced rural dwellers to relocate to cities where they encountered overcrowding and poor sanitation. The soldiers themselves suffered disproportionately from yellow fever, and heavy losses increased their vulnerability to attack. Although US leaders initially refrained from intervention, in February 1898 the *USS Maine* explosion prompted widespread calls for action. On 25 April 1898, after an enthusiastic response to a call for military volunteers, the United States declared war on Spain.

The conflict forced Spain to relinquish island territories in both the Caribbean and the South Pacific. While Cuba eventually became a sovereign nation, in December 1898 the United States annexed the island of Puerto Rico. (Its inhabitants, now over 3.5 million people, are United States citizens by virtue of their residence in the territory.) In the Pacific, the US attacked Spanish territories in the Philippine Islands and completed the annexation of Hawaii in July 1898. (Hawaii became the fiftieth US state in 1959.) By the end of the Cuba campaign, roughly 5,500 US soldiers had died in from disease—as opposed to about 700 casualties from war wounds—but the total number of Spanish dead since 1895 was ten times greater. An estimated 295,000 soldiers and civilians died during the Cuban insurrection, more than 95 per cent from disease and other noncombat causes.[27] As discussed in chapter 7, revolution and war also ravaged the Philippines, where contagious diseases including malaria broke out in the 1890s, and a cholera epidemic that began in 1902 killed an estimated 200,000 people.

In the Caribbean, yellow fever remained more powerful than any army, and its control was a central concern for the US force that occupied Cuba between 1898 and 1902. As soldiers continued to die, in the summer of 1900 the US Surgeon General dispatched a Yellow Fever Commission led by Major Walter Reed (1851–1902). While Reed was aware of Ronald Ross's research on malaria, he was more influenced by the work of Carlos Finlay (1833–1915), a Spanish researcher in Havana who had proposed that mosquitoes transmitted yellow fever. When Finlay made this claim in 1881, very few scientists contemplated a link between mosquito bites and human disease. Most of his colleagues remained persuaded by germ theories that did not involve insects. Although Finlay conducted numerous experiments, he did not account for the incubation period of the virus in mosquitoes, and his results, therefore, were inconclusive. Researchers also were unaware at the time that nonhuman primates host yellow fever's causal virus, and the only known means of advancing knowledge was human experimentation.

However, Reed's broad experience with the Army Medical Corps prepared him to accept Finlay's theory. Beginning in 1875, Reed served US soldiers and American Indian communities in western territories, and he then completed studies in bacteriology and pathology at the Johns Hopkins University Hospital in Baltimore. In 1898–99, immediately before his posting to Cuba, Reed led a commission that

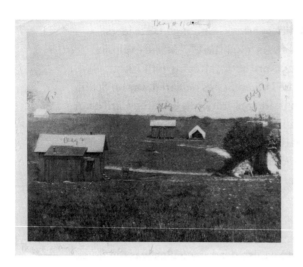

IMAGE 4.2 Camp Lazear yellow fever experiment huts. These huts were erected to test the spread of yellow fever under various conditions. The hut in the left foreground is illustrated in figure 4.2.

investigated an epidemic of typhoid at US military camps preparing for the war with Spain. There were an estimated 24,000 cases and 2,000 deaths from the disease among volunteer recruits in hastily constructed barracks. Bacteriological analysis soon indicated that flies carried typhoid bacteria from latrines to mess tents, a route that one medical officer called "a literal highway of disease."[28] The commission's landmark report explained how individuals contracted typhoid fever and also drew attention to the geographic diffusion of disease among regiments as they moved through a complex system of state and national camps.[29]

In Cuba, as leader of the Yellow Fever Commission, Reed could not isolate a yellow fever pathogen—YFV, unlike the typhoid bacteria, was too small for microscopes of the time—but he oversaw experiments to test its mode of transmission at a compound separated from the main American army camp. Beginning in November 1900, the commission's doctors exposed volunteers to infected mosquitoes and conducted subcutaneous injections of blood taken from yellow fever patients. Both procedures caused yellow fever cases in several volunteers. Reed then devised a further experiment to rule out the spread of yellow fever by fomites (objects that were contaminated by infected effluvia or blood). For this trial, he designed two small wooden huts that exposed volunteers to various conditions. In Building Number One, several groups of volunteers lived for twenty days with clothes and bedding that were soiled with vomit, sweat, and feces from yellow fever patients. In Building Number Two, three more volunteers occupied disinfected chambers separated by a wire mesh screen—one man in one room, two in the other (see figure 4.2). All the living conditions were identical except that the solitary man was exposed to mosquitoes that had fed on yellow fever patients. None of the men who lived with soiled items in Building One contracted yellow fever. In Building Two, one man fell ill after he was exposed to bites from infected mosquitoes for four days.

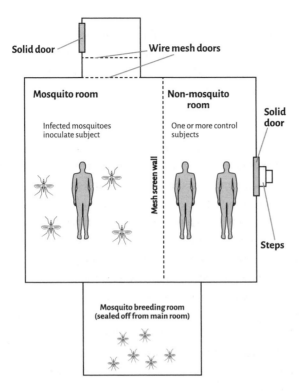

FIGURE 4.2 Building Number Two, "infected mosquito building"

There were other investigations as well, but the Yellow Fever Commission had demonstrated, as far as was possible, that surface exposure to yellow fever effluvia did not spread the disease and that mosquitoes were not only annoying but also dangerous.

In addition to its findings, the Yellow Fever Commission was notable for its thoughtful approach to the consent of research subjects. Human tests were essential but risky. One member of the commission, Jesse Lazear (1866–1900), died after exposing himself to infected mosquitoes, and another member, James Carroll (1854–1907), became seriously ill. As the experiments proceeded, the gentlemanly Reed insisted that volunteers receive information about the risks and benefits of the trial as well as financial compensation if they were not soldiers (a number of volunteers were recent Spanish immigrants). All of the subjects were guaranteed medical care, which the Spanish civilians found especially attractive because they were likely to contract the disease anyway. Eventually, a total of twenty-nine individuals contracted yellow fever, five died, and a sixth suffered lifelong disability. The Yellow Fever Commission's procedure for disclosing the risks of scientific investigation set a meaningful precedent for the human research standards that would be developed decades later.[30] However, as discussed in chapter 2, it did not mark the end of medical research that was conducted on vulnerable individuals, without consent, or under false pretenses.

The Commission's findings provided justification for an all-out assault on mosquitoes in Havana. Oversight of this task fell to medical officer William Gorgas (1845–1920), who imposed quarantines of infected areas and provided window screens to block mosquitoes. He also trained his sights on the mosquitoes' breeding grounds. Inspectors targeted every open source of fresh water. They drained puddles, fitted pipes with mesh, and poured a layer of oil on open water casks to prevent larvae from surfacing. Havana residents were ordered to drain their house gutters and eliminate standing water, and they were fined if mosquito larvae were found on their property. Gorgas's methods were unpopular but they worked. In the spring of 1901, only one case was reported in March and none at in April, May, and June. Yellow fever's causal agent still had not been identified; the virus evaded microscopic scrutiny and it passed through filters designed to strain out bacteria. However, the comprehensive sanitary measures loosened endemic yellow fever's grip on Cuba.

Disease, Race, and US Imperialism in the Caribbean

In the Spanish-American conflict, the United States emerged as a full-fledged imperial power. Mosquito control became a routine component of US military actions in the Caribbean and the Philippines. From an economic standpoint, the most significant venture was the US takeover of a strip of land in the isthmus of Panama and the completion of a trans-isthmian canal. As the Scots and the Spanish had found, occupiers of this strategic region exposed themselves to one of the most disease-ridden environments in the Americas. In the 1880s, a canal construction project overseen by French developer Ferdinand de Lesseps (1805–1894) had failed disastrously. Previously, de Lesseps had overseen the successful completion of the Suez Canal, which connected the Red Sea and the Mediterranean after 1867. In Panama, however, de Lesseps's company encountered mudslides, financial mismanagement, and, above all, yellow fever and malaria that killed well over 20,000 workers. After bankruptcy and a failed attempt to revive the project, in 1904 investors persuaded US officials to purchase the work site and nearby railroad for $40 million. The United States also supported the efforts of Panamanian rebels to secede from Colombia and negotiated a treaty to access the Canal Zone. This area of roughly 500 square miles was then designated as an "unorganized possession" under the direct control of a US government commission.

Between 1904 and the canal's completion in 1914, roughly 60,000 workers excavated over 230 billion cubic yards of dirt and rock. Alongside this remarkable feat, the quasi-colonial status of the Canal Zone enabled the US Army to enact extraordinary environmental measures in the service of disease control. Gorgas was appointed Chief Sanitary Officer, and he applied strategies similar to the Havana campaign, albeit with some refinement. In Panama City and Colon, where yellow fever endangered migrant workers (more so than the region's native inhabitants), Gorgas focused on controlling mosquitoes and larvae and invested less energy in quarantine than he had in Cuba. At the peak of the anti-mosquito campaign in 1906, the anti-mosquito brigades conducted more than 117,000 inspections and oiled larvae in 11,000 houses. Equally big steps were taken in the countryside to remove *Anopheles* mosquitoes that carried malaria. On either side of the canal, hundreds of square miles of wetlands were drained and deforested, and remaining bodies of water were doused with thousands of gallons of chemicals. The canal also required creation of a 154-square-mile artificial lake to enable ships to shift elevation as they moved across the isthmus. The economic impact of the Panama Canal is undeniable—roughly 5 per cent of the world's global trade by volume still traverses the channel—but the project also displaced tens of thousands of people and transformed the ecology of the region with consequences that have unraveled ever since.[31]

The Canal Zone administrators also attempted, ostensibly for public health reasons, to duplicate the race relations that had developed in the United States since the end of the Civil War in 1865. Particularly in the southeastern United States, a patchwork of "Jim Crow" laws and social norms enforced segregation and lower social status for African Americans. In the Canal Zone, social divisions were created by paying skilled workers (almost all white) in gold, while unskilled workers (almost all nonwhite) were paid in silver. West Africans and other "coloreds" were considered immune from yellow fever, but it was thought that their bodies might harbor the disease and endanger "gold roll" workers even if they did not display symptoms. As one administrator told a lecture audience in 1908, "to prevent the infection of the mosquitoes who have access to the men we are protecting, [it is necessary] simply to segregate the quarters of these men from those of the natives and colored laborers—a source of infection to the insects—a sufficient distance."[32] One result of this segregated regime was that African workers received much less care for other maladies such as pneumonia and dysentery.

Indeed, the public health campaigns in Panama illustrate how beliefs concerning race had shifted as colonial officials conducted public health initiatives around the world. Earlier Europeans had focused their frustration on an inhospitable tropical environment and the vulnerability of travelers to unfamiliar climates. Later, in an era marked by the awareness of bacteria, military officers and bureaucrats instead attributed disease to unsanitary habits among colonized peoples who might spread infections that affected them less severely than "whites." In the Philippines, where Americans conducted health campaigns that resembled those in Panama, US Army officers viewed the defeat of tropical diseases as part of the broader effort first to subdue and then to control Filipinos. As Alexandra Minna Stern has noted, public health officers also transplanted practices of racial hygiene to contexts in the United States, such as west coast Chinatowns, the US-Mexico border, and the policies of other state and local agencies.[33] American colonizers were not unique. As we saw in chapters 1 and 2, a similar ethos of segregation also informed white South Africans as they created a rationale for the apartheid regime that was formally instituted in 1948. Likewise, as British colonial officers combated plague and malaria in India, they criticized aspects of local society and culture that seemed incompatible with Western sanitary ideals.

Colonial public health officers such as William Gorgas believed that their efforts would make the tropics safe for whites, enabling civilized peoples to reclaim the regions where humanity had begun. In Panama, they shifted from a traditional emphasis on quarantine to focus upon vector control (mosquito eradication), and, after the 1920s, microbiologists also developed an effective yellow fever vaccine. However, neither vector control nor vaccination would tame the disease completely.

Controlling Yellow Fever: Two Steps Forward, One Step Back

In the early twentieth century, sanitary measures to control yellow fever and other diseases coincided with growing US military and economic ambitions. Since the United States was also the world's leading destination for immigrants, officials increasingly paid attention to the threat of disease from its southern neighbors. In December 1902, representatives from twelve American countries met in Washington to lay the groundwork for an International Sanitary Bureau to coordinate national

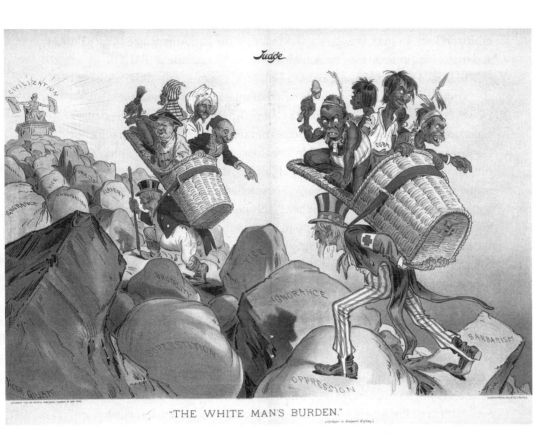

"THE WHITE MAN'S BURDEN."
(Apologies to Rudyard Kipling.)

IMAGE 4.3 "The White Man's Burden (Apologies to Rudyard Kipling)." This magazine cartoon by Victor Gillam was published in the British magazine *Judge* during the Spanish-American War (1899). It depicts imperialist ventures as altruistic, civilizing missions. The cartoon appeared less than two months after Kipling published a poem entitled "The White Man's Burden: The United States and the Philippine Islands." Kipling's verse encouraged US actions. One passage read: "Take up the white man's burden/ The savage wars of peace/ Fill full the mouth of famine/ And bid the sickness cease."

Gillam depicted personifications of Great Britain and the United States (John Bull and Uncle Sam) bearing less-civilized peoples of the world. The path toward a monument of "Civilization" is littered with boulders bearing labels such as "Vice," "Ignorance," and "Cruelty." Uncle Sam's red-cross armband symbolizes the perceived importance of vaccination, sanitation, and hygiene programs that were undertaken on a large scale. The condescending image also creates a racial hierarchy among colonized peoples: Britain's older colonies—including Egypt, India, and "China" (i.e., Hong Kong)—are depicted as more civilized than the crude caricatures of Cuba, Hawaii, the Philippines, and Puerto Rico in Uncle Sam's basket.

health policies. In 1923, the agency was renamed the Pan American Sanitary Bureau and thereafter (in 1958) the Pan American Health Organization (PAHO).

To some US officials, successes in Cuba and Panama raised the prospect that the burden of yellow fever could be eased dramatically or lifted altogether. However, the opening of the Panama Canal also greatly increased the danger of exposure for "unseasoned" populations around the world. In 1916, eradication of the disease was declared as a goal by the Rockefeller Foundation, a philanthropy funded with the enormous resources of John D. Rockefeller (1839–1937), the owner of the Standard Oil Company. Rockefeller's commitment to health-related philanthropy began in 1902 when he established the Rockefeller Institute in New York as a leading center for research in disease and biomedicine. The Rockefeller Foundation, chartered in 1913, funded public health training in the US and other countries, and it also sponsored field research and disease eradication programs worldwide. The Foundation burnished Rockefeller's image—and sheltered millions of dollars from taxes—but it also exerted leadership in the development of global health initiatives based on scientific research. For decades, Rockefeller public health philanthropy supported efforts to expand American influence abroad.

In its campaign against yellow fever, the Foundation dispatched teams to Ecuador (1918) and Nigeria (1925), while French scientists began investigations in Senegal (1927). These programs encountered some challenges. In Ecuador, a bacteria that was mistakenly believed to cause yellow fever became the basis for a vaccine that was injected into thousands of people. Fortunately, there were no catastrophic consequences but research continued to be hampered by efforts made by Rockefeller researcher Hideyo Noguchi to prove that yellow fever was caused by a spirochete.[34] Scientists at work in the field also determined that yellow fever virus circulated among other primates and several mosquito species. While this was an important finding, the discovery that yellow fever thrived in woodland ecologies apart from humans also indicated that complete eradication was impossible.

But laboratory investigation also yielded successes. In 1927, both French and American researchers in Africa isolated viruses that would be used to create live vaccines that conveyed long-lasting immunity. Vaccine development built on research by Max Theiler (1899–1972), who, in 1937, emulated the strategy of attenuation that was pioneered in the 1880s by Louis Pasteur (1822–1895). As discussed in the next chapter, Pasteur created weakened forms of pathogens by heating and drying material from infected animals. Theiler's team, instead, attenuated YFV by infecting successive generations of mice (a technique called "passaging") to produce a less virulent form of the virus. The resulting microbe provoked a human immune response but did not cause dangerous symptoms.

Between the 1930s and the 1970s, as regional and global public health initiatives expanded on many fronts, efforts to counter yellow fever incorporated both vaccination and mosquito eradication. In the mid-1930s, the "French vaccine" was made compulsory in France's African colonies and more than 80 million doses were administered. Administration of this vaccine was discontinued in 1980 amid concerns about neurological side effects, but a second vaccine—named "Asibi" for the man whose blood sample contained the initial virus—dramatically reduced urban yellow fever in regions outside of French influence, including South America. Mosquito control efforts also concentrated on South America. In 1947, the Pan American Sanitary Bureau targeted the A. aegypti mosquito for eradication. A. aegypti populations were dramatically reduced, in part through the use of pesticides but also through public education programs that encouraged homeowners to shelter water storage containers and local officials to eliminate standing water in dumps. By the late 1960s, A. aegypti had been eliminated from South America with the exception of regions in the northernmost countries (Colombia, Venezuela, and Dutch Guiana). Proponents of eradication such as Fred Soper (1893–1977)—the chief mosquito warrior for the Rockefeller Foundation—forecast that eradication would be a watchword for public health administrators of the future.[35]

However, only ten years later, many of the gains of both vaccination and mosquito-control programs had evaporated. France's African colonies became independent nations in the early 1960s and vaccinations lapsed owing to lack of funds, inadequate infrastructure, and political unrest that disrupted health programs. The United States and the Caribbean remained relatively free of yellow fever but A. aegypti reclaimed most of South America as its range. Experts have attributed this reinfestation to growing resistance to pesticides among the mosquitoes and also to the continual presence of A. aegypti mosquitoes in the Caribbean and the southern United States. While Caribbean nations such as Haiti did not have the means to conduct mosquito eradication programs, in the United States the programs received little money or political support. Mosquito control programs were labor-intensive and required a degree of surveillance that private landowners in the United States resisted. The availability of a vaccine, and the fact that only a few Texas and Florida counties hosted A. aegypti year-round, further discouraged aggressive action.[36]

The 1950s and 1960s were an era of unprecedented global collaboration in public health. But the successes of smallpox eradication and a permanent reduction in the incidence of polio would not be repeated with yellow fever.

Conclusion

Yellow fever has never taken hold in Asia. The reasons why are a mystery: roughly 2 billion people live in Asian countries inhabited by *A. aegypti*, and dengue already circulates in many regions. Some experts have suggested that, in the Asian context, dengue has "outcompeted" the yellow fever virus in the drive to inhabit mosquitoes. It may also be that human dengue infection affords some cross-protective immunity against yellow fever. However, the threat of an Asian outbreak has seemed more imminent as travel has increased between China and parts of Africa. In early 2016, China reported some of its first cases of yellow fever among travelers returning from Angola, where a localized outbreak developed into the most widespread African epidemic in decades. Continual importation of the virus into southern China or Thailand may one day initiate a major outbreak among large unvaccinated populations.[37]

Even without a catastrophic event, the global burden of yellow fever remains high: conservative figures published by the WHO estimate there are roughly 84,000–170,000 cases and 29,000–60,000 deaths annually, most of which are in Africa.[38] While long-term data are not available for much of Africa, it is certain that interrupted vaccination programs, steep population growth, and urbanization have transformed yellow fever morbidity and mortality in the last half-century. In 1900, many Africans survived mild cases of yellow fever as children, and the vast majority lived in rural settings where large outbreaks were impossible. In the twenty-first century, the growth of large cities, particularly in West Africa, has substantially increased the risk of epidemics of both yellow fever and dengue. Although South America has had fewer episodes, in Brazil one of the worst outbreaks of yellow fever in a century began in the summer of 2016 and killed more than 670 people in the next two years. Some cases occurred near large metropolitan areas, raising fears that an urban transmission cycle among infected humans and *A. aegypti* mosquitoes would cause a major epidemic.[39] As supplies of vaccine ran short, Brazilian health officials were forced to dilute the doses and solicit donations of vaccine from other parts of the world.

Will global warming contribute to more outbreaks of yellow fever? Increases in temperature and more extreme fluctuations in precipitation encourage the spread of *A. aegypti* to new habitats and explosive growth in mosquito populations during rainy weather. Worldwide, roughly 3.8 billion people live in regions that are also inhabited by *A. aegypti* mosquitoes. If current trends in climate change and population growth continue, in fifty years this number will grow by 2–2.5 billion. As global temperatures rise, regions in the middle latitudes of the United States and Europe will become suitable for seasonal habitation by the mosquito.[40] However, experts caution against predictions that do not account for many variables. Temperature, rainfall, and humidity all have a dynamic influence upon disease transmission and mosquito behavior. What has been observed for malaria also applies to yellow fever: the influence of climate change should not be viewed separately from the impact of ecological and social change, politics, and economics.[41]

While Europeans lamented the terrible effects of yellow fever in the Caribbean over the centuries, it is an irony that their nations created the conditions in which *A. aegypti* now thrives in the Americas. After 1500, the slave trade provided the means for *A. aegypti* mosquitoes to emigrate, and plantations created an ideal habitat for them that had not existed before. Colonial migration patterns created a landscape of differential immunity in which yellow fever eventually played an outsized role in revolutionary uprisings. European immigrants were more vulnerable than native-born Africans and Caribbeans to yellow fever and other tropical diseases. Shifting imperialist theories of environment and race used the difference to justify Western dominance. Well into the twentieth century, perceptions of tropical diseases and subordinate peoples bolstered theories of racial hierarchy and justified segregation measures in the Americas and elsewhere.

The emergent scientific discipline of tropical medicine also supported imperialist activity by the United States. However, the sweeping quarantines and anti-mosquito campaigns that the US Army orchestrated in Havana and the Panama Canal Zone could not be sustained. *A. aegypti* is as rampant now as it was in 1930, and today's mosquitoes spread a more virulent form of dengue fever as well as the Zika virus. Yellow fever's resurgence demonstrates that partial or temporary control measures can sow future challenges if the relationships among insects, climate, and humans shift. As chapter 9 will further explore, the measures taken against yellow fever underscore the dangers and difficulties that accompany campaigns against mosquitoes.

In addition to yellow fever's important role in political developments, in the nineteenth century it also influenced a wide-ranging debate over trade, quarantine, and public health. In this context it shared a stage with cholera, another disease with terrifying symptoms that revealed the dangers of international commerce. More so than yellow fever, however, cholera outbreaks struck at the heart of Europe, forcing a fundamental reassessment of the impact of industry and the causes of disease.

WORKSHOP: DEBATING THE SPREAD OF DISEASE IN REVOLUTIONARY-ERA PHILADELPHIA

The French Revolution has always been recognized as a watershed event that had repercussions beyond Europe. Recent scholars have attempted to place it more firmly in a framework of global history. Certainly, the half-century between 1775 and 1825 was tumultuous throughout the Atlantic world. In addition to Britain's American colonies, wars of independence convulsed the peoples of the Caribbean and Latin America who revolted against France and Spain. Nor were political ideology and revolutionary conflict isolated from biological forces: not only did yellow fever dramatically shape events in the Caribbean, further north in Philadelphia the severe outbreak of 1793 revealed political fault lines in the new American republic.

France had assisted the American rebels in their successful battle for independence, but after the bloody French Revolution that began in 1789, Americans contemplated how closely they wanted to be associated with France and with trading interests from the French Caribbean. Were the French useful allies and commercial partners or a source of dangerous ideology? For physicians and other observers, their perspective concerning French involvement often colored perceptions of the source of yellow fever. Federalists, who feared radical influences from abroad, tended to blame arrivals from Saint-Domingue for importing the disease. Republicans, who wished to support the lucrative Caribbean trade, often attributed disease to unsanitary conditions at the city's docks.

Among people of African descent, the social and intellectual turmoil of the French Revolution and the war of Haitian independence raised the issue of racial equality. French proclamations celebrated the inherent equality of "man" (although not of women and men), and the United States Declaration of Independence, in 1776, had declared it "self-evident" that "all men are created equal." For Philadelphia's men of African descent who knew of the Haitian revolution, it seemed possible that these sentiments could also apply to their social and political status. The question was especially pointed in Philadelphia, where many free black families cohabited with whites. Since Africans were deemed by some to be immune from the disease, they were encouraged to assist whites during the yellow fever outbreak. African individuals carried stretchers and tended the sick. The assessment of their service formed part of a broader discussion about the "sensibility" of African peoples and their capacity to act as equals of whites.

An Account of Rise, Progress, and Termination of the Malignant Fever ... in Philadelphia— Anonymous (1794)

The treatise including this passage was issued along with several other documents by the Philadelphia publisher Benjamin Johnson. The passage begins by implying that commercial prosperity had eroded the city's moral fabric. But it also offers a defense of Philadelphia's clean environment, as opposed to the contaminating impact of foreign (French) arrivals. The author relies upon a concept of contagion to suggest that infected persons brought yellow fever to Philadelphia either from Saint-Domingue or France.

At the period when the malignant fever made its appearance in Philadelphia, the city, by a series of prosperity in commerce, had grown to a state of opulence [*excessive wealth*] not recorded in the historic page. Her inhabitants indulged themselves in all the gratifications of luxury and dissipation to be procured in this Western hemisphere. Her streets were crowded by the gay carriages of pleasure going and returning in every direction; new and elegant buildings were seen rising in every quarter; and her port was thronged with shipping from every trading country in Europe and both the Indies.... This uncommon flow of prosperity had its too common effect. The citizens too generally had forgotten the fountain from whom all their blessings flowed; and impiously said or seemed to say: "by thy wisdom and by thy traffic, hast thou increased thy riches."

By the unfortunate divisions in St Domingo, one of the French Islands, many of its inhabitants, to avoid the fire and sword of their stronger antagonists, had fled from their homes; and, about the time the contagion took place in Philadelphia, a large number of them found refuge among us. Before they had left their own burned and bloodied shores their hearts had been appalled by scenes of the most atrocious cruelty, and by the sight of numerous bodies of the slain which had remained unburied for many days, so that the air must have become too polluted for healthful respiration, had they been permitted to stay. Many of these unfortunate refugees came in vessels exceedingly crowded, as well as poorly provided with the means necessary to preserve health. Had they even left their homes in a state of soundness, some of course arrived sickly.

About this time, likewise, the licensed plunderers of the Ocean, belonging to the same nation, brought in their prizes for ... sale. One of these freebooters, belonging to Marseille in France (the hotbed of pestilential disease), after a lengthy circuitous cruise, came into our port and brought with her the "Flora," a prize ship, both in a sickly condition. [*The allusion to Marseille as a pestilential "hotbed" recalls the outbreak of plague in the city more than seventy years earlier.*] HERE the inhabitants have generally agreed to fix the origin of the late dreadful visitation [*of disease*]. And in this opinion they have been confirmed by two physicians [*William Currie and Isaac Cathrall*] who visited the sick in the earliest and every succeeding stage of the disease.

[*The following passage is attributed to Currie and Cathrall.*] "From all the evidence we have been able to collect," say they, "the disorder made its first appearance in Water

Street, at Richard Denny's lodging house, who kept an ordinary frequented by a number of Frenchmen who had lately arrived in some of the suspected vessels.... [*The text then lists examples of people who died at the Denny boarding house and elsewhere in Water Street.*] From a comparative view of all the preceding circumstances—from the contagious nature of the disease, and from its resemblance of its leading symptoms to those of the yellow-fever of the West Indies—there can be no doubt that the contagion which gave rise to the disease here was imported. And [*almost certainly*] it was introduced and communicated by some of the crew or the passengers of the said vessels. That the fever originated from the rotten coffee, as has been suggested, is altogether chimerical [*i.e., completely implausible*]...."

[*The passage then criticizes the claims of Benjamin Rush, a physician of "very consider-able reputation" not mentioned by name, whose theory disagrees with the claims made above. The author suggests that visiting ships, not conditions at the docks, are to blame for the epidemic.*]

But this opinion hath been combatted by a physician of very considerable reputa-tion and practice.... He supposes that the contagion was generated from the stench of a cargo of damaged coffee which had been landed near the same place where it made its first appearance, on a suspicion that a vegetable putrefaction might produce such a disease. This gentleman has deservedly gained much credit by his noble and humane attention to unhappy patients of the contagion during its most perilous stages, but the majority of his fellow citizens think he has carried the spirit of discovery too far in tracing its origin.

It is certain that neither this disease, nor any other similar to it, has ever visited this city at any preceding time since it was founded unless it was undeniably traced to a foreign source.... The cleanliness of our streets and wharfs has been neglected more in former times than lately; they have, also, been worse affected by putrid vegetable substances; and we have had every diversification of seasons—wet and dry, hot and cold—that could assist in produc-ing such an effect; and as the learned doctor has not produced sufficient reasons to convince a number of his fellow citizens of the justness of his opinion in this instance, he must indulge them in the opinion that the deleterious miasmata was introduced from abroad, and from the sick on board one of the three vessels before mentioned.

[*In a later section, the text comments on the service rendered by people of African descent. It suggests that they acted bravely since it was not clear during the epidemic that they were immune to the pestilence. The text also replies to the charge that Africans took advantage of whites by charging high prices by commenting on the dangers of employment and suggest-ing that it was sensible to request some payment.*]

It is remarkable that the French who settled among us, and particularly those from the West Indies, were in a particular manner preserved from this sickness. Some few, however, took it and died. The black people, likewise, were exempted in a peculiar manner from the contagion. Very few of them were taken and still fewer died. Had it not been for the exertions and attentions of some of these despised people, the calamity and distress of the city would have been much aggravated....

Those who are acquainted with human nature will readily allow that the principle of self preservation must operate upon the blacks as strongly as upon other people. Now although experience has shown that they have almost universally escaped the contagion, yet at that time [*during the actual epidemic*] the fact was not absolutely established ... and as they were ignorant of the physical properties of bodies; and as even we, with all the advantages of education have not yet been able to develop [*i.e., determine*] the cause of their wonderful preservation, the idea which they may have had of the danger would very probably prevent many from undertaking such a difficult and hazardous employment.... It should be considered that their education has been such as to keep them in ignorance of the finer feelings of nature, that they generally have been imposed upon, that they are universally poor, and must possess, like others, an ambition of procuring something for future contingencies.

An Enquiry into ... the Causes and Effects of the Epidemic Disease Which Raged in Philadelphia—Jean Devèze (1794)

Devèze was a French physician who arrived in Philadelphia by ship very shortly before the outbreak commenced. His text advances traditional Galenic arguments in support of the view that miasmas were the source of disease. In this case, the downplaying of a possible contagious spread also deflected responsibility away from French/West Indian ship traffic.

A few days after my arrival at Philadelphia, the seventh of August 1793, it was reported that many people had lost their lives in consequence of a sore throat. The rapid progress of the disease gave reason to suppose that it had some contagious property annexed to it. The death of many persons in the same quarter, and nearly at the same time, gave sanction to the opinion that it was a proven certainty to be very dangerous to approach those who were attacked with it....

In short, the public papers inspired you with terror by pretending to declare the disease contagious. They went further—they advised marking those houses where the epidemic had already sacrificed some victims. This was, no doubt, one of the causes of the rapid destruction that spread devastation through this unfortunate city....

[*In a later passage, Devèze advances an alternate view of the causes of the epidemic.*]

I will examine these causes under two heads: general and particular. The general causes are known to all: the little cold during the previous winter and extreme heat of the succeeding summer, which was accompanied by the usual storms, to which may be added the fruit of the year being exceedingly bad.

Among the particular causes we may reckon burying grounds in the midst of the city. These places of interment are injurious from the vapors which exhale from them and corrupt the atmosphere, and also by the miasmata which the rain-water carries with it as it filters through the earth and passes into the wells…. Another cause of corruption in the city is the tan-yards and starch manufactories and also the quays, where at low water the mud is uncovered, from which a quantity of pernicious vapors arise; in short, the ditches with which the city is surrounded from the earth being taken out to make bricks; where the water, from stagnating during the summer, sends forth infectious exhalations….

All these causes united must necessarily corrupt the blood and give to the bile such a degree of acrimony as to become the principal cause of the epidemic.

A Narrative of the Proceedings of the Black People during the Late Awful Calamity in Philadelphia—Absalom Jones and Richard Allen (1794)

Absalom Jones and Richard Allen were leaders among a group of African American freedmen who saw an opportunity for charity and increased status during the yellow fever outbreak. Allen was also active in attempts to raise money for a Christian church to serve Philadelphia's African community.

Even more than the anonymous text above, Jones and Allen celebrate the bravery and altruism of black men. They object to rumors that "make us blacker than we are"—including allegations made by pamphleteer Matthew Carey—and they highlight black "sensibility," in contrast to the intemperance on display at the white-led emergency hospital at Bush Hill. They also dispute the claim that blacks were less vulnerable to yellow fever than whites and insinuate that some writers understated the risks to blacks in order to encourage their help. This tract was printed together with an open letter urging the abolition of slavery in the United States.

In consequence of the partial [*i.e., biased*] representation of the conduct of the people who were employed to nurse the sick in the late calamitous state of the city of Philadelphia, we are solicited by a number of those who feel themselves injured thereby, and by the advice of several respectable citizens, to step forward and declare facts as they really were….

Early in September, a solicitation appeared in the public papers to the people of color to come forward and assist the distressed, perishing and neglected sick; with a kind of assurance that people of our color were not liable to take the infection. Upon which we and a few others met and consulted on how to act on so truly alarming and melancholy an occasion....

In order to better regulate our conduct we called on the mayor the next day to consult with him how to proceed so as to be most useful. The first object he recommended was a strict attention to the sick and the procuring of nurses. This was attended to by Absalom Jones and William Gray; and, in order that the distressed might know where to apply, the mayor advertised the public that upon application to them they would be supplied. Soon after, the mortality increasing, the difficulty of getting a corpse taken away was such that few were willing to do it when offered great rewards. The black people were looked to. We then offered our services in the public papers by advertising that we would remove the dead and procure nurses. Our services were the production of real sensibility; we sought not fee nor reward until [*because of the amount of work*] we were not adequate to the service we had assumed. The mortality increasing rapidly obliged us to call in the assistance of five hired men in the awful discharge of interring the dead....

When the sickness became general and several of the physicians died, and most of the survivors were exhausted by sickness or fatigue, that good man Dr. Rush called us more immediately to attend the sick, knowing we [*Jones and Allen*] could both bleed [*i.e., perform bloodletting*]. He told us we could increase our utility by attending to his instructions and, accordingly, directed us where to procure the medicine duly prepared, with proper directions how to administer them, and at what stages of the disorder to bleed, and when we found ourselves incapable of judging what was proper to be done, to apply to him.... This has been no small satisfaction to us; for, we think, that when a physician was not attainable we have been the instruments, in the hand of God, for saving the lives of some hundreds of our suffering fellow mortals.

We feel ourselves sensibly aggrieved by the censorious epithets of many who did not render the least assistance in time of necessity, yet are liberal of their censure [*i.e., quick with criticism*] for us for the prices paid for our services when no one knew how to make a proposal to anyone they wanted to assist them. At first we made no charge, but left it to those we served in removing their dead, to give what they thought fit—we set no price until the reward was fixed by those we had served. After paying the people we had to assist us, our compensation is much less than many will believe....

We wish not to offend, but when an unprovoked attempt is made to make us blacker than we are, it becomes less necessary to be over cautious on that account; therefore we shall take the liberty to tell of the conduct of some of the whites.

[*After anecdotes of dishonest behavior by white nurses, the text describes the conditions at Bush Hill, a hospital and isolation station where numerous victims died.*]

Mr. Carey [*a critic of African workers*] tells us Bush Hill exhibited as wretched a picture of human misery as ever existed. A profligate abandoned set of nurses and attendants (hardly any of good character could at that time be procured) rioted on [*i.e., stole or misused*] the provisions and comforts prepared for the sick, who (except at the hours that the doctors attended) were left almost entirely destitute of every assistance. The dying and the dead were indiscriminately mixed together. The ordure and other evacuations of the sick were allowed to remain in the most offensive state imaginable. Not the smallest appearance of order or regularity existed. It was in fact a great human slaughter house where numerous victims were immolated [*burned alive*] at the altar of intemperance....

[*The text contrasts this with the fortitude of nurses who attended people privately.*]

We can assure the public that there were as many white as black people detected in pilfering, although the number of the latter employed as nurses was twenty times as great as the former.... [T]he people were glad to get any person to assist them; a black was preferred because it was supposed they were not so likely to take the disorder [*i.e., contract the disease*].... The case of the nurses, in many instances, were deserving of commiseration, the patient raging and frightful to behold; it has frequently required two persons to hold them from running away, others have made attempts to jump out of a window ... others lay vomiting blood and screaming enough to chill them with horror.

[*In a later passage, Jones and Allen refute the claim that people of African descent were not vulnerable to the contagion.*]

The public were informed that in the West Indies and other places where this terrible malady had been it was observed that the blacks were not affected with it. Happy would it have been for you, and much more so for us, if this observation had been verified by our experience.

When the people of color had the sickness and died we were imposed upon and told it was not with the prevailing sickness until it became too notorious to be denied. Then we were told some few died but not many. Thus were our services extorted *at the peril of our lives*, yet you accuse us of extorting *a little money from you.*

The bill of mortality ... will convince any reasonable man who will examine it that as many colored people died in proportion as others. In 1792, there 67 of our color [*were*] buried and in 1793 it amounted to 305; thus the burials among us have increased more than fourfold. Was not this in great degree the effects of the services of the unjustly vilified black people?

INTERPRETING THE DOCUMENTS

1. What is the attitude of the anonymous tract author toward French involvement in Philadelphia? Is any distinction made between French ships from the mainland and from the West Indies? Why might individuals in Philadelphia consider French mercantile activity with caution?

2. Compare the descriptions of the causes of yellow fever in the first two passages. What kinds of arguments and evidence do they use? Do you see any way that these contrasting approaches (or the ideas of miasma and contagion more broadly) could be reconciled, or does believing in one rule out belief in the other?

3. Both the anonymous writer and the Jones/Allen tract praise the actions of African Americans, but they do so in different ways. What claim about the status of black people lies behind the narrative in Jones/Allen's treatise? How do you think the author of the anonymous tract would respond to the claim that blacks were equal in "sensibility" to whites?

MAKING CONNECTIONS

1. Consider the opening of the anonymous tract and its description of Philadelphia's "opulence." What comparisons can you draw between this document and the connections drawn between commercialism and disease during other epidemics? How is the discourse concerning disease and human moral agency shifting and how is it staying the same?

2. Reread the passage from the Paris medical faculty's explanation of the causes of plague in chapter 1. How do the arguments there about the cause of disease compare to Jean Devèze's description of yellow fever miasmas in Philadelphia?

3. The belief that Africans and African Americans were immune to yellow fever contrasted with the observation that Indigenous peoples were particularly vulnerable to smallpox. How do you think white Europeans and Americans might have resolved this contradiction?

For further reading: J. Worth Estes and Billy G. Smith, *A Melancholy Scene of Devastation: The Public Response to the 1793 Yellow Fever Epidemic* (Philadelphia: Science History Publications, 1997).

Notes

1. The phrase was already an aphorism by Aristotle's time in the fourth century BCE. Harvey M. Feinberg and Joseph B. Solodow, "Out of Africa," *Journal of African History* 43, no. 2 (2002): 257.

2. Jeffrey R. Powell, Andrea Gloria-Soria, and Panayiota Kotsakiozi, "Recent History of *Aedes aegypti*: Vector Genomics and Epidemiology Records," *Bioscience* 68, no. 11 (2018): 854–60, at 854.

3. Paul Sutter, "'The First Mountain to Be Removed': Yellow Fever Control and the Construction of the Panama Canal," *Environmental History* 21, no. 2 (2016): 253.

4. J.E. Bryant and E.C. Holmes, "Out of Africa: A Molecular Perspective on the Introduction of Yellow Fever into the Americas," *PLOS Pathogens* 3, no. 5 (2007): e75.

5. Powell, Gloria-Soria, and Kotsakiozi, "Recent History," 854–57.

6. Mariola Espinosa, "The Question of Racial Immunity to Yellow Fever in History and Historiography," *Social Science History* 38, no. 4 (2014): 437–53.

7. David Birmingham, *Trade and Empire in the Atlantic, 1400–1600* (New York: Routledge, 2000), 6–15.

8. Philip Curtin, "Epidemiology and the Slave Trade," *Political Science Quarterly* 83, no. 2 (1968): 203.

9. John Thornton, *Africa and Africans in the Making of the Atlantic World, 1400–1680* (New York: Cambridge University Press, 1992).

10. Olaudah Equiano, *The Interesting Narrative of the Life of Olaudah Equiano, or Gustavus Vassa, the African* (London, 1794), 51–52.

11. J.R. McNeill, *Mosquito Empires: Ecology and War in the Greater Caribbean, 1620–1914* (Cambridge: Cambridge University Press, 2010), 106–19.

12. Francis Borland, *The History of Darien* (Glasgow, 1779), 69.

13. Robert Larin, *Canadiens en Guyane, 1754–1805* (Paris: Presses Universitaires Paris Sorbonnes), 129.

14. Peter McCandless, "Revolutionary Fever: Disease and War in the Lower South, 1776–1783," *Transactions of the American Clinical and Climatological Association* 118 (2007): 225–49.

15. Richard Grove, "The Great El Niño Event of 1789–93 and Its Global Consequences: Reconstructing an Extreme Climate Event in World Environmental History," *Medieval History Journal* 10, no. 2 (2007): 75–98.

16. Martin S. Pernick, "Politics, Parties and Pestilence: Epidemic Yellow Fever in Philadelphia and the Rise of the First Party System," *William and Mary Quarterly* 29, no. 4 (1972): 559–86.

17. McNeill, *Mosquito Empires*, 242–58.

18. Quoted in Rebecca Earle, "'A Grave for Europeans'? Disease, Death, and the Spanish-American Revolutions", *War in History* 3, no. 4 (1996): 376.

19. Erwin H. Ackerknecht, "Anticontagionism between 1821 and 1867," *Bulletin of the History of Medicine* 22, no. 5 (1948): 562–93. This essay's long-term impact is considered in Alexandra

Minna Stern and Howard Markel, "Commentary: Disease Etiology and Political Ideology: Revisiting Erwin H. Ackerknecht's Classic 1948 Essay, 'Anticontagionism between 1821 and 1867,'" *International Journal of Epidemiology* 38, no. 1 (2009): 31–33.

20. Peter Baldwin, *Contagion and the State in Europe, 1830–1930* (Cambridge: Cambridge University Press, 1999), 201–26.

21. M. Audouard, "The Negro Slave Trade Considered as the Cause of Yellow Fever," ed. and trans. Kaori Kodama, in *História, Ciências, Saúde—Manguinhos, Rio de Janeiro* 16, no. 2 (2009): 521–22.

22. Mark Harrison, *Contagion* (New Haven: Yale University Press, 2012), 7–15.

23. Margaret Humphreys, *Yellow Fever and the South* (Baltimore: Johns Hopkins University Press, 1992), 53.

24. William Coleman, *Yellow Fever in the North* (Madison: University of Wisconsin Press, 1987), 182–87.

25. Deborah J. Neill, *Networks in Tropical Medicine: Internationalism, Colonialism, and the Rise of a Medical Specialty* (Stanford: Stanford University Press, 2012), 14.

26. James L.A. Webb Jr, *Humanity's Burden: A Global History of Malaria* (Cambridge: Cambridge University Press, 2009), 128–29.

27. Matthew Smallman-Raynor and Andrew D. Cliff, "The Spatial Dynamics of Epidemic Diseases in War and Peace: Cuba and the Insurrection against Spain, 1895–98," *Transactions of the Institute of British Geographers* 24, no. 3 (1999): 332, Table 1.

28. Vincent J. Cirillo, "'Winged Sponges': Houseflies as Carriers of Typhoid Fever in 19th- and Early 20th-Century Military Camps," *Perspectives in Biology and Medicine* 49, no. 1 (2006): 55.

29. Matthew Smallman-Raynor and Andrew D. Cliff, "Epidemic Processes in a System of U.S. Military Camps: Transfer Diffusion and the Spread of Typhoid Fever in the Spanish-American War, 1898," *Annals of the Association of American Geographers* 91, no. 1 (2001): 71–91.

30. Molly Caldwell Crosby, *The American Plague: The Untold Story of Yellow Fever, the Epidemic That Shaped Our History* (New York: Berkley Books, 2006), 153–83.

31. Ashley Carse and Christine Keiner, "Panama Canal Forum Introduction," *Environmental History* 21, no. 2 (2016): 207–18.

32. Alexandra Minna Stern, "Yellow Fever Crusade: US Colonialism, Tropical Medicine, and the International Politics of Mosquito Control," in *Medicine at the Border: Disease, Globalization and Security 1850 to the Present*, ed. Alison Bashford (New York: Palgrave Macmillan, 2006), 50.

33. Alexandra Minna Stern, *Eugenic Nation: Faults and Frontiers of Better Breeding in Modern America* (Berkeley: University of California Press, 2016), 28–56.

34. J. Gordon Frierson, "The Yellow Fever Vaccine: A History," *Yale Journal of Biology and Medicine* 83 (2010): 78–79.

35. Fred L. Soper, "Rehabilitation of the Eradication Concept in the Prevention of Communicable Diseases," *Journal of Public Health Policy* 80, no. 10 (1965): 868.

36. Jean Slosek, "*Aedes aegypti* in the Americas: A Review of Their Interactions with the Human Population," *Social Science and Medicine* 23, no. 3 (1986): 249–57; Peter J. Hotez, "Zika in the United States of America and a Fateful 1969 Decision," *PLOS Neglected Tropical Diseases* 10, no. 5 (2016), https://doi.org/10.1371/journal.pntd.0004765.

37. Sean Wasserman et al., "Yellow Fever Cases in Asia: Primed for an Epidemic," *International Journal of Infectious Diseases* 48 (July 2016): 98–102.

38. WHO Yellow Fever Fact Sheet, May 2016. The statistics reflect models based on African data from 2013. http://www.who.int/mediacentre/factsheets/fs100/en/.

39. Catherine I. Paules and Anthony S. Fauci, "Yellow Fever—Once Again on the Radar Screen in the Americas," *New England Journal of Medicine*, 8 March 2017. https://doi.org/10.1056/NEJMp1702172.

40. Andrew J. Monaghan et al., "The Potential Impacts of 21st-Century Climatic and Population Changes on Human Exposure to the Virus Vector Mosquito *Aedes aegypti*," *Climatic Change* 146, no. 3–4 (2018): 487–500.

41. Paul Reiter, "Global Warming and Malaria: Knowing the Horse before Hitching the Cart," *Malaria Journal* 7, supplement 1 (2008), https://doi.org/10.1186/1475-2875-7-S1-S3.

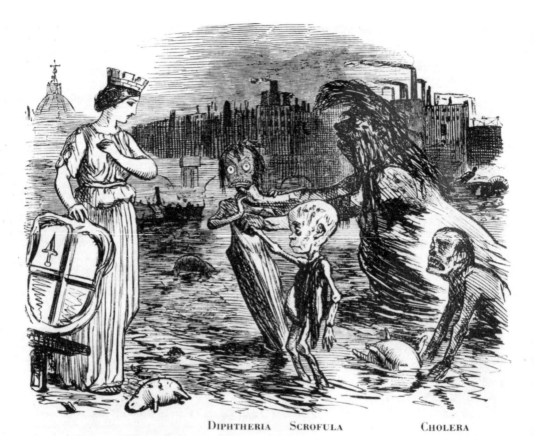

DIPHTHERIA   SCROFULA   CHOLERA

FATHER THAMES INTRODUCES HIS OFFSPRING TO THE FAIR CITY OF LONDON
(*A Design for a Fresco in the New Houses of Parliament.*)

IMAGE 5.1 "Father Thames introduces his offspring to the fair city of London." When this cartoon appeared in Britain's *Punch* magazine (1858), the belief that water was a source of infection for cholera and other diseases was just beginning to gain wide acceptance.

CHOLERA AND THE
INDUSTRIAL CITY

5

A fter days of rumbling, Mount Tambora on the South Pacific island of Sumbawa blew itself to pieces on 10 April 1815. This volcanic eruption, now considered the greatest in human experience, buried nearby villages in fiery ash and launched an estimated 9.8 cubic miles of rocky matter into the air. In the months that followed, the blanketing stratospheric cloud turned skies yellow thousands of miles away. 1816 was remembered as the year with no summer; many crops failed throughout the northern hemisphere, and farmers in the eastern United States reported frost in August. In 1817, the annual monsoon came early to India's Ganges River region and drenched the delta with torrential rain. A terrifying outbreak of disease caused people to vomit explosively, empty their bowels, and die with painful cramps. Communities gathered by the river to burn the dead. An English traveler recounted his horror at "the stench proceeding from the burning bodies, and the lurid gleams of the blazing fires reflected by the water."[1]

Did the unearthly weather of the preceding years cause this epidemic? James Jameson, a British physician in Calcutta (now Kolkata), thought so, although he drew no link between the weather and Tambora's eruption. In a comprehensive report he submitted in 1820 to Calcutta's authorities, Jameson detailed the effects of "distempered" weather in the previous five years and concluded that unusual humidity, drought, and winds had somehow spread the cause of the new, vicious cholera. A landmark document of its time, Jameson's report soon was left aside by Europeans who focused on sanitation and, eventually, upon the concept of

disease-causing germs. Current scientists, however, no longer dismiss his assessment, nor the idea that a new form of cholera was occasioned by the volcanic
fallout. Abundant evidence confirms that outbreaks of cholera are intimately
linked to ocean temperatures and other climatic conditions that shifted radically
in Tambora's wake.

Sixteen years after the eruption, observers anxiously watched another
outbreak of the disease sweep across Russia and eastern Europe. By the end of
1832, many thousands of Europeans had died from cholera, and it had crossed the
Atlantic to Quebec City, New York, and hundreds of smaller communities.
Mortality in India and other parts of Southeast Asia was even higher—the
surviving evidence only permits rough estimates, but it is certain that more than
1 million Indians had died from the disease since its initial outbreak in 1817. Even
in India, other diseases killed more people in the nineteenth century than cholera
but none imprinted more deeply in the imagination.

Cholera reflected the new technologies and emerging social tensions
brought by industrialization and the spectacular growth of cities. Railway lines
hastened cholera's movement through Asia and Europe. Frigates and steamships
brought it to Britain and the Americas in ballast-water tanks, as well as in the
bodies of migrants and soldiers who traveled in ever larger numbers. Once
cholera reached crowded industrial slums, the unsanitary living conditions and
contaminated water were ideally suited to spread the disease. Since Victorian
modesty demanded the concealment of bodily functions, sudden attacks of
vomiting and diarrhea represented a frightening loss of self-control. Outbreaks
of cholera were associated with filth and indecency. They encouraged upper-
class scrutiny of the poor and suspicion of recent immigrants. In turn, high
mortality among the poor fueled popular resentment and protest against the
moneyed and powerful.

The social response to the disease sharpened debates among doctors, scientific researchers, and government officials, not only about cholera but also the
foundations of pathological thinking. Before the mid-1870s, as with yellow fever,
clinicians and public health officers discussed quarantine, sanitary reform, and
variations on the concepts of miasma and contagion. Thereafter, researchers aided
by improved microscopes offered biological arguments with a specificity that had
been impossible before. After 1884, when Robert Koch claimed that the disease
was caused by a microbe, the offensive against cholera introduced a new conception of germs and fostered—for better and worse—a paradigm of infectious
disease based on the invasion of pathogens.

Etiology and Early History

The cholera microbe is a vibrio, a comma-shaped bacterium with a long tail that thrives in warm, salty water. There are more than 200 subspecies of *Vibrio cholerae* which are classified into serogroups according to their cell surface antigens. Most subspecies are innocuous, but several cause gastrointestinal diseases in humans, including the serogroups O1 and O139 that cause cholera. When these vibrios are ingested through contaminated water or seafood, their distinctive tails propel them into the host's intestinal lining. In a behavior known as **quorum sensing**, the vibrios emit signaling molecules that apparently allow them to detect both the number of other vibrios and the total number of bacteria in their environment.[2] This triggers the secretion of a toxin that ruptures the bonds between cells in the lining. The cells empty salts and water into the gut; profuse vomiting and diarrhea often ensue within hours of infection, spreading the bacteria further and causing death unless the fluids and salts are replenished. Widespread underreporting of cholera cases obscures the estimated global burden, but it is estimated that several million people contract cholera annually and roughly 100,000 die from the disease.

While much remains unknown about the factors that influence susceptibility to cholera, it is clear that not all people are equally vulnerable. Low levels of stomach acid and some nutrient deficiencies heighten the risk of infection, and individuals with blood type O face a greater risk of developing severe symptoms.[3] Some infected individuals do not fall ill or exhibit few symptoms; they, and individuals who are in recovery, may shed vibrios for days or weeks. Thus, the cholera microbe can either spread violently through uncontrolled bodily fluids or pass unnoticed from apparently healthy people. This dynamic confounded nineteenth-century public health measures and often thwarts efforts to control cholera today.

Ancient writings from around the world, including the Hippocratic texts and Sanskrit writings from India, refer to stomach ailments with symptoms that resemble cholera. But some evidence links its origins more firmly to the Ganges River delta that embraces northeast India and Bangladesh. Veneration of a cholera goddess, named Olavedi by Hindus and Olabibi by Muslims, dates back to antiquity. A recent genetic population study of the delta's inhabitants suggests that mortality from cholera has influenced demography in the region for many centuries.

In the decades before 1800, British observers reported a cholera-like malady among Hindus who made pilgrimages to the Ganges River. These outbreaks were relatively local, but in the summer of 1817 a wave of disease struck Calcutta in the Ganges Delta region and spread through much of Asia, including China and Japan. This outbreak subsided by 1823; thereafter, four more pandemics originated in India and circled the globe between 1826 and 1896. Most regions had cholera-free periods of several years or more, but outbreaks also accompanied large-scale human movements and conflicts such as the Crimean War. This, at least, was the overall pattern in Europe but elsewhere circumstances differed. In coastal Japan, for example, cholera was endemic for decades after 1858, when an American steamship apparently reintroduced the disease after the milder first outbreak. By the early twentieth century, public health measures and improved water supplies mostly protected Europe and North America but a sixth pandemic devastated India and other parts of Southeast Asia. Since 1961, when a new variant of the microbe emerged in Indonesia, cholera has never completely disappeared. In addition to occasional epidemics in the Americas, the disease remains prevalent in many parts of Southeast Asia and has found a persistent foothold in regions of sub-Saharan Africa.

For decades after the cholera microbe was identified, researchers puzzled over its attributes, especially its apparent ability to vanish and reappear. In the 1970s, marine scientist Rita Colwell identified *V. cholerae* in Chesapeake Bay on the east coast of the United States.[4] Numerous studies eventually concluded that human infection is only incidental to the organism's remarkable ecology. Vibrios can exist and reproduce either independently or in association with plankton, particularly tiny crustaceans known as copepods. They flourish in estuaries where fresh water and salt water mix. In this environment they can enter a dormant phase for months and reactivate when water temperature, salinity, and other conditions are ideal. Research has shown that rising water temperature fosters the growth of copepod populations and the vibrios that they host.[5] The investigation of vibrios as independent organisms has brought one additional, unwelcome conclusion: since cholera's causal microbes flourish in nature, the disease cannot be eradicated.

Europe's Pandemic of 1831–1832

Apart from its physical effects, cholera in the nineteenth century was a fearsome disease because observers could anticipate its arrival far in advance. In 1829 and 1830, the disease traveled north from India and branched out along overland trade routes and waterways. While observers did not agree on the way that cholera was transmitted, by all accounts its steady march resembled waves of plague from earlier centuries. Authorities in the Russian and German lands attempted the same quarantines, disinfection, and sanitary cordons that had halted plague, notably at Marseille in 1721. They also tried cures such as bloodletting and ingesting solutions of calomel (mercuric chloride). These treatments and others had no benefits, and effective therapies were not widely available until the twentieth century.

The fear of disease set many social controls in motion.[6] As cholera approached Moscow in September 1830, Russia's tsar sent soldiers to dig up roads and destroy ferries and bridges, limiting the city to only four entrances with checkpoints. The neighboring state of Prussia fortified its 200-mile border with Russia and Poland with more than 60,000 troops, including cavalry patrols and men stationed in wooden huts spaced 100 meters apart. Travellers were required to stay at quarantine stations for several days while their belongings were washed and fumigated. Letters were punctured or torn open. Even paper money was packed in oilcloth then unwrapped in soapy water and counted while wet. Across Europe, cities imposed curfews, canceled fairs, destroyed stray cats and dogs, and arranged for the swift disposal of corpses, a measure that violated customary burial practices and caused great resentment. Residents of a house where someone had died from cholera were ordered to stay inside, and sometimes even entire neighborhoods were placed under armed guard.

But cholera was not plague. Quarantines and disinfection of goods did little against a pathogen that traveled by water and often caused no visible symptoms. The measures frustrated merchants and angered lower-class city dwellers and peasants who bore the brunt of the mortality and were trapped in afflicted areas. In Russia and Hungary, where military and health authorities were often nobles, peasants attacked sanitary cordons and pillaged castles. City dwellers protested against higher prices, the disruption of livelihoods, and the destruction of property that officials considered contaminated. In Berlin, citizens complained that sanitary cordons were frightening and "are only enforced against the poorer class of people."[7] One of the largest outbursts took place in April 1831, when a police official in Paris instructed residents to collect garbage for a company with a contract for sanitation services. The intent was to clean the city but the order infuriated ragpickers who foraged garbage as their livelihood. Thousands of people took to the boulevards, burning property and erecting barricades in the heart of the city before police halted the riot.

As the historian Richard Evans has observed, this popular unrest contrasted with the violence that had accompanied plague epidemics.[8] Whereas plague-stricken communities had attacked Jews, alleged witches, or other marginal groups, cholera riots targeted authorities who were blamed for harsh sanitary measures or even for starting the epidemic. It is a mark of the deep distrust between classes that doctors were often suspected of colluding with elites to murder the urban poor. In Hungary, Germany, and Russia, rumors circulated widely that doctors suffocated cholera patients behind closed doors, or that chloride compounds and other disinfectants were actually used to poison wells. The suspicion took a different form in Britain, where independent surgical schools often secured subjects for dissection by underhanded means. In many cities, including London and Edinburgh, riots followed accusations that doctors were killing patients to provide cadavers. In Manchester, when a man discovered that his grandson had been buried headless, a crowd carried the coffin through the streets, attacked the cholera hospital, and burned the carts used to transport the dead.[9]

Outbreaks in North American cities began in the summer of 1832 and fanned out westward along rail lines and rivers. Here attention focused upon immigrants who were arriving by the tens of thousands every year. Many were physically weak and some were ill; a newspaper in Quebec City compared the immigrants to a vast army that tramped through, leaving the sick, wounded, and dead behind. As hundreds died from cholera in Quebec City and Montreal, the disease reached New York City from British passenger ships and via canals that had recently connected the Great Lakes and the Hudson River.[10] Irish immigrants, some of whom had worked to dig the canals, were singled out for particular disapproval. Observers agreed with the New York Board of Health that the Irish were "exceedingly dirty in their habits, much addicted to intemperance, and crowded together in the worst portions of the city."[11]

As this statement illustrates, in the 1830s imperatives of morality and hygiene were bound together, much as they had been during epidemics of plague or smallpox in earlier centuries. The ancient notion that a person's habits or constitution predisposed them to illness was updated to reflect the experience of nineteenth-century city dwellers. Faced with outbreaks that often were terrifying, religious leaders called for communal repentance and self-control. Preachers suggested that the laws of nature were also divine laws, and diseases such as cholera could be viewed simultaneously as natural occurrences and as a reflection of God's displeasure. To such critics, it was no surprise that people who ate immoderately, drank heavily, or indulged in other vices succumbed to a grisly end. Of course, these sentiments often were directed at poor or marginal people and stressed individual action instead of systemic forces such as living or working conditions.

Repeated waves of cholera aggravated tensions created by social disruption and growing urban poverty. However, during later pandemics European government officials mostly refrained from isolation measures or invasive disinfections that destroyed property. During the outbreak that began in 1848 many communities faced mortality far above the level of the early 1830s but there was less unrest directly related to cholera. Successive outbreaks also enabled doctors and researchers to investigate the origins and spread of the disease. Their observations inspired new theories but also breathed life into old ones.

Cholera and Industrial London

The debate over cholera and other health concerns was especially urgent in mid-nineteenth-century London, an epicenter of industry and the capital of a global colonial network. After decades of explosive growth, London had nearly 2 million inhabitants in 1840. The lower-class people who flooded into the city seeking jobs faced unhealthy living conditions. In factories and workshops they encountered smoke and clouds of dust, harmful chemicals and dangerous machinery. At home, families crowded into tenement buildings or windowless cellars with mud floors and no water. "We live in muck and filth," lamented a letter sent to the London *Times* in 1849. "We ain't got no priviz [privies], no dust bins, no drains, no water-s[up]plies and no drain or suer [sewer] in the [w]hole place ... We all of us suffer, and numbers are ill, and if the C[h]olera comes Lord Help Us."[12] Conditions were much the same among coal miners in Newcastle, weavers in Manchester, and dockhands in Liverpool, but London was especially notorious for its sprawling slums and the reeking fog that often enveloped the streets. The city sustained over 6,000 cholera deaths in 1832, and more than twice that number when the disease returned in 1848.

The water infrastructure in London and other growing metropolises was conducive to the spread of various waterborne diseases. Alongside cholera, these included **typhoid** (or typhoid fever), which is now attributed to infection with *Salmonella typhi* bacteria, and **dysentery**, a condition of intestinal inflammation that may be caused by various bacteria, viruses, or other pathogens. These and other diarrhea-causing conditions are a significant cause of disease and mortality today, and they undoubtedly accompanied cholera and spread on their own in many instances.

By the early nineteenth century, London had a sizable patchwork of under-ground sewers but the system was only designed to drain surface water from the street level. In dwellings, including multistory buildings, pits that held human waste could be several feet deep and had to be periodically emptied by removers of "night-soil" who carted refuse away by the ton. Running water was supplied to homes, often for only a short time each day, by one of several private companies. The better-off inhabitants who could afford this could also enjoy a new urban comfort: the flushing toilet, known as a water closet, which was installed in tens of thousands of London homes after the 1820s. Over the years, as the liquid volume of waste increased, overflow from cesspools collected in the streets with animal droppings and garbage, emitting loathsome odors that everyone assumed to be unhealthy.[13]

These unwholesome conditions captured the attention of social reformers who grappled with the challenges of urbanization. Led by an energetic lawyer named Edwin Chadwick (1800–1890), they began from the premise that govern-ment offices should oversee large-scale investments in public welfare. Alongside changes to Britain's poor-relief scheme, the reformers focused on health policy, especially as it became clear that illness was a great obstacle to productivity among the destitute. Chadwick and his associates targeted living conditions but mostly sidestepped discussion of the role that factories played in the social problems of the time. In this they differed from social critics such as Friedrich Engels (1820–1895), whose account of working conditions in Manchester during the 1840s offered a scathing critique of industrial capitalism.[14]

The reformers' arguments also reflected a growing interest in the use of data to study populations and the collective impact of poverty and disease. In 1838, Parliament created a General Registry Office (GRO) to record births, deaths, and marriages. Its Compiler of Abstracts, a former apothecary named William Farr (1807–1883), soon earned acclaim for his analyses of mortality and his attempts to standardize disease names that previously had been reported inconsistently. Although attention to this topic was not new—officials in London had tallied deaths from plague and other maladies for centuries—Farr's approach encouraged officials to draw conclusions from consistent reporting and to identify the most urgent social problems. In 1842, Chadwick used information from Farr and poor-relief officials across Britain to compile a sweeping exposé titled *Report on the Sanitary Condition of the Labouring Population of Great Britain*. This work combined maps, statistics, and first-hand reports to mount an impressive case for improve-ments to ventilation and drainage, street cleaning, and control of vagrants. Filth was expensive, Chadwick argued; poor living conditions encouraged immoral behavior and caused diseases that forced workers and their dependents to seek poor relief. In response, the British Parliament passed the Public Health Act for England and Wales (1848), which created a three-member General Board of Health and provided for the foundation of numerous local boards of health. In many respects, the legislation was a compromise—metropolitan London was exempted, ostensibly because of its size, and the Board had little power to compel action. However, the Board reflected an approach to public health that was proactive rather than reactive, and acknowledged the need for ongoing involvement of both local and national governments.[15]

What perceptions of disease underlay this sanitarian approach to public health? For the lawyer Chadwick and his medical advisor, Thomas Southwood Smith (1788–1861), the source of disease lay in the atmosphere. Piles of filth posed a danger because they created putrid vapors that mixed with air and were inhaled by nearby inhabitants. This view had ancient roots in miasma theories, and was considered conservative at the time, but the sanitarians were confirmed in their view by statistical data as well as their moral and political sensibility. The attack on filth demanded social improvement, more so than outward-looking quarantine policies that focused on border control.

Some officials disliked Chadwick's heavy-handed efforts to centralize public health authority. He was removed from the Board of Health in 1854 and the Board itself was abolished in 1858. Over decades, however, the sanitarian approach to public health encouraged activity by local authorities. It also provided a rationale for the funding of massive public works projects, especially sewer construction and water filtration, which dramatically reduced the incidence of certain diseases. The immediate impact was less salutary. Because Chadwick and his associates considered polluted water less dangerous than polluted air, they encouraged Londoners to empty their garbage into the rivers. A law passed in 1846 empowered city officials to enforce this measure, and thereafter builder Thomas Cubbitt observed the disastrous result: "The Thames is now made a great cesspool, instead of each person having one of his own."[16] The policy was especially damaging in regard to waterborne diseases because tidal surges in the Thames reversed the water current and pushed waste back upriver.

Chadwick and other sanitarians have been an easy target for historians who have criticized their backward-looking focus on miasmas and the soiling of the Thames. However, where cholera was concerned, most medical practitioners of the time shared their skepticism of pure contagion theory.[17] For a disease to be considered contagious, observers looked for proof of direct transmission between people or other objects. Smallpox, for example, was thought to spread via close contact, and it was easily transferred from one person to another by inoculation. Cholera offered no such proof; while the disease moved from region to region, within communities it often erupted in several locations at once and the victims fit no obvious pattern. People who tended the sick did not fall ill more than anyone else, and even some brave investigators who swallowed fluids from cholera victims did not contract the disease.

Some thoughtful observers, therefore, suggested that cholera belonged to a category of diseases, including yellow fever and typhoid, which were contagious only under certain circumstances. William Farr's treatise, *Report on the Mortality of Cholera in England, 1848–49*, published in 1852, provides an excellent example of a "contingent contagion" theory. In the GRO, Farr assembled statistics on mortality, including cholera deaths, for decades until his retirement in 1880. In the process, he became an acknowledged authority on vital statistics and a pioneer in medical surveillance. Farr's treatise analyzed information he collected from Britain's cities and also incorporated insights from Justus von Liebig, a German chemist who studied fermentation. This natural process was believed to be closely related to the growth of disease-causing material. The example of fermentation that received the most attention was the activity of yeast in bread dough or alcohol production. Von Liebig described yeast's interaction with sugar as a chemical process of decomposition or putrefaction, a breakdown that could produce poisons of the kind that were present in rotted vegetables or ill-cooked meat. As we will see, this view would soon be challenged, but, in the 1850s, Farr found von Liebig's approach to putrefaction instructive. He used the term "zymotic"—derived from a Greek word that meant "to ferment"—to describe diseases that seemed to spread in a similar fashion. Each zymotic disease had a catalyst—for cholera, Farr called it "cholerine," or "cholrine"—that could spawn an outbreak when it met the wrong local or atmospheric conditions.[18]

Farr could not isolate the catalyst for cholera, but his theory reconciled the traditional concept of miasma with his observations and mortality data. Farr firmly believed that the air closer to sea level was unhealthy because poisonous particles were suspended in the low clouds that often hovered over cities. Contaminants would also flow downhill in water and seep into poorly drained soil at lower elevations. In his *Report*, Farr gave special attention to London, and proposed a consistent relationship between the elevation of houses above sea level and the frequency of cholera deaths. Farr's associates, who hailed his study as a major work, believed that the theory explained why cholera and other diseases struck certain neighborhoods so quickly. Once contaminated air encountered dirt and hunger, all it needed was a spark to ignite an outbreak among the poor people who were susceptible to the poison. In 1849, the Board of Health suggested that "a single infected person ... may act on that population zymotically, that is, as the leaven which sets in action the fermenting mass."[19] Doctrines of "contingent contagion" incorporated different kinds of arguments and lent support to stereotypes concerning the role of the poor in the spread of disease.

John Snow and London's Water

Such theories plausibly explained the spread of cholera and provided a rationale for many sanitary measures, but ultimately they remained unproven. As cholera approached Britain for the third time in 1853, answers to the key questions—what caused cholera and how to cure it—remained elusive. "We know nothing," sighed an editorial in The Lancet medical journal. "We are at sea, in a whirlpool of conjecture."[20]

By this time, a young doctor named John Snow (1813–1858) had joined the debate. Born to a laborer's family in York, by 1844 Snow had moved to London and obtained qualifications as a surgeon, apothecary, and physician. He was fascinated by the behavior of gases and human respiration. In 1846, after Snow witnessed a demonstration of ether's use as an anesthetic, he fashioned an inhaler in his home laboratory. He also studied the behavior of a more potent gas, chloroform. As an authority in this new field, Snow administered chloroform to Queen Victoria when she gave birth to Prince Leopold in April 1853. Before this procedure, many Britons had objected to anesthesia on both medical and religious grounds. Royal endorsement, and Snow's repeated success with the birth of Princess Beatrice, encouraged the British elite to accept the practice.

Snow's work with gases also encouraged him to question the belief that cholera spread primarily through the air. Snow first saw cholera as a young surgeon's apprentice in 1831. By the time of the second outbreak in 1848, he knew that a gas such as chloroform could kill when a person received a concentrated dose but that the gas diffused over a short distance to become harmless. Snow could not see how inhaling offensive miasmas on a city street could spread disease, especially since many workers such as tanners or butchers breathed in noxious fumes daily but did not get sick. Instead, he connected cholera's transmission to its pathology: the gastrointestinal symptoms of cholera indicated that it affected the alimentary canal, which led to the stomach instead of the lungs. Snow surmised that cholera was ingested, not inhaled, meaning that the source of disease was water contaminated by the feces of cholera victims. His work included investigations in Surrey, thirty miles from London, where cholera outbreaks had struck row houses with cesspools that were near the water supply. Snow argued his thesis in *On the Mode of Communication of Cholera* (1849), and he further suggested that the flushing of water closets into the Thames had worsened the recent epidemic.[21]

Snow's theory received polite interest from London's medical community—Farr noted it in his own treatise in 1852—but most observers found theories of contingent contagion more persuasive. Snow continued his work in anesthesia and general practice until the summer of 1853, when cholera returned to London. Thereafter, Snow's reading of weekly mortality reports (issued by Farr from the GRO) suggested to him a unique opportunity to test the role of water quality. Two companies, Southwark & Vauxhall and Lambeth, supplied water to parts of south London. Some neighborhoods received water from one company and some neighborhoods received water from both. In 1848, both companies drew their water from a part of the Thames that was affected by the tidal flow. Four years later, the British Parliament passed the Metropolis Water Act, which ordered London's water companies to move their intakes north of the city above the tidal influence. By 1853 the Lambeth Company had complied but Southwark & Vauxhall had not. The neighborhoods they supplied provided the conditions for a natural experiment: in areas serviced by just one company, Snow could compare the incidence of cholera in 1848 with that of 1853; in areas serviced by both companies, he could compare the incidence of cholera in 1853 among houses that had different water supplies but otherwise identical environments.

These investigations required Snow to interview thousands of South London residents for information on cholera cases and their water supply. This he did, in his spare time, for months in 1854. For cases when residents did not know which company piped water to their house, Snow devised a test for a water sample. He interrupted this project at the end of August 1854 to investigate a violent outbreak of cholera in his own Soho neighborhood. As nearby residents died by the hundreds, Snow raced from house to house, using addresses provided by the GRO to track down associates of the deceased. With help from a local pastor, Henry Whitehead, Snow determined that the source of the outbreak was a pump on Broad Street where many cholera victims had obtained their water. At Snow's request, the neighborhood parish council removed the handle from the pump, and afterward the outbreak abated. In 1855, Snow published a revised version of his work that included evidence from this outbreak and his larger study. The high cholera mortality among Southwark & Vauxhall customers—more than eight times the rate of Lambeth customers in the area served by both companies—indicated to Snow that the spread of cholera was entirely due to contaminated water.[22]

Historians have often cited this treatise as a founding work in the history of epidemiology. At the time, however, the burden of proof rested with Snow, and many questioned his arguments. Officials agreed that water supply probably influenced the spread of disease—the Metropolis Water Act is evidence of that—but they stopped short of Snow's insistence that contaminated water was the *sole* cause of cholera. Careful readers pointed out weaknesses in the data that Snow presented in the larger study. Moreover, at Broad Street the outbreak was winding down before Snow approached the parish council and, as he conceded himself, no one could prove that removing the pump handle had a meaningful impact on mortality. Although Snow used a microscope to examine samples of water from the Broad Street pump and noted the presence of "white, flocculent particles," these observations added little to the other circumstantial evidence. As it happened, in the summer of 1854 an Italian researcher named Filippo Pacini (1812–1883) published observations and drawings of a cholera-causing microbe and even suggested that "vibrions" spread through water and diarrhea.[23] But Snow, who died in 1858, was unaware of Pacini's research. His own writings referred to an unspecified "morbid poison" and did not connect cholera to any kind of microbe.

By the late 1850s, it was still unclear how cholera spread, but the mounting evidence that water played a role—and the fact that polluted rivers looked and smelled awful—persuaded city governments across Europe to invest in sewer infrastructure. In 1859, the London engineer Joseph Bazalgette (1819–1891) began construction of more than 1,100 miles of sewer lines, pumping stations, and embankments to route the city's sewage away from inhabitants. Paris undertook a similar program in 1855, and a quarter century later its sewer system extended over 350 miles. Other metropolises, ports, and river communities followed suit by the end of the nineteenth century. In 1866, when cholera struck London again, the converts to a waterborne theory included William Farr. By this time, Farr was one of the few experts who was acquainted with Pacini's microscopic observations as well as Snow's mapping studies. In his report on the outbreak, Farr criticized the East London water company that caused most of the mortality by allowing unfiltered water from London's Lea River to reach its customers. Farr did not abandon his theory of miasmas and elevation entirely, but his attention to Pacini's vibrions signaled a shift among investigators: they increasingly assigned responsibility for disease to living beings that had just become visible.[24]

The New Science of Microbes

In the 1860s, few observers were as well informed as Farr, but important changes were afoot in both scientific research and the political context in which it took place. As new, more powerful microscopes yielded exciting discoveries, scientific expertise increasingly symbolized a nation's cultural vitality. The fight against cholera became deeply interwoven with national and international politics as the impact of colonial trade and global transportation networks increased.

Concerns over cholera, yellow fever, and other diseases prompted European nations to discuss quarantine and sanitation at a series of international summits. Four such conferences convened between 1851 and 1874.[25] Although most participants agreed that cholera spread from India through human activity, they reached no consensus on its causes, mode of transmission, or what public health measures were needed. Some participants were sympathetic to the views of Max von Pettenkofer (1818–1901), a respected German professor of hygiene at the University of Munich, who advocated sanitary improvements over quarantine. Pettenkofer allowed that there might be a cholera microbe of some kind. However, similar to contingent contagion theorists such as William Farr, he denied that microbes could cause the disease by themselves and he dismissed what he called "English water mania." There had to be something more: whereas Farr had suggested that elevation influenced the incidence of cholera, Pettenkofer claimed that soil of a particular quality was required to incite a microbe's poisonous quality. He expressed his concept in a simple formula: a cholera microbe (x) encounters low, porous soil separated from groundwater (y) that triggers the germ to release a poisonous miasma (z). Such multicausal theories were more convincing, or more politically acceptable, than Pacini's simpler claim that microscopic vibrions attacked the human intestines.

Nonetheless, the concept of a "germ"—a microbe that grew or multiplied under certain conditions—influenced perceptions of disease as microscopic analysis reshaped scientific understandings of nature.[26] The researchers attracted to this growing field included the French chemist Louis Pasteur, who developed strategies for observing and culturing microbes in the 1850s and 1860s. A gifted investigator, Pasteur was also an astute opportunist who appreciated the practical value of microbial science for agricultural fields that were a key part of the French economy. Pasteur's early work focused on the molecular structure of acids, but he took a greater interest in microbiology after he joined the University of Lille in 1854. Local distillers asked him to investigate fermentation and spoilage in the production of beetroot alcohol. With this project, Pasteur entered one of the most heated debates in the new scientific arena: was fermentation caused by a chemical reaction, as Justus von Liebig had asserted, or by microscopic organisms, as others had claimed? With careful measurements, Pasteur demonstrated that the yeast involved in alcohol manufacture increased in weight when it was combined with sugar and ammonia. Von Liebig had described fermentation as a chemical decomposition of sugar that involved yeast but was not caused by it; Pasteur suggested, instead, that yeast cells broke down sugar as they multiplied, and this physiological process yielded by-products that included alcohol and carbon dioxide.

Pasteur's use of the microscope and his focus on microbes as living beings opened new avenues of inquiry and enabled remarkable discoveries. In 1865, he patented a process for heating wine to destroy bacteria and mold. Beer and eventually milk were also "pasteurized," reducing human exposure to disease-causing agents. In 1865, Pasteur entered a new arena when he was called to investigate a mysterious epizootic of silkworms, a looming threat to the profitable textile industry in southern France. It emerged that more than one malady was at work; Pasteur not only identified particular signs of diseases, he trained farmers in the use of microscopes to select healthy worms and eggs. In the late 1870s, now an acclaimed scientist, Pasteur and his colleagues focused upon methods to induce immunity to common pathogens. This research was encouraged by a chance discovery that a culture of the bacteria that caused fowl cholera (a disease unrelated to human cholera) could weaken over time and lose its ability to produce disease. Chickens that were inoculated with the weakened (or attenuated) pathogen became resistant to a fully virulent strain. In a paper submitted to the French Academy of Sciences in 1880, Pasteur described the process as "vaccination," in homage to Edward Jenner's cowpox inoculations to prevent smallpox.

Along the way, Pasteur developed a knack for dramatic demonstrations that displayed the power of invisible microbes and his control of them. In May 1881, Pasteur applied the attenuation technique to anthrax, a disease of livestock that received fresh attention after Robert Koch described the behavior of its causal microbe in 1876. For his experiments Pasteur used procedures developed by a rival, a veterinary surgeon named Jean-Joseph-Henri Toussaint (1847–1890). Confidently inviting reporters to witness, over several days Pasteur gave twenty-five sheep successive inoculations of attenuated anthrax culture and then administered a fully virulent strain both to these sheep and to twenty-five additional sheep that had not been inoculated. The sheep who had received attenuated anthrax survived, the others died, and Pasteur (without crediting Toussaint) cemented his reputation.[27] Livestock were soon vaccinated by the millions; and soon thereafter Pasteur developed a vaccine that prevented swine erysipelas, a bacterial infection of pigs that causes fever and arthritis and is often lethal.

Some of the most far-reaching innovations involved tools and methods. In 1884, one of Pasteur's assistants, Charles Edouard Chamberland (1851–1908), devised a method of purifying water by squeezing it through the tiny pores in a tube of unglazed porcelain. Procedures with the "Chamberland filter," which initially were performed to filter bacteria from a water supply, soon laid the groundwork for the study of organisms that were too small for microscopes of the time to render visible. The existence of such microbes, soon known as "filterable viruses," was inferred from their ability to pass through the porcelain in ways that the larger bacteria could not. Not all of the early research involved humans directly—some of the first studies with a Chamberland filter, in the early 1890s, established that a tobacco plant disease was caused by a virus. Within a few years, however, Chamberland filters were used to isolate the agents (both toxins) that caused diphtheria and tetanus in humans as well as the virus that causes foot-and-mouth disease in cattle.

In July 1885, Pasteur oversaw another high-stakes experiment to cure rabies. Few people contracted this disease but it inspired fear and morbid fascination. After possible infection from an animal bite there was a terrifying interval of several weeks before symptoms emerged. Thereafter, rabies was always lethal; the sufferers seemed robbed of humanity as they fell into a violent delirium that was often accompanied by vomiting or excess salivation. Unlike the causal agents of anthrax or fowl cholera, the rabies virus could not be cultured because it was much smaller and invisible to the microscopes of the time. However, rabies had a lengthy incubation period, which meant that there was time to attempt treatment before the gruesome onset of disease. Over several years, Pasteur and a collaborator, Émile Roux, had tested an inoculation procedure on dogs and on two human subjects. Although the results were inconclusive, an opportunity for a dramatic human trial arose when Pasteur was approached by the anxious parents of a young boy, Joseph Meister, who had been mauled by a rabid dog. Although he was not himself a physician, and therefore could not legally treat patients, Pasteur prepared a series of thirteen inoculations using material from the spinal cords of rabies-infected rabbits. Each inoculation contained spinal cord samples that were dried for successively longer periods to weaken the virulence of the infected material. Meister survived, and within months hundreds of patients (many of whom, most likely, had not actually contracted rabies) traveled to Paris to receive the remarkable treatment. As enthusiastic reports circulated around the world, Pasteur was showered with honors and financial support for vaccines and other research. Between 1888 and Pasteur's death in 1895, he served as the director of the Pasteur Institute, which soon led many efforts to investigate infectious diseases.

Pasteur's experiments were in the tradition of Edward Jenner's cowpox vaccinations. However, there were important differences not only between Pasteur's methods and Jenner's but also among Pasteur's own experiments. Jenner vaccinated with cowpox to prevent smallpox—using material from one disease to induce immunity to another—while Pasteur, in his fowl cholera and anthrax trials, used attenuated strains of a pathogen to induce immunity to stronger strains of the same pathogen. As Andrew Mendelsohn has suggested, much of Pasteur's work centered around an emergent concept of the virulence of microbes and his attempts to modify it so that human bodies could mount a successful response.[28] In these experiments, Pasteur also demonstrated that microbe cultures that were suitable for vaccination could be produced in a laboratory. It was, therefore, unnecessary to pass diseased material directly from one person to another in the way that smallpox vaccinators had frequently relied on children. Pasteur's experiments with rabies were far more speculative—he never cultured the rabies virus, or even saw it, and in his trial with Joseph Meister he wagered that his injections would provide effective therapy after Meister had been bitten. None of Pasteur's experiments illuminated what happened within human bodies that enabled them to respond to the attenuated microbes that he had produced. The workings of his vaccine, like Jenner's smallpox vaccine, remained a mystery.

In short, Pasteur's intuitive leaps led to spectacular results but left important unanswered questions. Some refused to be awed by his success. Pasteur's critics included Koch, twenty years younger, who shot to prominence almost overnight. In the early 1870s, Koch was an obscure medical officer working among farmers in Posen, a rural region in the north-German state of Prussia. In a modest home laboratory, Koch inoculated mice, dogs, and pigs; he cultured bacteria in drops of

Microscopes and the Origins of Microbiology

Until the mid-nineteenth century, most people found the idea that minuscule creatures influenced human affairs to be implausible or even ridiculous. Microscopes enabled a profound shift in thinking that transformed medicine and the fundamental understanding of the natural world.

The first microscopes relied on the fact that light bends as it passes through materials of varying transparency and thickness. The development of optical microscopes (and also telescopes) began around 1600, when glassworkers in the Netherlands developed two types of devices. Compound microscopes focused light with two lenses, an eyepiece and an objective, while simple microscopes used a tiny glass sphere mounted on a metal plate held close to the eye. The latter were perfected by the singular genius of Antonie van Leeuwenhoek (1632–1723), a cloth merchant in Delft. The best of his microscopes magnified objects over 250 times and could resolve (i.e., distinguish) objects less than a micron—a millionth of a meter—apart.

Microscopes that used multiple lenses eventually surpassed van Leeuwenhoek's devices but only after certain challenges were overcome. Early compound microscopes produced images with blurred edges and color distortions because light refracted into different-colored rays once it penetrated the objective lens. By 1830, inventors in several countries had designed objectives that combined different types of glass to correct the aberrations (figure 5.1).

Initially, microscopes were dismissed as playthings for enthusiasts. After 1865, however, improvements to their construction and innovation in other fields made the technology too powerful to ignore. In the German city of Jena, physicist Ernst Abbe (1840–1905) collaborated with instrument maker Carl Zeiss (1816–1888) to research the theoretical basis of light refraction. Abbe's calculations greatly improved the manufacture of microscope objectives, which previously had been a trial-and-error-process. Abbe designed a lens assembly, called a condenser, which focused light before it passed through the specimen. He and others also developed immersion lenses, which used drops of water or oil to increase resolving power. Robert Koch was the first physician to combine the new technology with photography as he researched anthrax in the 1870s.

The magnifying and resolving limits of the optical microscope, which are imposed by the wavelength of light, were reached by 1900, but microscopy advanced in many directions during the twentieth century. In the 1930s, Frits Zernike (1888–1966) developed the phase-contrast microscope, which adjusted the pattern of light waves to reveal transparent structures that are invisible to other optical instruments. This removed the need for staining, which killed living cells, and enabled scientists to observe the behavior of bacteria. At the same time, researchers developed microscopes that used streams of electrons and substituted electromagnets for lenses. First used in 1931, electron microscopes vastly increased resolving power and enabled the viewing of viruses, which vary in size but are often 100 times smaller than most bacteria. Although scientists had already confirmed the existence of some viruses by other means, it was now easier to investigate them and identify new ones.

Currently, optical and electron microscopes remain useful for clinical evaluations and the detection of new pathogens. Other methods generate data about molecules that is not in picture form but can be used to generate computer models. In X-ray crystallography, researchers analyze how molecules scatter a beam of X-rays to yield a higher level of detail than electron microscopes can provide. Atomic force microscopes position a tiny probe next to a molecule and measure how the attractive and repulsive forces between them move the probe up and down. As research descends to the level of a nanometer—a billionth of a meter—one important challenge is to investigate how viral proteins interact with DNA in natural conditions. Microscopy has advanced far beyond its optical roots, but it remains an interdisciplinary undertaking that now combines biology, physics, computer science, and nuclear engineering.

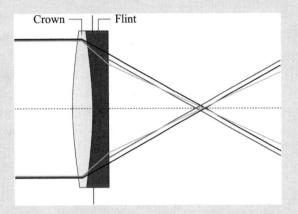

FIGURE 5.1 Correcting chromatic aberration. Light refracts at various angles as it passes through different types of glass. Nineteenth-century microscopes combined crown and flint glass to bring light to a focal point. This corrected aberrations and enabled greater magnification and resolution.

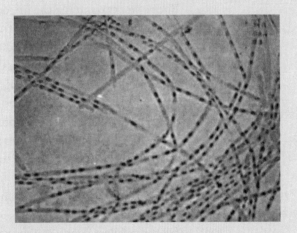

IMAGE 5.2 Robert Koch's anthrax bacillus. This photograph, published in 1877, illustrated the microbe's life cycle, which included the development of long filaments and small durable spores (the dark ovals). The first printed photographs of bacteria provided powerful evidence for the existence of microscopic organisms.

aqueous humor (eyeball fluid) from rabbits and bulls. As noted above, it was Koch who first explained the persistence and transmission of anthrax in the farm environment. Previous researchers had debated the cause of anthrax disease and, in 1868, a Parisian investigator named Casimir Devaine (1812–1882) had argued that a microbe was the sole responsible agent. Whereas Devaine had speculated that flies spread anthrax pathogens to cause outbreaks, Koch's detailed study revealed that the microbe produced spores that could lie dormant in soil for years. Their persistence explained why livestock contracted anthrax without exposure to infected animals, a riddle that had perplexed anxious farmers all over Europe. Because the spores were rod-shaped, Koch called them "bacilli," from a Latin word for "little wands."

In 1876, Koch's landmark essay on anthrax made him the first scientist to convincingly explain how a specific microbe caused a specific disease. He further demonstrated that culture-bred microbes, free of any animal contamination, would have the same effect as material passed directly from one animal to another. More so than Pasteur, Koch eventually emphasized that various microbes were discrete species of organisms; they had distinctive life cycles, they could be recognized by consistent biological and chemical traits, and they caused unique clinical symptoms that could be distinguished under the microscope. Thus, Koch's work countered the lingering belief that diseases such as plague and cholera somehow sprang from the same source or were the same disease with symptoms that changed depending on environmental conditions.

As his circle of collaborators widened, Koch innovated numerous methods for culturing microbes and staining them with different colors to increase visibility. Anxious to communicate his results, Koch labored over photography methods, which also prodded him to improve the preparation of specimens. Koch's images of anthrax, first published in 1877, were the first photographs of microbes ever to appear in print. Koch believed that photographs offered important proof for his claims, and he always stressed that they should not be retouched to alter the image in any way. As he wrote in 1881, "the photographic image is not only an illustration, but above all a piece of evidence, on the credibility of which must not fall the smallest doubt."[29] Nonetheless, drawings remained important for Koch and other scientists—not only did sketches permit the depiction of color, they also allowed authors to highlight important structures and omit others that were deemed unimportant or distracting.

In 1880, Koch joined the Imperial Health Office in Berlin. As discussed further in the next chapter, Koch's team quickly devised methods for culturing microbes that served as the basis for the discipline of microbiology. In a paper published in 1881, Koch described in detail his techniques for photomicroscopy and culturing. Building on the work of Edwin Klebs (1834–1913) and Jacob Henle (1809–1885), the team at the Imperial Health Office refined a set of procedural steps to discern the role of microbes in disease. While they were later known as "Koch's Postulates," the steps were first presented in a paper published in 1883 by Friedrich Loeffler (1852–1915). In order to demonstrate a causal relationship, a microbe must be constantly present in diseased tissue; it must be isolated and grown in a pure culture; the culture, when introduced into another animal, must be shown to induce the disease; and an identical microbe should then be isolated again.

This procedure, combined with technical improvements to microscopes, charted a new course for the international circle of researchers who investigated disease. Koch received worldwide acclaim in the spring of 1882 when he proposed that the much-feared respiratory ailment known as "consumption" was caused by a living microbe. The era soon dubbed the "golden age of bacteriology" had begun.[30]

Cholera and International Politics

By 1883, Koch and Pasteur exerted great influence on the direction of scientific research in their respective countries. Their interests ran in different directions, although their scientific approaches may not have been as far apart as some accounts suggest.[31] Pasteur, who had the training of an industrial chemist, developed an ecological approach to microbes and he attempted to exploit their properties for human health and other purposes. Koch, a physician, viewed microbes primarily as pathogens that must be eliminated to prevent disease. Nationalist sentiments amplified the rivalry between these ambitious men and the research communities that grew around them. During the Franco-Prussian War in 1870–71, Prussia had wrested territory from France and joined with other regional states to form the German Empire. Bitterness on both sides and renewed pride among Germans encouraged leaders to promote Koch and Pasteur as national champions of scientific prowess and cultural vigor. Their personal animosity intensified when Koch's students published essays that criticized Pasteur's methods in the anthrax experiments. The rift widened even further in September 1882 when Koch attended a lecture by Pasteur at a conference in Geneva. Koch did not understand French, and a mistaken translation by a colleague led him to believe that Pasteur's remarks insulted his work. For generations, their personal competition and contrasting research interests deeply influenced European approaches to vaccination and the control of infectious diseases.

In an era of rapidly expanding international commerce, economic objectives influenced the approaches to contagious disease that various nations favored. At the international sanitary conferences, French and Italian representatives, who recalled the impact of plague, had pressed for vigorous quarantine regulations. The agendas of other delegates blunted their initiative. German interests in trade and territorial expansion heightened as the nation consolidated in the wake of victory over France. More pointedly, British public health authorities in India, particularly the sanitary commissioner J.M. Cuningham (1829–1905), maintained that quarantine would not address local environmental conditions that were the most significant cause of cholera.[32] One particular bone of contention was the opening, in 1869, of the Suez Canal that connected the Mediterranean and the Red Sea. As chapter 7 will discuss in greater detail, this maritime artery enabled a more rapid spread of diseases as well as commerce. The danger was recognized to some extent, but British officials opposed maritime quarantines that would lengthen the sailing time between Bombay and London. Delegates from Muslim regions voiced similar concerns, warning that burdensome quarantines would anger millions of pilgrims to Mecca.

Patriotism, colonial politics, and personal ambition came to a head in July 1883 when a telegram from Egypt announced to British officials that cholera had erupted in the Mediterranean port of Damietta. Europeans were concerned because cholera had entered the region through Egypt in 1865. France, Germany, and Britain sent scientists to investigate. The French delegation included two members of Pasteur's laboratory, and Koch himself arrived with the Germans. For the British, who controlled the nearby Suez Canal, an admission that cholera was transmissible threatened terrible economic consequences. The British team lacked an expert in microscopy—perhaps on purpose—and its members soon left Egypt after claiming that unusual weather patterns, not a shipborne infection, had caused an unimportant local outbreak. The French and German teams observed various microbes but neither could induce cholera in an inoculated animal. As Egypt's outbreak waned, one member of the French team died from cholera and the others returned home. But the German team followed the trail to India, which for most non-British observers was the presumed origin of the Egyptian outbreak.

Koch's activities in India were eagerly followed by the German popular press as well as public health officials. In a report from Calcutta that was published in February 1884, Koch described a comma-shaped microbe, which he called the "cholera bacillus," in the intestines and stool of cholera victims, as well as on their clothes and bedding. His team also conducted autopsies on individuals who had died from other intestinal conditions such as dysentery. Since the microbe appeared in great numbers in cholera victims and in no one else, Koch argued that it produced the disease regardless of conditions inside or outside the body. A few weeks later, the German team investigated an outbreak centered on a small pond in Calcutta's outskirts and they found the same microbe in the water and the bodies of cholera victims. As John Snow had done, the German team had traced the spread of cholera to a defined water supply, this time with the benefit of microscope techniques that could identify a culprit.

Koch's claims came as a revelation to most observers. The Prussian elite hailed his work as a triumph for German science, and he returned to a hero's welcome in Berlin. Koch advocated firm control of river traffic, isolation of the infected and potentially infected, attention to water supplies, and ongoing surveillance of sanitary conditions by state authorities. These practical suggestions dovetailed with the interests of imperial officials who were eager to promote the influence of the German government. In 1891, Koch was installed as the director of a new Institute for Infectious Diseases, an answer to the French Pasteur Institute founded a few years earlier. However, lingering doubts remained about Koch's theory of cholera transmission. By his own standards of proof, the evidence from India was not definitive. Not all people infected with the bacteria fell ill, and the German team never induced the disease in an animal with a bacterial culture. British medical officers in India, humiliated by Koch's exploits in the colony, publicly rejected his results. Other experts, including Pettenkofer, vehemently denied that a microbe could cause cholera by itself and argued for the influence of factors, such as soil quality, that varied with local conditions.

But Koch's views were vindicated in 1892, when a disastrous cholera outbreak struck Hamburg, a major industrial port near the mouth of the Elbe River.[33] Hamburg was ruled by a hereditary merchant elite as an independent city within the Prussian-led German Empire. In the era of steamships, the city's population had exploded to over half a million. Hamburg's water and sewer system, which had been constructed in the 1840s, did not include a filtration process. To most observers, the cholera outbreak apparently arose from living conditions experienced by migrants from Russia who were fleeing famine and religious persecution. As they arrived in Hamburg by the thousands, many of them seeking ship passage to the United States, city officials warehoused them in barracks at the harbor. After sewage contaminated the water supply in August, more than 8,000 people died of cholera in four months and ships carried it across the Atlantic to New York. The situation contrasted starkly with Altona, a neighboring city controlled by Prussia, which had installed a sand filtration system and had much lower mortality.

The outbreak laid bare Hamburg's neglect of city infrastructure and the gaping inequality between its wealthy merchants and large industrial underclass. Many streets had no running water and crowded, unsanitary conditions that resembled London a half-century before. Koch arrived to lead the emergency response and toured the city's poorest neighborhoods. His verdict on Hamburg's squalor echoed through Germany: "Gentlemen, I forget that I am in Europe."[34] At heart, the cholera crisis revealed that Hamburg's patricians were incapable of representing the citizens' interests and governing a complex, industrialized city. Under Prussian authority, a disinfection program commenced, construction began on a water filtration system, and the slums were soon dismantled. Within a few years, Hamburg expanded voting rights and introduced sweeping administrative reforms, including a paid professional staff organized along the lines of the imperial bureaucracy.

This was one of the last major outbreaks of cholera in Europe and it presaged the importance of microbe theories of disease for public health measures in years to come. However, Koch's germ theory did not bring about change by itself, and its swift acceptance was not due solely to the strength of the evidence. Before the Hamburg outbreak, most European cities had already improved water supplies and sanitation. Officials could agree on these measures even when the causes of disease were in doubt. After 1884, many found Koch's view of microbes politically expedient as well as scientifically sound. His claim that the cholera microbe always behaved the same way—and, therefore, required the same measures everywhere—appealed to observers who lobbied for greater intervention by national governments and higher status for medical professionals. Prussian officials were willing to overlook the weaknesses in Koch's arguments and they increasingly ignored Pettenkofer, who argued for the importance of variable environmental factors. Measures against cholera, like those undertaken to combat bubonic plague, offered an opportunity for advocates of national governments to strengthen their hand against resistance by local forces.

The concept of "germs" eventually overturned miasma theories, but Koch and other theorists also reinforced an essentially political argument that sanitarians had made for decades: forceful government action was necessary to prevent disease and counter its effects. European countries mostly continued to draw on the repertoire of quarantine, sanitation, and disinfection measures that they had used throughout the nineteenth century. How they did so varied according to forces at work in each country, and also shifted over time, but the clear trend was toward increased control of health measures by national governments. This also entailed a change in attitude toward the role of poverty and "filth" in the spread of disease. In the 1830s, the spread of disease among the poor was frequently attributed to immoral or unhealthy habits that predisposed them to disease. Sixty years later, it was Hamburg's irresponsible elites who were scorned for allowing citizens to be exposed to a water supply that contained a harmful pathogen. As diseases were linked to specific microbial causes that could be identified with expert methods, governments increasingly asserted the authority to enforce compliance with public health laws by rich and poor alike.

Pandemic without End? Cholera in the Non-Western World

By the turn of the twentieth century, most Europeans and North Americans were protected from cholera by developed water infrastructure. The same could not be said for many other regions around the world, especially the Indian subcontinent. Between 1865 and the end of British rule of India in 1947, colonial officials reported 23 million deaths from cholera, a figure that almost certainly understates the disease's full impact.[35] By the end of the nineteenth century, cholera in India was primarily a rural disease since larger cities such as Madras and Calcutta implemented sanitary reforms similar to the British ones. As evidence for germ transmission mounted in Europe, colonial officials persisted in the view that India's environment uniquely abetted the spread of cholera. Recent climate research suggests that their observations may have been partly correct: intense periods of warm rainfall, such as monsoons, change the temperature and salinity of estuaries and can trigger renewed growth among cholera vibrios that previously were dormant. The observation that large-scale Hindu pilgrimages to the Ganges River often occasioned major outbreaks added a cultural dimension to British claims that cholera was a permanent fixture among Indian peoples. Moreover, as noted earlier, the opening of the Suez Canal in 1869 discouraged any talk in India of the spread of cholera by contagion.

Colonial policies exacerbated India's challenges with cholera, as well as with malaria and plague. From the 1860s forward, more than 30,000 miles of irrigation canals and channels were constructed under British direction, many without drainage ditches. In farming areas with poor sanitation, flooded fields readily transported contaminated fecal matter and provided breeding grounds for malaria-carrying mosquitoes.[36] British famine relief policies also encouraged the spread of diseases. During periods of widespread death in the 1870s and the 1890s, starving families were gathered by the thousands in relief camps that often had inadequate sanitation or water supplies, contributing to high rates of cholera in districts that were already under stress. We have seen (in chapter 1) the damaging effects of British anti-plague measures and the limited usefulness of germ theory before the role of rodent vectors was understood. It may not be possible to quantify the impact of colonial policies, but there is no doubt that British intervention contributed to the burden of disease among India's diverse communities.

Although the global incidence of cholera diminished in the 1920s, another chapter in its history began in 1961, when a relatively novel vibrio subspecies touched off a pandemic that has continued into this century. Compared to "classical" cholera, which caused the fifth and sixth pandemics, the variant known as "El Tor"—named for the Egyptian quarantine station where it was first observed—had a lower fatality rate, produced more asymptomatic human hosts, and caused hosts to excrete vibrios for longer periods. El Tor replaced classical cholera in outbreaks across the developing world between the 1960s and the early 1990s. One of the largest outbreaks, which began in the coastal cities of Peru in 1991, eventually spread throughout Latin America and caused hundreds of thousands of cases. The current pandemic has lasted over fifty-five years, more than twice as long as any previous cholera wave, and shows little sign of abating.

The 1991 outbreak prompted scientists to reflect on the relationship between cholera and other aspects of changing ocean ecosystems. Cholera was found all along the nearly 2,000 kilometers of Peruvian coastline. Researchers linked its emergence to the growth of coastal algae blooms and other shifts in water conditions that were spurred by rising temperatures caused in the short term by El Niño fluctuations and more profoundly by global warming.[37] Will higher ocean temperatures encourage the evolution of more harmful vibrios? Some investigators have suggested that vibrios are exchanging DNA fragments more frequently, increasing the likelihood of a new El Tor strain or another harmful pathogen. Recent research in the North Atlantic has linked rising surface sea temperature to the spread of vibrios and small outbreaks of related human disease.[38] But such relationships are difficult to measure. Ocean data have not been collected for long periods, and measurements related to large-scale El Niño events cannot account for the local factors that may influence vibrios and disease in a given region. Much remains mysterious; with this research, scientists have returned, ironically, to the nineteenth-century interest in climate and environment, although they have left aside culturally freighted judgments on the Indian subcontinent and its peoples.

The emerging interest in climate's impact on cholera outbreaks has not replaced the more traditional concern with the spread of infection by humans. The 2010 outbreak in Haiti, on the Caribbean island of Hispaniola, illustrated how routine air travel now enables cholera anywhere in the world to threaten a vulnerable society. Cholera erupted after a powerful earthquake damaged Haiti's water and sanitation infrastructure, which was already the weakest in the western hemisphere. This was Haiti's first documented cholera outbreak in history, and evidence pointed to a remote origin: early cases were found near an encampment of United Nations (UN) peacekeepers from Nepal, where cholera had been present a few weeks before. None of the peacekeepers were sick, but later genomic analyses supported the conclusion that a strain of cholera had been imported from Southeast Asia, perhaps by a single asymptomatic carrier.[39] Belatedly, the UN acknowledged its role in the crisis; cholera became endemic in Haiti, and since 2010 has infected at least 750,000 people (roughly 7 per cent of the national population) and caused at least 10,000 deaths. In Hispaniola's other nation, the Dominican Republic, tens of thousands of cholera cases were reported, but a more robust water infrastructure forestalled a catastrophic outbreak.

Vaccines and treatment have reduced cholera's impact but do not address its underlying causes. The first cholera vaccine injections were developed before 1900 by researchers influenced by Pasteur. Since the 1980s, oral vaccines using killed bacteria have replaced injections. Current vaccines convey partial immunity for only two to three years. They are administered selectively, either to help contain major outbreaks or for visitors to regions where cholera is common. More attention, therefore, has focused on providing oral rehydration treatment (ORT), clean water mixed with the proper proportion of sugar and salts. ORT packets are inexpensive and can be widely distributed; they are effective for many diarrhea-causing conditions and annually save the lives of more than 1 million people, mostly children. However, vaccinations and therapy cannot substitute for a consistent supply of clean drinking water that is separated from human and animal waste. In regions with no modern sanitation, public health advocates have sought simple ways to filter water that are rooted in local cultural practices. In India, for example, it has been found that pouring water through several layers of inexpensive sari cloth can filter microbes and substantially reduce the incidence of cholera.

Conclusion

Cholera is a disease of both poverty and climate change. While the precise effects of temperature shifts on vibrio-caused disease remain to be clarified, it is certain that climate change has influenced levels of coastal flooding, monsoon patterns, and episodes of extreme rainfall. These developments disrupt marine ecosystems and increase the burden on dams, sewers, and other water engineering systems. Such shocks disproportionately affect less affluent societies and the inhabitants of crowded cities with relatively little sanitary infrastructure. Histories of cholera usually describe its impact as a series of waves, but health experts now reckon with a world in which an epidemic of cholera is a permanent possibility.

To many observers this global challenge is reminiscent of the problems that beset European cities as they mushroomed in size during the nineteenth century.[40] Industrialization not only provided the means for cholera to spread, it also created urban conditions that propelled cholera outbreaks into catastrophes and fostered the diffusion of other waterborne pathogens. However, urbanization in the twenty-first century far outstrips both the speed and the scale of earlier transitions. In 1900, the world's urban dwellers made up less than one-fifth of the population (and by some criteria less than 15 per cent) in a world inhabited by less than 2 billion people. Today's global population exceeds 7 billion; roughly half of the world's inhabitants live in cities, and hundreds of millions experience inadequate housing, poor water supplies, or unsafe sanitation infrastructure.[41] Vast, underresourced urban environments not only facilitate the spread of familiar pathogens, they encourage adaptations by microbes or animal vectors that give rise to new diseases. In conflict zones, wholesale destruction enabled by modern warfare has also increased the scale of suffering. In Yemen during 2017–18, hundreds of thousands of

suspected cholera cases were reported
during a devastating civil war that
disrupted water systems and food
supplies.[42]

In the nineteenth and early twentieth
centuries, many regions of Africa and
Southeast Asia became more vulnerable
to cholera as they were connected to
global trade networks in unequal colonial
relationships. In the twenty-first century
cholera remains persistent in sub-
Saharan Africa. The high prevalence of
malnutrition and infections such as
malaria and AIDS that depress immune
system functions undoubtedly contribute
to the incidence of cholera in this region.
The assessment of cholera's burden in
Africa relies on incomplete reporting, but
estimates of the annual incidence of

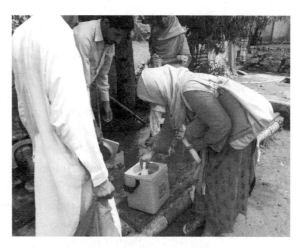

IMAGE 5.3 Investigation of a cholera outbreak in Pakistan. A health researcher collects a water sample at the village of Pir Pighwal in summer 2014. In addition to taking water samples, experts interviewed households and educated the community on the control and prevention of cholera. Water sources were subsequently chlorinated.

cholera on the continent ranged upward of 1.3 million cases in the early
2010s.[43] On the Indian subcontinent, the reshaping of the agricultural landscape for colonial economic interests encouraged the spread of cholera and
malaria. The challenge now is to replace models of "development" that
benefited colonizing powers with investments in water and sanitation that
take account of local social and cultural patterns. This is especially pressing
for cholera-prone coastal regions, including parts of Pakistan, Bangladesh,
Indonesia, and Mozambique that will experience increased flooding as ocean
levels rise.

The changing perception of cholera in Europe during the nineteenth
century reflected a profound shift in scientific thinking that was enabled by
new microscope technology and the rising status of laboratory investigation.
Through the mid-nineteenth century, engineers and the bureaucrats who
employed them led the fight against disease. Their approach to cholera married
ancient concepts with increasingly sophisticated techniques for examining the
forces that influenced populations. After 1875, European scientists demonstrated that the immediate human cause of anthrax, cholera, and other
scourges was a living microbe. As presented by Robert Koch, the concept of

germs replaced vague, multicausal theories with a clear, disarmingly simple narrative: specific pathogens caused specific diseases when they entered the human body, and to prevent disease it was necessary either to stop the microbes from entering or prepare the body to resist them. Sanitary measures remained important thereafter, but authority passed increasingly to doctors and research-ers with specialized tools and knowledge of a microbial world that remained invisible to the average person.

Research on the behavior of microbes casts nineteenth-century explanations of disease in a new light. It is true that the details of miasma theories did not withstand microscopic scrutiny. And theories that highlighted aspects of the environment, especially those of British colonial officials, sometimes were colored with self-interest. However, theories of contingent contagion pointed toward a truth that recent science has reaffirmed: cholera epidemics result not just from the *actions* of microbes but from their *interactions* with environmental, biological, and social factors. As Alfredo Morabia has observed, Max von Pettenkofer's soil theory was incorrect in its specifics, but his x,y,z equation pioneered a theoretical concept of interaction in an epidemiological context.[44] Today, although a great deal is known about the genetic properties of cholera vibrios, scientists are just beginning to unravel the manifold interactions that influence cholera's behavior in individuals, communities, and ecosystems. Much the same is true for the relationships among microbes: researchers now empha-size interactions within complex bacterial communities (**microbiomes**) in various environments.[45]

The so-called golden age of bacteriology focused on a simpler cast of characters. In the last quarter of the nineteenth century, scientists convinc-ingly characterized microbes as invaders within the body. Public health measures expanded in their scope but also became more targeted against the invisible threats rather than broader social and environmental conditions. The triumph of germ theories involved persuasion as well as proof—both Robert Koch and Louis Pasteur staged dramatic demonstrations, highlighted the significance of their findings, and downplayed uncertainty as they advocated particular health measures and scientific research agendas. As the next chapter will explore, when concepts of germs moved from the laboratory into the broader Western culture they influenced not only government campaigns against disease but also everyday approaches to health, hygiene, and the natural world.

WORKSHOP: WILLIAM FARR, JOHN SNOW, AND THE ORIGINS OF EPIDEMIOLOGY

The story of the Broad Street pump is one of the most famous episodes in the history of modern science. In many accounts, it is a tale of medical progress, of miasma theories of disease which were replaced by a concept of contagion that led toward the new paradigm of germ theory. Its protagonist, John Snow, is cast as a distinctively modern hero: a farsighted scientist whose innovative use of data challenged the mistaken beliefs of his time and founded the modern field of epidemiology.

But this simple narrative is misleading. The story changes, and other lessons emerge, when we consider John Snow in relation to his associate, the statistician William Farr. Although the two men worked independently, both investigated cholera during multiple outbreaks and both relied on data concerning the incidence of disease in various locations. Snow, the physician, connected the gastrointestinal symptoms of cholera to the distribution of mortality in order to argue that cholera was spread by contaminated water supplies. This hypothesis was correct, but Snow's insight would have been impossible without the informa- tion provided by Farr's surveillance system, which included the names and addresses of cholera victims whom Snow could interview for information on particular cases. Indeed, Snow credited Farr's work with alerting him to the importance of water supply for the incidence of cholera in South London. As a recent historian has observed, Farr and Snow performed a "scientific duet," as their complementary ideas and methods converged in a new approach to a deadly disease.

Farr's initial hypothesis about the spread of cholera was superseded along with other claims that emphasized the role of the atmosphere or airborne particles. However, the importance that he assigned to the environment resonates today when we consider how factors such as temperature or water quality, as well as human living conditions, influence the spread of cholera and other diseases. Moreover, Farr exemplified an important analytical skill that is often in short supply: the ability to modify one's beliefs when additional data or changing research methods yield new conclusions. After Snow's death, it was Farr who endorsed the idea that microscopic beings were responsible for cholera's symptoms, years before Robert Koch identified the causal microbe in 1884.

"Influence of Elevation on the Fatality of Cholera"—William Farr (1852)

As a statistician, Farr was convinced that many patterns in nature, including the spread of disease, could be expressed in mathematical terms. In 1852, he believed that cholera particles of some kind were carried through the air. Houses at lower elevations were at greater risk because the particles settled into clouds close to the ground and filth flowed downstream to collect in valleys. Farr accurately described a correlation but was mistaken about the cause; the lower-class neighborhoods closest to the Thames suffered the most cholera not because of their lower elevation but because their water supplies were more contaminated.

[T]he mortality from cholera in London bore a certain constant relation to the elevation of the soil, as is evident when the districts are arranged by groups in the order of their altitude. We place the districts together which are not on average twenty feet above the Thames, and find that on this bottom of the London basin the mortality was at the average rate of 102 in 10,000.... By ascending from the bottom to the third terrace, the mortality is reduced from 102 to 34; by ascending to the sixth terrace it is reduced to 17. It will be observed that the number representing the mortality on the third terrace is one-third of the number 102, representing the mortality on the first; and that the mortality on the sixth terrace is one-sixth part of the mortality on the first. And a series approximating nearly to the numbers representing the mortality from cholera, is obtained by dividing 102 successively by 2, 3, 4, 5 and 6.... [*The data in the preceding passage are summarized in* figure 5.2.]

Cholera has not only been most fatal in the low, and least fatal in the high parts of the country, but the fatality has reduced proportionally as the dwellings of the population have been raised above the sea level. The epidemic began and was most fatal in the ports on the coast; and in ascending the rivers step by step, we saw it grow less and less fatal. This made it probable that a certain relation existed between elevation and the power of cholera to destroy life....

Elevation of the land involves several conditions which have an important effect on life and health. As we ascend, the pressure of the atmosphere diminishes, the temperature decreases, the fall of water increases, the vegetation varies and successive families of plants and animals appear in different zones of elevation.... As the rivers descend, the fall of their beds often grows less, and the water creeps sluggishly along, or oozes and meanders through the alluvial [*marshy*] soil. The drainage of the towns is difficult on the low ground, and the impurities of

Mortality from Cholera in London	
Mean Elevation of the Ground above the Thames High Water Mark	**Mean Mortality from Cholera per 10,000 People**
0	177
10	102
30	65
50	34
70	27
90	22
100	17
350	7

[*Farr observed that for each increase in elevation of 20 feet, the decline in mortality roughly followed the series 1/2, 1/3, 1/4, 1/5, 1/6. For example, the reported mortality for houses at an elevation of 50 feet was exactly 1/3 the mortality at 10 feet, and the mortality at 100 feet was exactly 1/6 the mortality at 10 feet. The correlation between mortality ratios and elevation was not always exact, but Farr believed the relationship was close enough to be significant.*]

FIGURE 5.2 William Farr's correlation of elevation and cholera mortality the earth lie on the surface, or filter into the earth. The wells and all the waters are infected. Where the houses are built on hill-sides and elevations, as in London, the sewage of each successive terrace flows through the terrace below it, and the stream widens, the ground becomes more charged, every successive step of the descent, until it is completely saturated in the parts lying below the high-water mark.

[*Farr's elevation theory also reflected his beliefs concerning the effect of environment on human societies in general. In this passage he adds arguments about the civilizations that have lived at higher elevations.*]

The people living on land of a certain elevation above the plains are not only safe from the attacks of cholera, remittent fever, yellow fever, and plague, but they are in a remark-able degree exempt from other maladies. Their functions are healthy, and their faculties are energetically developed. They present the finest type of the human race. This is evident not only in Cashmere, Georgia, and Circassia, but in all the hill-tribes of India.... The Arabs and the Abyssinians too, on the elevated lands of the desert, and on the sides of the mountains from which the Nile descends, present a striking superiority over the people of Lower Egypt; their fiery life, love of liberty, and warlike genius, place them immeasurably above the Fellahs....

The people bred on marshy coasts and low river margins, where pestilence is generated, live sordidly, without liberty, without poetry, without virtue, without sciences. They neither invent nor practise, the arts; they possess neither hospitals nor castles nor habitations fit to dwell in; neither farms, freeholds nor workshops. They are conquered and oppressed by successive tribes of the stronger races, and appear to be incapable of any form of society except that in which they are slaves....

On the high lands men feel the loftiest emotions. Every tradition places their origin there. The first nations worshipped there. High on the Indian Caucasus, on Olympus and on other lofty mountains, the Indians and the Greeks imagined the abodes of their highest gods; while they peopled the low underground regions, the grave-land of mortality, with infernal deities. These myths have a deep signification. Man feels his immortality in the hills.

On the Mode of Communication of Cholera—John Snow (London, 1855)

Snow used several types of evidence to argue that the cholera poison was waterborne: anecdotes about victims, data and a map from an outbreak in the Golden Square neighbor-hood, and a large-scale comparison of districts with different water supplies. The following passage discusses mortality during the Golden Square outbreak in 1854, which Snow investigated with data provided by William Farr at the GRO. Snow's famous map (see map 5.1) illustrated his claim that cholera spread to the neighborhood through water from the Broad Street pump.

The most terrible outbreak of cholera which ever occurred in this kingdom is probably that which took place in Broad Street, Golden Square, and the adjoining streets, a few weeks ago. Within 250 yards of the spot where Cambridge Street joins Broad Street, there were upwards of 500 fatal attacks of cholera in ten days. The mortality in this limited area probably equals any that was ever caused in this country, even by the plague; and it was much more sudden, as the greater number of cases terminated in a few hours....

I requested permission to take a list, at the General Register Office, of the deaths from cholera, registered during the week ending 2nd September, in the subdistricts of Golden Square, Berwick Street, and St. Ann's, Soho, which was kindly granted ... and I made inquiry, in detail, respecting the eighty-three deaths registered as having taken place during the last three days of the week.

On proceeding to the spot, I found that nearly all the deaths had taken place within a short distance of the pump. There were only ten deaths in houses situated decidedly nearer to another street pump. In five of these cases the families of the deceased persons informed me that they always sent to the pump in Broad Street, as they preferred the water to that of the pump which was nearer. In three other cases, the deceased were children who went to school near the pump in Broad Street. Two of them were known to drink the water; and the parents of the third think it probable that it did so....

In some of the instances, where the deaths are scattered a little further from the rest on the map, the malady was probably contracted at a nearer point to the pump. A cabinet-maker, who was removed from Philip's Court, Noel Street, to Middlesex Hospital, worked in Broad Street. A boy also who died in Noel Street, went to the National school at the end of Broad Street, and having to pass the pump, probably drank of the water. A tailor, who died at 6, Heddon Court, Regent Street, spent most of his time in Broad Street. A woman, removed to the hospital from 10, Heddon Court, had been nursing a person who died of cholera in Marshall Street....

As there had been deaths from cholera just before the great outbreak not far from this pump-well, and in a situation elevated a few feet above it, the evacuations [*i.e., feces*] from the patients might of course be amongst the impurities finding their way into the water, and judging the matter by the light derived from other facts and considerations previously detailed, we must conclude that such was the case.... [*An associate of John Snow, Henry Whitehead, later claimed that the first case of cholera in the neighborhood was an infant who came down with cholera a few days before the main outbreak. A cesspool where her mother emptied soiled diapers lay only a few feet from the Broad Street pump.*]

Whilst the presumed contamination of the water of the Broad Street pump with the evacuations of cholera patients affords an exact explanation of the fearful outbreak of cholera in St. James's parish, there is no other circumstance which offers any explanation at all, whatever hypothesis of the nature and cause of the malady be adopted.

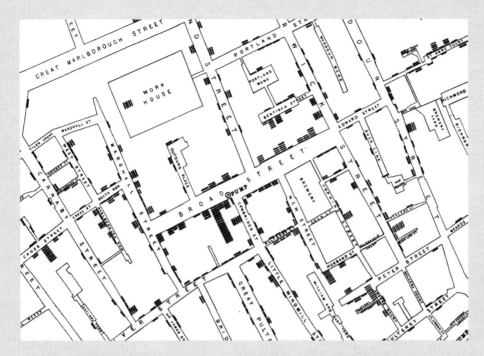

MAP 5.1 Detail of John Snow's cholera map and the Broad Street pump. This map (part of a larger one titled "Cholera in Golden Square, August–September 1854") demonstrated that cholera deaths in the Golden Square neighborhood, indicated by the black bars, correlated strongly with proximity to the Broad Street pump. Snow also found it significant that the nearby workhouse to the north had only a few deaths among several hundred occupants and the brewery to the east had none at all. Both facilities had their own pumps that provided uncontaminated water.

[*In a later passage Snow rejects Farr's elevation theory and cites his larger study of water districts to support the claim that cholera spreads in water.*]

Dr. Farr discovered a remarkable coincidence between the mortality from cholera in the different districts of London in 1849, and the elevation of the ground; the connection being of an inverse kind, the higher districts suffering least, and the lowest suffering most from this malady. Dr. Farr was inclined to think that the level of the soil had some direct influence over the prevalence of cholera, but the fact of the most elevated towns in this kingdom, as Wolverhampton, Dolais, Merthyr Tydfil, and Newcastle-upon-Tyne, having suffered excessively from this disease on several occasions, is opposed to this view, as is also the circumstance of Bethlehem Hospital, the Queen's Prison, Horsemonger Lane Gaol [*prison*], and several other large buildings, which are supplied with water from deep wells on the premises, having nearly or altogether escaped cholera, though situated on a very low level, and surrounded by the disease.

I expressed the opinion in 1849 that the increased prevalence of cholera in the low-lying districts of London depended entirely on the greater contamination of the water in these districts, and the comparative immunity from this disease of the population receiving the improved water from Thames Ditton [*i.e., water from the Lambeth Company*] during the epidemics of last year and the present, as shown in the previous pages, entirely confirms this view of the subject; for the great bulk of this population live in the lowest districts of the metropolis.

"Report on the Cholera Epidemic of 1866 in England"—William Farr (1868)

By 1868, Farr was persuaded that contaminated water was the main source of London's cholera. His statements reflect the influence of Filippo Pacini's observations as well as John Snow's analysis of water supplies. Farr suggests that the cholera "particles" or "corpuscles" are living beings, which explains why their impact on London is temporary. Despite his emphasis on the role of water, Farr does not give up on the concept of airborne transmission entirely.

Thus, by the year 1866, from the observation of the three great plagues, we had learned enough of the causation of cholera to justify us in believing that in London it could be confined within narrow limits—in the first place, by preventing any extensive distribution of the cholera-stuff through water, as the companies, in compliance with the water act of 1852, had, it was believed, since 1854 carried out all their purifying filtering works; and, in the second place, by the organization of the Health Officers, who could secure attention to the early treatment of premonitory diarrhea and to the destruction by disinfectants of the cholera flux....

It may appear at first sight impossible that the cholera flux of one or more patients should produce any effects in the waters of a river like the Thames. But living molecules endowed with the power of endless multiplication are inconceivably minute, and may be counted by millions in a drop of water. Pacini, an excellent microscopic observer, has found that the germs of vibrions (molecule vibrionali) are less than 1/25000 of an inch in diameter ... it is evident that a cubic inch might hold millions of cholera particles and one cholera patient might disseminate in water millions of millions of zymotic molecules....

The infection-power of cholera liquid is essentially transitory; it is developed in given circumstance in its intense form, and in a community as well as in an individual—in India as well as England—it grows as well as declines by a law of its own: it is epidemic only for a time and by periods of years. It has its seedtime and its harvest in each locality; and the air or water which one day is poisonous may a few days afterwards be harmless. There is thus an essential difference between zymotic venom and a metallic poison like arsenic.

[*In a later passage, Farr suggests that economic interests have contributed to a misunderstanding of cholera and argues again that contaminated water is the primary cause of the East London outbreak. Note the approving reference to the ancient Hippocratic text* Airs, Waters, Places.]

Hippocrates in his great work sought the causes of epidemics in earth, air and water. The discoveries of the nature of air by Boyle [*seventeenth-century English scientist Robert Boyle, who conducted well-known investigations on the properties of air*] and others fixed attention on that element in the last century; in recent times air has had its sectaries [*supporters*] and so has water; but as the air of London is not supplied like water to its inhabitants by companies the air has had the worst of it, both before parliamentary committees and royal commissions. For air no scientific witnesses have been retained, no learned counsel have pleaded; so the atmosphere has been freely charged with the propagation and the illicit diffusion of plagues of all kinds; while Father Thames, deservedly reverenced throughout the ages, and the water-gods of London, have been loudly proclaimed immaculate and innocent. If diseases spread they did it not, it was the air....

The population of London probably inhaled a few cholera corpuscles floating in the open air, and more rising from polluted waters and from the sewers, but the quantity thus taken from the air would be insignificant in its effects in comparison with the quantities imbibed through the waters of the rivers or of ponds into which cholera dejections [*i.e., vomit and sputum*], either in the diarrheal stage or the stage of collapse, had found their way and been mingled with sewage by the churning tides. During the height of the cholera explosion in East London nothing unusual was there visible in the atmosphere; the air was transparent and often bright in the sunshine; but the river Lea, close to the Old Ford reservoirs, and to the ponds from which the water was distributed in those fatal days, looked black, foul, contaminated ... only a very robust scientific witness would have dared to drink a glass of the waters of the Lea at Old Ford after filtration.

INTERPRETING THE DOCUMENTS

1. How does Farr's 1852 text describe the relationship between environment and culture? What do you think his attitude was toward the poor people of London? In general, how did perceptions of the poor shape the elite response to cholera in the nineteenth century?

2.   John Snow's analysis of the Golden Square outbreak includes points plotted on a map and interviews with the associates of cholera victims. How do the different types of information reinforce Snow's claim about the Broad Street pump?
3.   The Golden Square map includes sites with only a few cholera cases or none at all. Why was the absence of cholera just as important as its presence for Snow's argument?

MAKING CONNECTIONS

1.   By 1850, the notion that disease spread through the air was very old. Why did William Farr think he had solid evidence to support this view? How does his discussion of miasma or "zymotic" forces compare with the arguments made about yellow fever or earlier diseases?
2.   Compare Farr's perceptions of high elevations to European notions about tropical environments and peoples (see chapter 4). What served as the basis for racial stereotypes in each social and scientific context?
3.   Cholera epidemics were enabled by industrial technology and the new urban landscape of nineteenth-century cities. Can you give other examples of social or technological changes that influenced the spread of disease?

For further reading: John M. Eyler, "William Farr on the Cholera: The Sanitarian's Disease Theory and the Statistician's Method," *Journal of the History of Medicine and Allied Sciences* 27, no. 2 (1973): 79–100; Alfredo Morabia, "Snow and Farr: A Scientific Duet," *Sozial-Und Präventivmedizin* 46, no. 4 (2001): 217–24.

Notes

1. Quoted in Gillen D'Arcy Wood, *Tambora: The Eruption That Changed the World* (Princeton: Princeton University Press, 2014), 84.
2. Steven T. Rutherford and Bonnie L. Bassler, "Bacterial Quorum Sensing: Its Role in Virulence and Possibilities for Its Control," *Cold Spring Harbor Perspectives in Medicine* 2, no. 11 (2012): 13, https://doi.org/10.1101/cshperspect.a012427.
3. Eric Nelson et al., "Cholera Transmission: The Host, Pathogen and Bacteriophage Dynamic," *National Review of Microbiology* 7, no. 10 (2009): 2–3.

4. Guillaume Constantin de Magny and Rita R. Colwell, "Cholera and Climate: A Demonstrated Relationship," *Transactions of the American Clinical and Climatological Association* 120 (January 2009): 123–25.

5. P.R. Epstein et al., "Health and Climate Change: Marine Ecosystems," *The Lancet* 342 (1993): 1216–19.

6. Peter Baldwin, *Contagion and the State in Europe, 1830–1930* (Cambridge: Cambridge University Press, 1999), 41–59.

7. Richard J. Evans, *Death in Hamburg: Society and Politics in the Cholera Years* (New York: Penguin Books, 2005), 262.

8. Richard J. Evans, "Epidemics and Revolutions: Cholera in Nineteenth-Century Europe," *Past and Present* 120 (August 1988): 123–46.

9. Pamela K. Gilbert, *Cholera and Nation: Doctoring the Social Body in Victorian England* (Albany: SUNY Press, 2009), 57.

10. Ashleigh R. Tuite, Christina H. Chan, and David N. Fisman, "Cholera, Canals and Contagion: Rediscovering Dr. Beck's Report," *Journal of Public Health Policy* 32, no. 3 (2011): 320–33.

11. Charles Rosenberg, *The Cholera Years: The United States in 1832, 1849 and 1866*, rev. ed. (Chicago: University of Chicago Press, 2009), 62.

12. James Benedickson, *The Culture of Flushing: A Social History of Sewage* (Vancouver: UBC Press, 2011), ix.

13. Steven Johnson, *The Ghost Map: The Story of London's Most Terrifying Epidemic—and How It Changed Science, Cities, and the Modern World* (New York: Penguin, 2006), 7–11.

14. Friedrich Engels, *The Condition of the Working Class in England*, ed. David McLellan (Oxford: Oxford University Press, 2009).

15. Christopher Hamlin and Sally Sheard, "Revolutions in Public Health: 1848, and 1998?" *British Medical Journal* 317, no. 29 (1998): 587–91.

16. Quoted in Johnson, *Ghost Map*, 120.

17. Margaret Pelling, *Cholera, Fever and English Medicine, 1825–65* (Oxford: Oxford University Press, 1978), 70–79.

18. John M. Eyler, "William Farr on the Cholera: The Sanitarian's Disease Theory and the Statistician's Method," *Journal of the History of Medicine and Allied Sciences* 38, no. 2 (1973): 79–100.

19. Quoted in "Reviews," *Monthly Journal of Medical Science* New Series 3, ed. George E. Day, Alexander Fleming, and W.T. Gairdner (London, 1849): 919.

20. Quoted in Stephen Halliday, *The Great Stink of London: Sir Joseph Bazalgette and the Cleansing of the Victorian Metropolis* (Cheltenham: History Press, 2001), 96.

21. Peter Vinten-Johansen et al., *Cholera, Chloroform and Medicine: A Life of John Snow* (Oxford: Oxford University Press, 2003), 199–230.

22. Vinten-Johansen et al., *Cholera*, 254–317.

23. Marina Bentivoglio, "Filippo Pacini: A Determined Observer," *Brain Research Bulletin* 38, no. 2 (1995): 161–65.

24. Eyler, "Farr," 95–100.

25. Norman Howard-Jones, "The Scientific Background of the International Sanitary Conferences" (Geneva: World Health Organization, 1975), 9–41.

26. Alfredo Morabia, "Epidemiologic Interactions, Complexity, and the Lonesome Death of Max von Pettenkofer," *American Journal of Epidemiology* 166, no. 11 (2007): 1233–35.

27. Gerald L. Geison, *The Private Science of Louis Pasteur* (Princeton: Princeton University Press, 1995), 145–76.

28. Andrew Mendelsohn, "Biology, Medicine and Bacteria," *History and Philosophy of the Life Sciences* 24, no. 1 (2002): 3–36.

29. Thomas Schlich, "Linking Cause and Disease in the Laboratory: Robert Koch's Method of Imposing Visual and 'Functional' Representations of Bacteria," *History and Philosophy of the Life Sciences* 22, no. 1 (2000): 43–58.

30. Steve M. Blevins and Michael S. Bronze, "Robert Koch and the 'Golden Age' of Bacteriology," *International Journal of Infectious Diseases* 14 (2010): e744–51.

31. Mendelsohn, "Biology, Medicine and Bacteria," 13–15.

32. David Arnold, *Colonizing the Body: State Medicine and Epidemic Disease in Nineteenth-Century India* (Berkeley: University of Berkeley Press, 1996), 191–95.

33. Evans, *Death in Hamburg*.

34. Quoted in Paul Weindling, "A Virulent Strain: German Bacteriology as Scientific Racism, 1890–1920," in *Race, Science and Medicine, 1700–1960*, ed. Waltraud Ernst and Bernard Harris (London: Routledge, 2002), 218.

35. Arnold, *Colonizing the Body*, 161.

36. Sheldon Watts, *Epidemics and History: Disease, Power and Imperialism* (New Haven: Yale University Press, 1999), 204–207.

37. Epstein et al., "Health and Climate Change," 1216–19.

38. Luigi Vezzulli et al., "Climate Influence on *Vibrio* and Associated Human Diseases during the Past Half-Century in the Coastal North Atlantic," *Proceedings of the National Academy of Sciences* (8 August 2016): E5062–71.

39. R.R. Frerichs et al., "Nepalese Origin of Cholera Epidemic in Haiti," *Clinical Microbiology and Infection* 18, no. 6 (2012): E158–63.

40. Elliott D. Sclar, Pietro Garau, and Gabriella Carolini, "The 21st Century Health Challenge of Slums and Cities," *The Lancet* 365 (2005): 902–903.

41. Carl-Johan Neiderud, "How Urbanization Affects the Epidemiology of Emerging Infectious Diseases," *Infection Ecology and Epidemiology* 5, no. 1 (2015), http://dx.doi.org/10.3402

/iee.v5.27060; WHO, "Facts: Urban Settings as a Social Determinant of Health" (2018), http://who.int./social_determinants/publications/urbanization/factfile/en.

42. WHO, "Outbreak Update—Cholera in Yemen, 8 November 2018," http://www.emro.who.int/pandemic-epidemic-diseases/cholera/outbreak-update-cholera-in-yemen-8-november-2018.html.

43. M.A. Mengel, "Cholera Outbreaks in Africa," *Current Topics in Microbiological Immunology* 379 (2014), https://doi.org/10.1007/82_2014_369.

44. Morabia, "Epidemiologic Interactions," 1233–38.

45. Julian Davies and Dorothy Davies, "Origins and Evolution of Antibiotic Resistance," *Microbiology and Molecular Biology Reviews* 74, no. 3 (2010): 428.

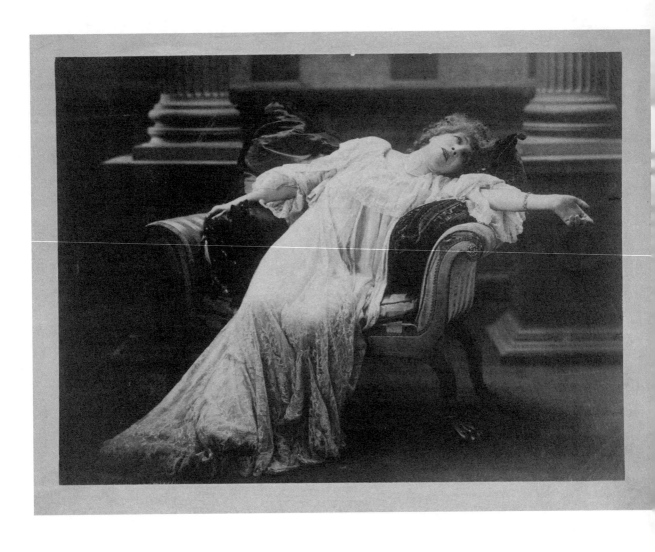

IMAGE 6.1 Actress Sarah Bernhardt in *La Dame aux Camélias* (ca 1890)

TUBERCULOSIS, SOCIAL CONTROL, AND SELF-CONTROL

6

No one died on stage like Sarah Bernhardt (ca 1844–1923). In 1880, the renowned French actress took the leading role in *The Lady of the Camellias* (*La Dame aux Camélias*, 1852), a play by Alexandre Dumas Jr, that depicted the exploits, redemption, and death from consumption of a Paris courtesan named Marguerite. For thirty years, in more than a thousand performances around the world, Bernhardt's passionate speeches, swoons, and coughs moved audiences to tears and thunderous applause. In 1911, she reprised the role in an early silent film that was well received in the United States as well as in France.

Bernhardt was a unique personality—she claimed to lie in a coffin as she prepared her lines—but many artists exploited the drama that was intrinsic to the malady that killed more people in the nineteenth century than any other. Cristóbal Rojas's sickbed portrait *Misery* (*La Miseria*, 1886), Giacomo Puccini's opera *The Bohemian* (*La Bohème*, 1890), and Thomas Mann's novel *The Magic Mountain* (*Der Zauberberg*, 1924) were all extraordinary works that evoked an ordinary reality for people around the world. Consumption was considered a "social disease," and its apparent causes—poverty, malnutrition, and overwork, compounded by hereditary or constitutional weakness—reflected widely held anxieties about the unhealthy effects of urban life. For many artists, the visibility and slow progression of its symptoms told a story of human vulnerability that was more apparent in some but common to all.

However, by the time Bernhardt's image flickered across a movie screen, the popular image of her signature malady was shifting. In the decades after Robert

Koch's discovery of a disease-causing microbe in 1882, the idea of a bacterial infection—tuberculosis—began to replace the ancient perception of a consuming, wasting affliction. Warnings about "germs" provided fodder for an emergent advertising culture that proclaimed the value of clean living for the growing middle classes of Western countries. The multilayered discourse about germs is a revealing instance of the transfer, and the transformation, of scientific knowledge as it entered the arenas of government, consumerism, and popular culture.

Etiology

Few things about tuberculosis are simple and none are fast. Most bacteria divide within minutes; *Mycobacterium tuberculosis* requires hours. Outbreaks of other diseases may last a few days or weeks, but epidemics of tuberculosis are measured in years or much longer. Today, over 2 billion people—between one-quarter and one-third of the global population—have been exposed to tuberculosis bacteria at some point in their lives. The WHO has estimated that 1.6 million people died from tuberculosis in 2017, including 0.3 million infected with HIV.[1]

M. tuberculosis is classified in a genus with nearly 200 species of mycobacteria. Some of these organisms live on dead or decaying matter, but about a dozen bacterial species—classified in the Mycobacterium tuberculosis complex (MBTC)—cause the symptoms of tuberculosis in animals. These pathogens infect cats, horses, and seals; they include a bacterial strain that affects cattle, *M. bovis*, which has long been recognized as a source of human tuberculosis. The bacteria that causes leprosy is also classified as a mycobacterium (*M. leprae*).

Tuberculosis has adapted to inhabit almost every organ in the human body. Pulmonary tuberculosis, which affects breathing and blood circulation in the lungs, is by far the most frequent form of infection. In spinal tuberculosis, the bacteria damage tissue between the vertebrae. This may cause a spinal curvature that, by the later eighteenth century, was named Pott's disease (for an eighteenth-century British surgeon, Percivall Pott). This characteristic deformity is a key clue for identifying tuberculosis in mummified corpses and other ancient remains. In the nervous system, the bacteria can cause meningitis, an inflammation of membranes that surround the brain and the spinal cord. Bacteria may also multiply in the lymph nodes and cause a large mass on the neck, a condition that for centuries was identified as scrofula. Weakness, dramatic weight loss, and night sweats accompany active infections, and these symptoms fueled a popular notion that tuberculosis destroys by consuming the body from within.

The course of pulmonary tuberculosis illustrates the pathogen's exquisite survival strategies and the challenge it poses for disease control. Bacteria are launched from one set of lungs to another by sneezes, coughs, or a conversation. In the lungs' tiny air sacs (alveoli), the bacteria reproduce slowly—dividing every twenty hours or so—while protected by sturdy cell walls that resist bodily acids and proteins. The body's first line of immune defense is to dispatch **macrophages**, cells designed to engulf and dissolve harmful microbes. In some cases, these cells destroy the bacteria; in others, macrophages and the rest of the immune system cannot contain the infection and active tuberculosis develops within one to three years. However, for the majority of infected persons, macrophages engulf the bacteria but do not destroy them. Instead, the bacteria enlist the body's own signaling proteins (cytokines) to summon additional cells to the site. The clustered cells form a cocooning nodule—called a granuloma, or tubercle—where infection can remain latent for many years.

These walled-off pathogens are dormant but not dead. The bacteria may reactivate and spread in individuals with weakened immune systems, including those who contract HIV. Recent research has shown that tuberculosis bacteria can feed on the remains of dead macrophage cells, replicating in the shell of their former attacker before escaping when conditions are ripe.[2] Therefore, efforts to control tuberculosis cannot merely halt new infections. They must also address the social factors that contribute to weakened immunity in the pool of latently infected persons. Why do some people develop this dreaded disease while others in similar social circumstances do not? This was a pressing question in the past and its answer remains elusive today.

Early History

Tuberculosis has been characterized as a "crowd disease" that, like measles or smallpox, became established as some human communities began to form large permanent settlements and domesticate livestock. As noted in chapter 3, however, not all current evidence clearly links smallpox's origins to early urbanization, and the same is true for tuberculosis. The ancestors of mycobacteria originated several hundred million years ago. Some genomic evidence suggests that mycobacteria began to co-evolve with humans in Africa about 70,000 years ago, and that tuberculosis found its human niche long before cattle were tamed. Cows may have humans to thank for tuberculosis rather than the other way around.

Distinct human strains of tuberculosis have evolved around the world for the last several thousand years or longer.[3] However, the ancient trail is blurred by the behavior of these bacteria over time. Mycobacteria have jumped from one species to another; this makes it difficult to track pathogens back to a common ancestor or to determine how humans and animals have traded and transformed them. In the last few centuries a strain of human tuberculosis that was prevalent in Europe spread to the Americas and Africa. This more virulent strain has supplanted other pre-existing ones and removed the traces of early mycobacteria in later populations. To understand the origins of tuberculosis, future research must reconcile findings from microbiology with what is known concerning early human settlements and migration patterns.[4]

In addition to ancient DNA and other physical remains, descriptions of maladies with tuberculosis-like symptoms survive in ancient Chinese, Ayurvedic (Indian), and Greek writings. In the second millennium BCE, Greek authors used the term *phthinein* to evoke a chronic wasting away or a process of being consumed. For a Hippocratic writer (ca fifth century BCE), the term *phthisis* referred to conditions that probably included pulmonary tuberculosis alongside pneumonia, various anemias, cancers, and other infections.[5]

Because leprosy and tuberculosis are now understood as mycobacterial cousins, historians have explored the relationship between these two diseases in Europe's later Middle Ages. This topic illustrates the challenge that arises when we apply modern disease categories to earlier social contexts. Beginning in the late eleventh century, many communities established leprosaria to serve as hospices for individuals who were disfigured and infirm. Hundreds of such facilities were founded after 1179, when Christian religious authorities formally mandated the separation of known lepers from the wider society. Starting in the fourteenth century, however, this movement waned. "Galloping consumption" emerged as a feared killer that was frequently observed by the sixteenth century while references to leprosy declined. Since tuberculosis is older in evolutionary terms than leprosy, and also more virulent, historians have suggested that tuberculosis progressively replaced leprosy as European cities increased in size and population density. Some research has also shown that infection with tuberculosis confers a degree of cross-immunity to leprosy. Increased incidence of tuberculosis, therefore, may have reduced the population that was susceptible to leprosy or caused high mortality among people who contracted both.

However, the imputed leprosy-tuberculosis relationship becomes less tidy when we consider other factors that influenced leprosaria in the medieval world. Europeans contributed to these institutions for reasons of religious piety as well as health, and often had an expansive definition of whom could be called a "leper." Evidence from ancient DNA analysis has confirmed that some individuals had leprosy in the modern sense (a mycobacterial infection), but others—how many is impossible to know—suffered from a range of chronic, disfiguring afflictions that other people simply wished to avoid. Widespread attitudes toward suspected lepers also shifted in the later Middle Ages. As Greco-Arabic medicine grew in influence during the thirteenth century, medical experts subjected these unfortunates to increased scrutiny. Authorities isolated and stigmatized them more aggressively, and the number of confirmed cases of the disease declined. Finally, individuals infected with *M. leprae* may have been more vulnerable to the Black Death and successive waves of plague, which, in any case, caused high mortality and reinforced fears about the spread of disease. In sum, the replacement of one mycobacteria by another may have hastened leprosy's decline in some instances, but this does not completely explain changes in social institutions or mortality patterns.[6]

By the mid-seventeenth century, "consumptions"—various conditions observed to cause wasting in the lungs—were considered a leading cause of death in European cities, and they would remain so for well over 200 years. According to the London Bills of Mortality in the 1660s "consumption and tissick" accounted for 2,000–3,000 deaths annually. Only plague was considered more lethal in that decade, and that was solely because the devastating epidemic of 1665 was held responsible for more than 60,000 deaths in the city. By the early nineteenth century, conditions were at least as bad, if not worse: in metropolises with populations in the hundreds of thousands, it is likely that the vast majority of inhabitants had latent infections. Perhaps one-fifth of all urban mortality was caused by tuberculosis, although conditions varied over time and by location. In times of food shortage or other deprivation, the residents of lower-class communities were primed for outbreaks. As the scale of industrial production increased, many people worked in occupations that increased their susceptibility to lung diseases by exposing them to coal dust, particles of cloth fiber, or toxic chemicals.

Unlike plague, smallpox, or diarrheal conditions that led swiftly to either death or recovery, consumptive illness unfolded gradually over months and years. It was everywhere—for the sick and their families, the true challenge was living with the malady rather than surviving it. Accordingly, there was incentive to frame chronic suffering in ways that made it more meaningful and easier to bear. Medical authorities held that consumption was caused by internal rot and decay, but other observers in the eighteenth and nineteenth centuries found more uplifting stories to tell.

"Consumptive Chic" and Social Criticism

There is nothing inherently alluring about bloody sputum, rattling coughs, emaciated bodies, or the other symptoms that many consumptives experienced. Nonetheless, as consumption emerged as a great scourge of urban life, perceptions of the malady intertwined with shifting notions of morality, civility, and even beauty. Before the eighteenth century, commentators idealized the "good" death as a struggle: a victory of virtue over evil in a contest for the soul, fortitude in the face of suffering, or a triumph over pain. While none of these concepts was explicitly rejected, eighteenth- and nineteenth-century sensibilities celebrated a more serene passing marked by contemplation and an acceptance of fate. Consumption's more violent symptoms were set aside to favor depictions of a slow, wasting ailment that softly bore people to their graves.

The privileging of what one recent scholar has termed "consumptive chic" derived from a venerable medical tradition.[7] Nineteenth-century physicians were still guided by the description of Aretaeus (ca first century CE) who described emaciated sufferers with coughing, sputum, and a persistent "febrile heat." Burning from within, the consumptive had a haunted appearance: "Nose sharp, slender; cheeks prominent and red; eyes hollow, brilliant and glittering...." Aretaeus found consumption most often in slender individuals whose shoulder blades "protrude like folding doors, or like wings; in those who have prominent throats; and those which are pale and have narrow chests."[8] Ancient doctors attributed such symptoms to humoral imbalance. Nineteenth-century physicians offered other explanations. Physician James Clark's influential manual *A Treatise on Pulmonary Consumptions* (1835) pointed to nervous excitability, especially in the young, as a contributing cause. Clark (1788–1870) and his contemporaries found that "consumptives" were often highly sensitive and intellectually precocious; their restless mental activity heightened their susceptibility to disease. The belief that certain people naturally were predisposed to the disease because of heredity or other innate qualities exerted influence into the twentieth century.

Perceptions of consumption mapped neatly onto notions of youthful passion that had roots in the Renaissance, and they also tapped into a network of images that linked love, death, and disease. Already in 1598, in the poem *Alba: The Months Minde of a Melancholy Lover*, English author Robert Tofte had represented consumption as a voracious fire in a pining lover: "Thus do I burne, and burning breath[e] my last, And breathing last, to naught consume away."[9] Nineteenth-century writers described the fires of creative genius in similar terms. A friend of the Romantic poet John Keats (1795–1821) remarked that Keats's early demise was written in his exquisitely refined features. To this observer, it was clear that "the flame burning within would shortly consume the outward shell [Keats's body]."[10] In other contexts, a consumptive malady signaled an effeminate spirit or constitution. Apart from high-strung male artists, it was women who were deemed most vulnerable. Dumas's story of a woman redeemed by love before her death inspired not only *The Lady of the Camellias* but also the acclaimed Italian opera *The Fallen Woman* (*La Traviata*, 1853) by composer Giuseppe Verdi (1813–1901). This cultural framing of tuberculosis was not limited to Western nations. As William Johnston and Fukuda Mahito have shown, in the late nineteenth century Japanese poets and novelists presented a similarly idealized vision of the fragile, graceful tuberculous person. The popular novel *The Cuckoo* (*Hototogisu*) by Kenjirō Tokutomi, printed numerous times after 1899, depicted a woman's affliction with tuberculosis as she faced family strife and wartime turmoil.[11]

For European and American audiences that were versed in Christian religious tropes, narratives of redemptive suffering also evoked humanity's rescue by the suffering of Christ. Authors exploited this analogy for didactic purposes in many works of fiction and nonfiction. In the United States, Harriet Beecher Stowe's wildly popular antislavery novel *Uncle Tom's Cabin* (1852) featured Eva, an angelic slave owner's daughter who dies of consumption after befriending the pious slave Tom. The novel contrasted Eva's own spiritual purity, and her dying wish that Tom be freed, with the immoral enslavement of one Christian to another. For other writers, the drawn-out symptoms of consumption invited engagement with a centuries-old tradition of saintly suffering. This theme guided a young French nun, Thérèse of Lisieux (1873–1897), whose autobiographical *Story of a Soul* (*Histoire d'une âme*, 1897) chronicled her painful demise among her convent sisters. Bedridden and racked with painful coughs, Thérèse embraced her trial as a path to become a true bride of Christ. In such works, the good death from consumption affirmed feminine purity and the primacy of the spiritual realm, while rejecting material pleasure, fallen sexuality, and social injustice.

Social reformers rejected such affectations. Poverty might be ennobling, but consumption's miseries were not: they symbolized a society in which the urban masses toiled and died in a heartless, unhealthy world. The novelist Charles Dickens testified to London's inhumane conditions in works such as *Nicholas Nickleby* (1838) and *A Christmas Carol* (1843) that critiqued the exploitive relationships created by capitalism. Karl Marx (1818–1883) famously linked consumptive disease, working conditions, and capitalism in *Capital* (1867). Marx cited statistics indicating that workers required 500 cubic feet of space to ensure good health. Since factory labor made this impossible, he concluded, "consumption and other lung diseases among the workforce are necessary conditions to the existence of capital."[12]

The relationship of poverty and respiratory illness has been a theme among historians of disease ever since Marx's day. However, explanations of consumption underwent a profound change in the 1880s, as the emerging field of microbiology radically altered perceptions of the entire natural world. Although medical treatments changed little at first, over time the introduction of germ theories prompted important changes at every level of society.

A New World of Germs

In the history of Western medicine, few turning points are clearer than Robert Koch's presentation to the members of the Berlin Physiological Society on 24 March 1882. His research team had isolated a rod-shaped microbe that Koch initially named *Tuberkelvirus*. Unlike Edward Jenner and some other predecessors, Koch used the term "virus" to mean "infective agent" (no one yet firmly distinguished between bacteria, viruses, and other microbes). Koch's team had cultivated the microbe, inoculated guinea pigs with it, isolated more samples from the diseased animals, and performed the cycle again. In his presentation, Koch did more than talk: he brought microscopes with hundreds of stained slides, inviting his astonished audience to judge with their own eyes. After Koch published his findings less than three weeks later, news of the discovery was rapidly translated and circulated around the world.

Koch was not an isolated genius. Already in the late seventeenth century, some physicians had referred to tubercles—from *tuberculum*, a Latin word for hump or little hill—to refer to the nodules that were a principle symptom of the disease.[13] In 1877, Edwin Klebs had suggested that tuberculosis was caused by a microbe. Koch also acknowledged a debt to the French researcher Jean Antoine Villemin (1827–1892), who tested the transmissibility of tubercular material with cows and rabbits during the 1860s. But Koch's confident pronouncements vaulted him to worldwide fame and, likewise, elevated the significance of bacteriology to a new plane. In a world where, by his own estimate, one in seven people died from consumption, Koch offered a disarmingly simple explanation: living microbes entered the body, multiplied, and attacked to cause disease.

This claim had far-reaching implications. Koch offered a powerful explanation both for the etiology of diseases (i.e., their initial causes) and for their spread. First, with regard to etiology, the identification of the tuberculosis bacteria unified seemingly disparate ailments. Although previous researchers had linked scrofula, Pott's disease, and various lung consumptions, Koch convincingly explained that all of these maladies were caused by one species of microbe. Conversely, distinct species of microbes caused different ailments. Cholera, pneumonia, plague, typhoid—all would soon be understood as a result of infection with a particular pathogen. Second, Koch reframed debates concerning the spread of disease and the respective roles of miasma, contagion, and heredity (or "predisposition"). According to Koch, the chief aim of disease control was to prevent living microbes from entering the body or multiplying inside the body. This focus promised to reorient medicine and public health. More broadly, the new bacteriology revealed a realm of existence that was invisible to everyone except a few elite researchers with the right equipment and training.

Koch's laboratory at Germany's Imperial Health Office developed cornerstone methods for the emerging field of research. One early task was to find a solid medium in which researchers could isolate pure cultures of bacteria. Experiments with egg whites and potato slices proved inadequate. Gelatin, a meat extract, was also tried, but its melting temperature was too low and some bacteria could eat through it. In 1881, lab assistant Angelina Fanny Hesse (1850–1934) suggested an algae extract, agar-agar, which cooks used to thicken soups and jellies. "Frau Hesse's medium" was remarkable. It was inedible for bacteria; it remained firm at temperatures up to 85 degrees Celsius but, when cooled, it did not congeal until falling to about 40 degrees Celsius. The agar gel could be inoculated with bacteria when cool and would remain firm at the higher temperatures necessary to incubate the bacteria. Additives improved the gel's performance. In 1887, another Koch assistant, Julius Richard Petri (1852–1921), devised a container with an overhanging lid—the Petri dish—that would prevent contamination of bacterial samples. Refinements continued, but by 1890 the essential methods were available to study a wide range of microbes.

SCIENCE FOCUS

Dye Another Day: Stains in Microbiology and Medicine

Innovations in one realm of science often have remarkable applications in another. Staining agents were first invented to color cloth for a growing textile industry, but they now perform many valuable functions in medical chemistry. Researchers and physicians have used them to observe and classify microbes and sometimes even to treat diseases.

In the later nineteenth century, researchers derived numerous organic chemical compounds from coal tar, which was a common by-product of the processes used to manufacture steel. One of these compounds, aniline, provided a basis for many stains that are used in microbiology, including methylene blue (as well as many other products such as foam rubber, tape, and plastics). Robert Koch's team used methylene blue to stain samples containing tuberculosis. When this dye was combined with a counterstain, the tuberculosis bacteria glowed bright blue against a dull background. Because stains illuminated microbes for untrained observers, they were a powerful tool of persuasion as microbiologists communicated with other scientists and the public.

A staining procedure devised in 1882 by the Danish researcher Hans Christian Gram (1853–1938) enabled later researchers to classify bacteria according to differences in their cell walls. In "Gram-positive" bacteria, the cell walls have a thick layer of sugars and amino acids (peptidoglycans) outside of a membrane (figure 6.1). This layer will retain a violet stain even after the bacteria are treated with a decoloring chemical such as ethyl alcohol. In "Gram-negative" bacteria, the peptidoglycan layer is thinner and sandwiched between two membranes. The outer membrane includes complex molecules (lipopolysaccharides) that help the bacteria resist antibiotics. Gram-negative bacteria that are treated with a decoloring chemical will not retain the violet stain, but they will hold a red (safranin) stain with a different chemical makeup. Although refinements continue, the Gram stain procedure is still used for the initial analysis of tissue samples.

Early microbiologists, notably Paul Ehrlich, also recognized that dyes could inactivate or kill certain species of microbes. Ehrlich focused on trypanosomes, single-celled parasites that cause sleeping sickness and various animal diseases. In 1891, Ehrlich demonstrated that

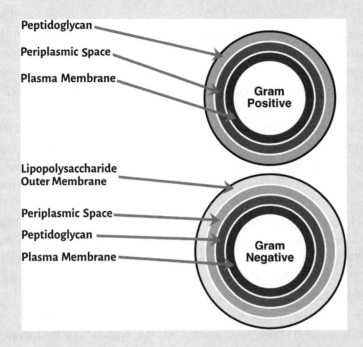

FIGURE 6.1 Gram-positive and Gram-negative bacteria. The Gram-negative bacteria include *Escherichia coli*, *Yersinia pestis*, and *Neisseria gonorrhoeae*. The lipopolysaccharides in the outer membrane have a toxic action that elicits a response from animal immune systems and defends against some chemical agents.

methylene blue could treat malaria, and a decade later he tested more than 100 synthetic dyes as treatments for diseases that afflicted horses and cattle. Although Ehrlich did not develop a sleeping sickness treatment himself, other researchers continued his line of inquiry and conducted tests of thousands of chemical compounds. In 1917, scientists at the Bayer Company synthesized Bayer 205, later renamed suramin, which remains a treatment for the early stages of one form of sleeping sickness. German chemists also synthesized quinacrine, a yellow dye that, in the 1940s, became a widely used antimalarial drug. In 1935, a red dye marketed as Prontosil became the first widely available sulfonamide, a group of synthetic medicines that cured a wide range of infections caused by bacteria including syphilis, strep throat, and meningitis.

Indeed, drugs derived from dyes may become more important as other medications lose their potency. In the 2010s, malaria researchers turned to methylene blue with renewed interest because malaria parasites had developed resistance to other drugs. Investigation confirmed that the dye prevents parasites from metabolizing hemoglobin in the human blood stream. In 2017, a study in Mali found that the dye contributed to effective treatment when it was added to other medications. All the results were promising except for one minor drawback: the dye turned the patients' urine blue.[14]

Simultaneously, Koch experimented with techniques to help researchers distinguish the innumerable organic forms that became visible with a microscope. He and other researchers turned to aniline dyes—chemicals produced from coal tar—that German textile producers used to color fabric. Koch had stained his anthrax samples for photography, but the tuberculosis microbes were much smaller and they did not respond to the first attempts to color them. Koch's team used methylene blue dye to confirm that a particular bacteria was always present in sick animals but not in healthy ones, and that the bacteria's appearance preceded the formation of tubercles. The presence of the microbe, not tubercles or other symptoms, signaled tuberculosis, regardless of where it manifested in the body. Koch had begun his career as a physician, but his meticulous, technical research—and his perspective on the cause of disease—now focused on the actions of microbes rather than the characteristics of the human bodies that they invaded. In 1890, Koch published a refined version of the procedural steps his team had developed that later were known as "Koch's Postulates."

The limits of Koch's approach would soon be clear, and some theorists continued to argue that the "soil" (the context within which germs spread) was as important as the microbial "seed" itself. A few even maintained that germs were merely a by-product of diseases that had other environmental or hereditary causes. Nonetheless, German microbiology enjoyed a remarkable run of success in the decade after Koch published his anthrax photographs in 1877. As noted in chapter 2, Albert Neisser isolated the gonorrhea bacteria in 1879. Albert Fraenkel identified *Streptococcus pneumoniae* in 1886, thus helping to distinguish pneumonia from tuberculosis. Among Koch's close associates, in 1883–84 Loeffler cultured the diphtheria pathogen (*Corynebacterium diphtheriae*) that Edwin Klebs had recently identified, and another Koch pupil, Georg Gaffky (1850–1918), confirmed the bacteria that causes typhoid (*Salmonella typhi*). The most spectacular coup was Koch's victory against French and English teams in the global race to identify the cholera bacteria, *V. cholerae*, in 1884 (see chapter 5). Koch received accolades from the German government, and he was awarded a professorship in hygiene at the University of Berlin.

These were stellar achievements, but Koch felt pressure to produce something more. The ultimate goal, after all, was to prevent or cure disease. Although Koch's claims speedily gained the attention of public health officials, effective vaccines and treatments proved elusive. In 1885, Koch's archrival Louis Pasteur seized the spotlight with the spectacular treatment of young Joseph Meister and other rabies patients. To Koch, this was a biting humiliation: not only was Pasteur a Frenchman, he offered a different vision of disease-causing microbes. Pasteur claimed that a pathogen's virulence could be attenuated, and he had used a procedure of successive injections to cure disease. This seemed to contradict Koch's claims that bacterial species were distinct and displayed unchanging characteristics, although, as Mendelsohn has shown, Koch was not inherently opposed to the idea of variable virulence and even complimented Pasteur on the discovery.[15] What may have annoyed Koch the most was that Pasteur secured financial support to create an independent research institute while Koch, now a university professor, was burdened by teaching and administrative tasks that he disliked.

The desire for swift success contributed to Koch's greatest failure, an abortive attempt to produce a cure for tuberculosis. After months of work in secret, Koch announced in August 1890 that he had found a substance that halted the growth of tubercle bacilli in guinea pigs. The findings were tentative, but Koch was soon besieged with pleas for help and he promised to release the remedy, soon called tuberculin, in November. Simultaneously, he negotiated with the Prussian Ministry of Culture, attempting to found a research institute while retaining the profits from tuberculin for several years. After numerous patients received injections, by early 1891 there were signs that tuberculin's beneficial effects were wildly overblown and that it sometimes even caused harm. When Koch revealed that tuberculin was little more than a glycerin extract of the tubercle bacilli, critics accused him of fraud. More tests confirmed that injections of small amounts of tuberculin caused immune reactions (in cattle as well as humans) and that this procedure could identify individuals who had been exposed to the bacteria. The diagnostic value of "Koch's lymph" was soon recognized, and it became an important tool for public health surveillance. But it was not the longed-for cure; instead, tuberculin demonstrated that the relationship of human bodies and bacterial pathogens was influenced by many physiological and environmental factors. A disease could not be explained or cured merely by isolating a microbe. The failure of tuberculin forced Koch to settle for a position as director of the Berlin Institute for Infectious Diseases rather than found an institute with greater independence from the Prussian government.

In Koch's circle, the first dramatic breakthrough in therapy came in the early 1890s from research on diphtheria led by Emil Behring (1854–1917). Once known as the "strangling angel," diphtheria is caused by highly contagious bacteria that spread through respiratory droplets. A common symptom is a thick, gray coating on mucous membranes that blocks the trachea and causes suffocation. Diphtheria was a leading cause of infant mortality in the nineteenth century, particularly after an epidemic that spread worldwide from Europe in the late 1850s. Research at the Pasteur Institute demonstrated in the 1880s that diphtheria's symptoms were caused by a toxin emitted by the bacteria rather than the bacteria themselves. In 1891, Behring injected increasing doses of diphtheria toxin into animal subjects and found that infected guinea pigs, sheep, and horses naturally produced material (called antibodies by later scientists) that neutralized it. With help from Ehrlich and the chemical company Hoechst, Behring used sheep and horses to produce a serum that he called "antitoxin." After Ehrlich published results of a clinical trial in 1894, many German cities introduced the new treatment and diphtheria mortality dropped in the country by more than 50 per cent in one year. Serum treatments also had some success in trials against tetanus and bubonic plague.

Some recent historians have pointed out that the new therapy did not cause the dramatic decline in diphtheria mortality all by itself. As bacteriological testing became more routine, many infected individuals were isolated and prevented from spreading the disease. Other childhood diseases such as scarlet fever, measles, and whooping cough were also waning, so it is possible that diphtheria antitoxin merely hastened a broader change that was already underway.[16] But to many people in the early 1900s, the antitoxin was a remarkable advance that illustrated the promise of public health strategies that targeted disease-causing microbes. Even when diseases could not be cured, officials armed with microscopes could now identify infected individuals and protect the community. Such sentiments also reinforced the response to the influenza pandemic of 1918, although at the time no effective vaccines or treatment for influenza were available.

In both the public sphere and domestic settings, new hygiene practices and products reflected a novel desire to avoid germs. As public health campaigns proclaimed crusades against invading microbes, measures to treat and cure "TB" held a special place in the quest for a healthy, well-regulated morality. Whereas earlier sanitary campaigns had emphasized public infrastructure, after 1890 public health authorities increasingly stressed the linkage between hygienic behavior, membership in society, and obedience to the state.

The Healthy Citizen and the Healthy State, 1880–1920

Health and hygiene received particular attention at international borders, which became increasingly busy after 1850. Millions of people migrated within Europe as industrialization displaced some workers and created opportunities for others.

Greater still was the tide of immigration across the Atlantic that brought more than 20 million people to ports in the United States and Canada between 1880 and 1920. The new arrivals were more diverse than the British islanders who had comprised the majority of immigrants earlier in the nineteenth century. Poles, Ukrainians, Italians, and Scandinavians sought factory jobs in eastern cities or farmsteads in the prairies. In the West, thousands of Chinese families found opportunities in coastal cities or in labor camps for railroad construction and mining. Just as Irish immigrants had been targets of suspicion, the newcomers were often presumed to be of inferior hereditary stock. Alongside concerns about ethnic diversity, the pandemics of cholera and bubonic plague in the 1890s provided more justification for stringent border control.

Before 1930, the majority of US immigrants entered the country at Ellis Island, New York, where the federal government opened a port of entry in 1892. In the shadow of the Statue of Liberty, an encounter with public health officers introduced lower-class travelers to the degree of regulation they could expect in their new country. While first- and second-class passengers were exempted from rigorous inspections or interviewed in their ship cabins, steerage passengers faced the prospect of being called out of line to disrobe, endure poking and prodding, and sometimes give samples of blood or urine. The conditions during the trans-Atlantic crossing served to reinforce biases that were rooted in ethnic and class distinctions. After several weeks in a crowded ship's hold with poor food, scarce water, and improper sanitation, it is no surprise that many travelers emerged weak, dirty, and sick. Although bacteriological examinations were infrequent before 1915, Ellis Island officials performed more than 20,000 laboratory tests in 1921.[17] At west-coast ports such as Angel Island near San Francisco, Asian immigrants often faced deportation after examination for **trachoma**, an eye disease that (officials claimed) was especially common among Chinese because of the shape of their eyelids. Some would-be immigrants were detained for weeks or sent home. For the rest, the spectacle of medical examination demonstrated the state's intention to enforce standards of health and obedience for the nation's workers and citizens.

Many US cities grew sharply in size, especially New York. By 1900, the combined population of its five boroughs was 3.4 million, over twice the number of the nation's second largest city, Chicago. In part because of the arrival of so many seemingly "unwashed" immigrants, public health advocates expressed alarm over the risks of disease among jostling crowds in public spaces and large families crammed into small, squalid dwellings. The earlier sanitarian focus on neighborhood planning, street cleaning, and sewer systems was now accompanied by recommendations concerning individual behavior. The prescriptions often had a moralizing tone. In metropolises such as London, Paris, or New York, nothing inspired greater outrage than the practice of spitting. Writers brooded over a habit they regarded as repulsive and potentially deadly. In a medical dissertation published in 1908, one Paris researcher even counted 875 wads of spit (*crachat*) on the boulevard between the Opera and the famed Rue Montmartre.[18] At gatherings of workers and employers, officials cautioned against the germ-filled "homicidal crachat" that lay in wait to contaminate the sole of a shoe. Some advocated for a complete ban on public spitting. Since most people considered this impractical—smokeless tobacco was popular among men at the time—experts instead vilified spitting on the floor and demanded spittoons filled with sawdust for public places.[19] Tuberculosis patients were encouraged to use personal spittoons, although some objected that it was undignified to use them in public or to wash them out.

Another focus of attention was drinking water, an urban amenity that benefited not only human travelers but also horses and cattle that traveled long distances. Many nineteenth-century cities offered fountains or wells with a cup for general use that was attached by a chain. In the United States, voices were raised to defend such "common cups" after public health officials warned that they might spread disease. Railway operators suggested that passengers would be inconvenienced without them; advocates of alcoholic temperance fretted that men in need of a drink would find one at a saloon instead. As common cups began to disappear, some buildings installed vending machines with paper cups, but even a minimal charge was a hardship for the poor and an annoyance for everyone else. After many states banned common cups in the 1910s, some cities installed public drinking fountains, or "bubble fountains," that pushed a stream of water straight up from a pipe. Later designs added a mouth guard to the nozzle and angled the stream to prevent contaminated water from falling back to the basin.[20]

As national governments increased the regulation of consumer products, some contentious questions concerned cows rather than people. As discussed in chapter 7, in the mid-nineteenth century the health of European livestock received increased attention after waves of cattle disease decimated herds and prodded governments into action. In 1890, after Koch's experiments demonstrated tuberculin's diagnostic properties, veterinarians immediately began testing cattle for bovine tuberculosis. They found substantial rates of infection in many herds, but officials disagreed on the necessary countermeasures.

Scandinavian countries and parts of Germany adopted the view of Danish veterinarian Bernard Bang (1848–1932), who advocated tuberculin testing of all animals, isolation of those that tested positive, and slaughter of cattle that showed signs of advanced disease. Other countries were more cautious; the tuberculin test was not always accurate and its repeated use was disruptive for animals on the farm. In 1901, Koch himself sowed controversy at an international conference when he suggested that bovine tuberculosis posed little risk to humans and pulmonary tuberculosis should remain the focus of attention. Although Koch eventually modified his view, the confusion caused years of indecision and delay, particularly in Europe. The United States began a national campaign for tuberculin testing of cattle in 1917 and Canada followed suit in 1923, but similar measures were not initiated in Germany until after World War II or in Great Britain until the 1960s.

The **pasteurization** of milk was another topic of heated debate. By 1910, studies of American cities estimated that roughly 10 per cent of the deaths among infants and young children—especially from diphtheria and typhoid— were caused by tainted milk.[21] Opponents of pasteurization objected that heating milk changed the taste and diminished its nutritional value. Dairy farmers protested against the procedure's expense. Questions lingered concerning the temperature and length of time the procedure required in order to reap safety benefits. However, support for pasteurization grew steadily among physicians and the public, particularly as the scale of milk distribution grew and supplies from many dairies were pooled in regional storage facilities. In 1908, Chicago became the first American city to require pasteurization and New York began to enforce a previously adopted ordinance in 1914. The procedure became widespread in the United States during the 1920s, France in 1935, and Britain in 1960.[22]

As the previous examples suggest, the United States took the initiative in various public health arenas as its population and industrial capacity rapidly expanded. But elsewhere, too, often beginning at the local level, governments took steps to cleanse streets of animal waste, inspect factories, impose building codes and require repairs, and assert quality control over water, food, and drink. These public health and sanitary measures did more to reduce mortality, particularly in cities, than cures and other targeted medical interventions.[23] The enforcement of regulations not only improved the health of citizens, it provided a source of legitimacy for state authorities and a foundation for intervention in other arenas. The growing middle classes in Europe and North America matched state-sponsored measures with attempts to control the spread of germs among individuals and in homes.

Sanitoria and the Reform of Behavior

From the 1880s forward, the trend toward germ theories—and the shift from "consumption" to "tuberculosis," in particular—presented new puzzles for public health advocates, medical practitioners, and the sick. On one hand, germ theories explained the cause and spread of various diseases in ways that had broad repercussions for hospital procedures. Greater attention was paid to the dangers posed by microbes and the need to isolate the sick, although many reforms took decades to implement. On the other hand, germ theories offered few improvements in treatment. Especially for tuberculosis, the remission of symptoms still seemed dependent on many individual factors, and total cure seemed a remote prospect. Thus, the standard treatment repertoire harkened back to ancient times: nourishing food and drink, combined with suitable rest and exercise in fresh air and sunshine. As the prestige of scientific medicine increased, such regimens of care fell under the authority of trained practitioners. These now increasingly included nurses, who asserted that their expertise with hygiene and bodily regimens could influence the progress of disease in individuals and also lessen spread of tuberculosis in populations.[24] In the absence of effective treatment for tuberculosis and other infectious diseases, authorities considered prevention the most effective weapon.

In hospitals, facilities for surgery and postoperative care were among the sites to revise procedures in response to germ theories. Traditionally, patients who underwent operations such as amputations or the setting of compound bone fractures faced extraordinary danger of systemic illness caused by invading microbes. This was true not only in harsh environments such as battlefields but also in surgical wards. Doctors and nurses circulated freely between different parts of the hospital (and the morgue). While some attended to the cleanliness of hands and tools, no steps were systematically taken to reduce the risk of contamination by health workers. This began to change after 1860, as surgeons incorporated findings by Louis Pasteur and others. In a lengthy paper published over several issues of *The Lancet* medical journal (1867), the influential British surgeon Joseph Lister (1827–1912) advanced the claim that surgical infections were caused by minute organisms that floated in the air. Lister's meticulous writings stressed attention to detail and the manual skills that **antiseptic** surgery demanded.[25] At first, he recommended chemical disinfection of surgical tools by dipping them in carbolic acid—already in use to preserve cadavers—and the use of wound dressings soaked in the disinfectant. He later devised a long-handled pump that sprayed carbolic acid solution into the air. Initially an object of ridicule, by the 1880s Lister's "donkey engine" symbolized a widely accepted principle: surgeons ought to follow antiseptic procedures to prevent germs from penetrating a wound and causing infection.

Listerian antisepsis offered procedures that combined the new science of microbes with the earlier sanitarian approach to clean environments. As discussed previously, the identification of numerous pathogens in the 1880s quickly shifted attention to their direct, local effects. By 1890, even Lister acknowledged that chemical sprays in the air were relatively ineffective and that more targeted measures were necessary. Progressive institutions such as the Johns Hopkins Hospital in Baltimore attempted instead to provide **aseptic** surgical environments that were entirely free of germs. Steam and heat were substituted for chemicals as the means of sterilizing equipment. In various European and North American hospitals, practitioners experimented with surgical gowns and masks. Nurses at Johns Hopkins were among the first to use thin rubber gloves, which were provided by the Goodyear Rubber Company after a special request from the hospital's chief surgeon, William Halsted (1852–1922).[26] After 1900, survival rates from surgical procedures markedly improved. As hospitals adopted germicidal procedures, they began to shed their reputation as gateways to death for the poor and disadvantaged.

Germ theories had less immediate impact upon practices in **sanatoria**, facilities that were dedicated to the treatment of tuberculosis. These facilities reflected widely held sentiments that medicine and morality went hand in hand and industrial cities were unhealthy for people with frail constitutions. Beginning in the mid-nineteenth century, practitioners had experimented with cures in peaceful alpine and forest retreats. Provisions to fund sanatorium treatment were included in Germany's national insurance scheme after 1884 and in Britain's National Insurance Act of 1911. By 1920 there were roughly 130 such institutions in Germany and 175 in England and Wales.[27] This model spread across the Atlantic to American patients who previously had sought open-air cures in mountain resorts or the warm, dry southwest. Many US and Canadian facilities were inspired by Edward Livingston Trudeau (1848–1915), whose cottages in the idyllic setting of Saranac Lake, New York, provided cures and a training ground in sanatorium methods. In 1900, 34 institutions in the United States offered nearly

4,500 beds; a quarter-century later, 536 institutions treated nearly 675,000 people, a total that approached 0.6 per cent of the nation's population.[28]

Some of these facilities, particularly in Germany, were publicly funded while others were sponsored by large companies or workers' unions. Conditions in them varied widely. A few institutions offered a pampered existence to the wealthy, attended by servants as they lay swaddled in blankets on open-air porches, took carefully regulated strolls, and checked their temperature at intervals. More often, sanatorium patients faced a humdrum, carefully monitored routine in a ward where they were expected to follow a doctor's instructions and sometimes to participate in "graduated labor" such as housekeeping or office work. One anonymous author in Melbourne, Australia, described the rigid environment in the sanatorium as akin to a religious convent.[29] This is, perhaps, not surprising: both institutions separated their inhabitants from the broader world and provided an atmosphere in which personal bodily care was to merge with morally uplifting behavior. Unlike convents, however, sanitoria were conceived as temporary institutions from which patients were expected to depart with new skills of self-maintenance for their chronic, infectious condition.

Armed with the tuberculin diagnostic test, public health advocates also focused their energies on the prevention of tuberculosis in children. After 1908, when the tuberculin test procedure was promoted at an international congress in Washington, practitioners increasingly referred to a new category of "pre-tubercular" individuals who did not display symptoms of disease but whose tests revealed exposure to the bacteria. Beginning in Farmingdale, New Jersey (1909), dozens of institutions known as "preventoria" provided strict regimens of rest, food, and outdoor activity for children who were deemed at risk. Such facilities were run almost entirely by nurses, who were charged not only with the children's well-being but also with home visits to ensure that the children would return to healthy, well-regulated environments. "Our purpose," one Farmingdale administrator wrote, "is to *permanently* save every child that comes to us."[30]

Despite such ambitions for social improvement, not everyone could enter such a facility. Poor individuals often could not afford an extended period away from work and family. In France, where suspicion of German methods fostered indifference to such institutions, home-based care was coordinated by dispensaries that were sponsored by various charities and government offices. These storefronts provided laundry services, food, and milk; some conducted home visits to advise patients on hygiene and routine for the tuberculous patient. Dispensaries treated patients as a source of infection and encouraged protective measures for family and friends. "[T]he cure of a consumptive is a meritorious work," noted one Paris observer in 1908, "but ... it is still better to prevent the healthy from contracting the disease."[31] After a slow beginning in the 1910s, by the early 1920s hundreds of facilities provided a watchful presence in French and British cities.

In some cases, surveillance of the sick was more overt. Cities in Belgium and France compiled *casiers sanitaires*, dossiers that cataloged the sanitary conditions and cases of disease in various neighborhoods. In 1893, New York City's health department started a similar register, and in 1897 it required doctors to report the names and addresses of all new tuberculosis cases. Dozens of American cities followed suit, despite protests from some patients and physicians. Since public health departments often shared information with other agencies, many individuals faced discrimination as they sought housing, insurance, and employment.[32]

Alongside charities and workers' associations, anti-tuberculosis leagues also assisted the public with fund-raising and awareness campaigns. After France founded a national anti-tuberculosis association in 1891, the idea spread to numerous other nations in the next two decades. Like the dispensaries, such leagues aimed to educate tuberculosis sufferers and their caregivers in hopes of protecting the general public. Central to this mission was the belief that householders could obtain the knowledge and

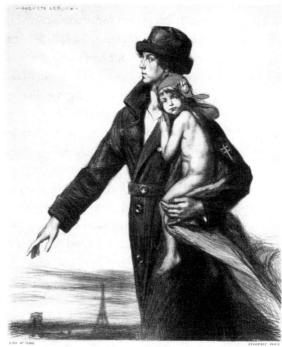

LA VISITEUSE D'HYGIÈNE VOUS MONTRERA LE CHEMIN DE LA SANTÉ ELLE MÈNE UNE CROISADE CONTRE LA TUBERCULOSE ET LA MORTALITÉ INFANTILE. SOUTENEZ-LA !

IMAGE 6.2 French public health awareness poster: "The public health nurse will show you the path to health. She leads a crusade against tuberculosis and infant mortality. Support her!" In this poster from ca 1920, created by Jules Marie Auguste Leroux, the woman's military bearing evokes the call to defend the French in battle during World War I. Personal and family hygiene are linked to national objectives. The public health nurse is cast as a figure of courage and authority.

skills necessary for disease control. As historian Nancy Tomes has put it, reformers proclaimed a "gospel of germs" that linked an individual's moral responsibility for hygiene to the common good. In 1900, James Loudon, the president of Toronto University (as it was then known), proclaimed a version of this ideal at the opening meeting of the city's anti-consumption association: "Every man's home should be a sanatorium, and I am glad to know that with the means now at our command it is possible for one to have consumption fairly well treated in the house."[33] In the United States, regional associations joined forces in 1904 under prominent medical authorities on the east coast, including Lawrence Flick (1856–1938) from Philadelphia, Hermann Biggs (1859–1923) of New York, and two clinicians from the Johns Hopkins University in Baltimore, William Welch (1850–1934) and William Osler (1849–1919). Their organization, first named the National Association for the Study and Prevention of Tuberculosis, and later the American Lung Association, signaled its approval of sanatorium methods by selecting Edward Livingstone Trudeau as its first president.

But what did it mean for "every home to be a sanatorium"? For the tuberculous themselves, it meant disciplined attention to body temperature, weight, and routines of diet, exercise, and rest. It meant refraining from activities that posed a risk, which might include boisterous singing that spread germs, a late-night outing that interfered with rest, or physical intimacy such as a kiss on the lips. But the exercises in restraint could have an acquisitive side as well. As Graham Mooney has explained, for some middle-class households, the "TB lifestyle" included the purchase of specialized products available through medical journals and mail-order services. Patients could buy a bed screen for privacy or to block light, an awning so they could sleep with head and shoulders outside in fresh air, or a footrest that doubled as a fire screen.[34] The excesses of this material culture of malady were occasionally ridiculed. For example, in *The Magic Mountain* (1924), Thomas Mann (1875–1955) mockingly described a wealthy patient who ponders whether he should purchase a thermometer with a velvet case to match his wallet and social class.[35]

Germ concepts also encouraged fresh approaches to domestic spaces and routines. To some extent, the new attitudes reflected older sanitarian calls to avoid decaying, dirty matter, but the focus on microscopic particles also directed attention to household articles and furnishings. Decorators turned away from a Victorian preference for heavy, folded draperies and thick fabrics toward a simpler aesthetic that offered fewer refuges for contaminating dirt and dust. Housekeeping manuals and advertisers recommended cleansers containing carbolic acid and lye. Above all, the gleaming white of a porcelain toilet signified a personal space where drinking water and sewage were separated and waste was flushed away. Such standards of cleanliness implicitly linked morality and social standing. Unlike the residents of crowded tenement buildings, people who could afford indoor plumbing would exert the necessary self-control to avoid disease through proper cleaning regimes and hygienic personal habits.

The attention to individual comportment even extended to fashion and hairstyle. Writers criticized floor-length skirts, once considered a badge of feminine decorum, as dangerous magnets for dust and grime. Unsuspecting housewives, it was asserted, would bring contaminants from foul city streets home to their families. Germ fears also focused on masculine traits—the full beard and moustache—that were now suspected vehicles for the spread of infection. A 1903 article in the US magazine *Harper's Weekly* distilled this shift in sentiment with a wry commentary on "the passing of the beard." A half-century before, the article noted, a beard was thought to purify air before it reached a person's respiratory tract. Not any more: "Now that consumption is no longer consumption, but tuberculosis, and is not hereditary but infectious, we believe that the theory of science is that the beard is infected with the germs of tuberculosis, and is one of the deadliest agents for transmitting the disease to the lungs."[36] New scientific concepts encouraged shifts in behavior, as well as deference to expert researchers and doctors who had privileged information about threatening microbes and how to avoid them.

Alison Bashford has used the phrase "hygienic citizenship" to evoke the range of beliefs, practices, and legal requirements that characterized the control of tuberculosis in the early twentieth century.[37] The primary task, as it had been a century before, was still to live with disease rather than to cure it. However, "life with TB" in the West was now structured according to concepts and values that were imposed by modern medicine and, in particular, by an increasing popular awareness (however imprecise) of germs.

In the West, rates of tuberculosis began a sustained decline around 1900 that continued after World War I and accelerated after World War II. This trend did not take place to the same extent in other parts of the world. Some isolated Pacific island and Inuit communities suffered high morbidity rates in the 1920s as they first encountered Europeans who brought the pathogen with them. However, the impact of "virgin soil" outbreaks should not be overstated. As recent genomic analysis has shown, strains of tuberculosis were already present worldwide, and rising levels of disease were triggered by large-scale shifts in living and working conditions. Broadly speaking, starting in the later nineteenth century, rates of tuberculosis rose as nations industrialized and workers faced the cramped, deprived living standards of factory towns. There were regional variations. For example, as Japan rapidly industrialized in the 1870s, conditions in the factories of a growing textile industry affected predominantly female workers.[38] Mineworkers in southern Africa contracted silicosis, caused by inhaling dust that aggravated all sorts of lung diseases.

In the decades after 1920, international coordination of anti-tuberculosis campaigns became more pronounced. As new tools were developed, the primary goal of medical intervention shifted, sometimes to emphasize prevention of the disease with a vaccine and sometimes to attempt cure with new antibiotics. Regardless of approach, the challenges posed by tuberculosis around the world did not diminish radically. They still haven't—in some respects, the challenges posed by tuberculosis are even more complex than they were a century ago.

Prevention and Treatment in the Twentieth Century

Although hundreds of millions of people (mostly children) received the small-pox vaccine during the twentieth-century eradication campaign, it is not the vaccine that has been administered the most worldwide. That distinction probably belongs to a less-successful prophylactic: the Bacillus Calmette-Guérin tuberculosis vaccine (BCG), named for the French biologists Albert Calmette (1863–1933) and Camille Guérin (1872–1961) who developed it in the early twentieth century from the causal bacteria of bovine tuberculosis, *M. bovis*. BCG is a live-attenuated vaccine, created by culturing bacteria through numerous generations to reduce their virulence. After it was first administered in 1921, skepticism greeted Calmette's reports of success in early trials that involved about 1,000 infants. In 1930, an accidental contamination of the vaccine in Lübeck, Germany, resulted in the deaths of more than seventy infants. At that point, the vaccine was almost discarded; the fact that it was not, and that instead BCG has now been administered to more than 4 billion people, says a great deal about the hunger for an effective weapon against tuberculosis. In the 1930s, this desire was especially acute among Indigenous communities in the remote "Indian country" of the rural western United States and in Canada. From these unlikely sites, research emerged that would, to a degree at least, renew faith in BCG's effectiveness.

In the late nineteenth century, Indigenous North Americans faced military conflict, forced migration, and deprivation that increased susceptibility to many diseases. In the United States, the end of the Civil War in 1865 freed up military resources for aggressive campaigns against Indigenous communities, while further north more focused attempts to control Indigenous people followed the enactment of Canadian Confederation in 1867. Moreover, by the 1870s, mass introduction of longhorn cattle from Texas had hastened the collapse of once-vast bison herds that sustained Indigenous societies of the Great Plains. Widespread hunger heightened the impact of epidemics, and the cattle themselves introduced pathogens that caused anthrax, Texas tick fever, and bovine tuberculosis. The latter disease could spread to humans who consumed infected organs and cuts of meat. James Daschuk suggests that this contributed to a steep increase in reports of tuberculosis during the 1870s. Thereafter, tuberculosis was the most visible health threat to Indigenous Americans, particularly among those who were forced into isolated, underresourced communities (called reservations in the United States and reserves in Canada) where they faced overcrowding, malnourishment, and a lack of basic necessities.[39] Further north, although European incursion was less sweeping, endemic tuberculosis nevertheless found a firm foothold as far north as Baffin Island by the 1860s. Into the twentieth century, tuberculosis frequently aggravated the impact of other diseases. Measles, influenza, and pneumonia would break out among isolated populations and then recede in a pattern that differed from the course of epidemics to the south.[40]

Although white public health officials viewed these developments with growing concern, they continued to approach tuberculosis among "Indians" as a racial problem. "The Indians are creatures of the environment," one Nebraska doctor wrote in 1921, with instincts that resisted the proper habits of hygiene and inclined them to vice.[41] It was claimed that Indigenous populations had developed less resistance to tuberculosis than more urbanized (and therefore civilized) peoples of European descent. In Canada, the problem was amplified by government policies that forced many thousands of children to attend residential schools where they encountered poor food, overcrowding, and other forms of abuse and neglect.[42]

Alarming rates of infection among Indigenous communities offered an impetus for long-term trials of BCG that influenced perceptions of the vaccine among experts around the world. In the fall of 1933, doctors in Saskatchewan began tests that involved roughly 600 infants. In 1936, American researchers commenced a study with 3,000 children scattered across several reservations in the West and southeastern Alaska. The US study, published by Joseph Aronson and Carroll Palmer in 1946, suggested that BCG offered "marked protection" from tuberculosis.[43] The conditions of the study prevented researchers from assessing the vaccine's impact apart from other factors that influenced morbidity and mortality. Although Aronson raised cautions about his results, international observers optimistically concluded from this study and others that BCG might reduce new cases of tuberculosis by as much as 80 per cent.[44]

With the exception of Britain, by the mid-1940s European countries had already initiated BCG programs with vaccine strains that were curated in various national laboratories. However, the North American studies were important: despite their limitations, they provided statistical evidence that BCG might reduce tuberculosis in marginal, impoverished populations. Ironically, US and Canadian officials never promoted BCG vigorously, but outside of North America a global rollout of the vaccine ensued. Among other anti-tuberculosis campaigns, between 1952 and 1962 a program that partnered the WHO and the United Nations International Children's Fund (UNICEF) administered more than 130 million vaccinations in developing countries.

Although the scope of these efforts was remarkable, on occasion they inspired mass resistance. For example, in southern India, vaccine protesters invoked Gandhi's suspicion of the practice and advocated for improved sanitation instead.[45] Critics included Chakravarti Rajagopalachari (1878–1972), an influential leader in Madras State who had been an associate of Gandhi. As he objected to "mass experimentation," Rajagopalachari questioned the vaccine's effectiveness and speculated that it might even cause disease because it used live (albeit attenuated) bacteria. Characteristics of the disease itself did not improve the campaign's image. Since tuberculosis was a slow-moving, wasting affliction that mostly affected adults, it did not inspire sympathy toward vaccinators as small-pox's devastating symptoms would later. Moreover, the lack of obvious symptoms among many infected people ruled out the possibility of the targeted surveillance and containment strategy that smallpox vaccinators eventually used. Although resistance to BCG did not halt vaccinations entirely, criticisms in India demonstrated that local elites would not always accept the priorities of global health advocates at the WHO and elsewhere.[46]

BCG remains the only tuberculosis vaccine and it is still administered in many populations. But how well has it worked? After much debate since the 1950s, there is still no easy answer. Several variables influence the vaccine's effectiveness. First, and most importantly, BCG was designed to prevent new infections and it does not cure dormant infections that might reactivate under certain conditions. Second, the various strains of vaccine have different properties and seem to vary in their interaction with *M. tuberculosis* and related bacteria. Some experts have suggested that the prevalence of non-disease-causing mycobacteria, which are especially widespread in tropical environments, may affect vaccine performance. Third, in contrast to the smallpox vaccine, it seems that the immunity BCG provides can be overwhelmed in individuals who are malnourished and repeatedly exposed to infection.[47] On balance, evidence from many studies suggests that BCG helps protect against some forms of tuberculosis, especially for children who have not yet been exposed to mycobacteria. But BCG's overall effect on rates of pulmonary tuberculosis has been modest. Unlike the smallpox vaccine, BCG has been administered not in hopes of eradicating tuberculosis but, rather, because other treatment options are considered impractical (i.e., too expensive) or ineffective.

During BCG's peak in the 1940s and 1950s, another innovation had an even more sweeping impact: the introduction of penicillin, streptomycin, and other drugs that enabled the treatment of many bacterial infections. In the late 1930s, the development of sulfonamides, followed by penicillin (see chapter 2), had raised hopes and inspired further research. At a college in Rutgers, New Jersey, a team led by Selman Waksman (1888–1973) ran thousands of tests with actinomycetes—soil bacteria that grow in microscopic, branching networks—in search of killer compounds. Among other discoveries, in 1943 Waksman's student Albert Schatz (1920–2005) isolated and named streptomycin, a chemical that affected a remarkably wide range of pathogens. Penicillin only treated infections caused by "Gram-positive" bacteria, microbes with a relatively porous cell wall. Streptomycin killed a wider range of pathogens, including *M. tuberculosis* and *Yersinia pestis*, the bacterium that causes plague. Waksman repurposed a term previously used as an adjective—"antibiotic," which literally means "against life"—and used it instead to denote a class of microbial substances that inhibit the growth of microorganisms.[48] Waksman's protocol for screening bacteria also provided an investigative model to identify more antibiotics.

Streptomycin's impact, like penicillin's, was swift. Administered by intramuscular injection, the drug cured many people within months. In particular, children with tuberculosis-related meningitis revived in ways that seemed miraculous. At the population level, in the United States between 1945 and 1955 annual tuberculosis mortality decreased from 39.9 deaths per 100,000 people to 9.1 deaths per 100,000.[49] Likewise, in western Europe, the incidence of tuberculosis declined 7–10 per cent per year in the 1950s. These figures had been declining already and would continue to fall until 1980, but streptomycin helped bring about the steepest drops in new tuberculosis cases and related deaths. Other infections that were often deadly, such as pneumonia or endocarditis (an infection of the heart lining), could now be cured quickly and effectively.

This success helped breed a change in attitude among public health officials in the United States and elsewhere after World War II. As Randall Packard and others have noted, leaders in the postwar order favored the use of technology to solve problems and foster growth in underdeveloped regions. The introduction of antibiotics coincided with other global health initiatives to alleviate suffering and encourage recovery. The BCG campaign, widespread use of DDT to kill mosquitoes, increased smallpox vaccinations, new anti-malarial drugs—all pointed to the potential for scientific knowledge to improve lives. Although a great deal was accomplished, the targeted measures that were favored also discouraged broad-based approaches to health promotion.[50] In the last part of the twentieth century, this narrowed focus would be tested as new challenges arose in the struggle against tuberculosis and divisions widened between wealthy and poor nations.

The Emergence of Antibiotic Resistance

From the start, researchers recognized that bacteria could develop resistance to the new antibiotics. In 1940, Ernst Chain had already identified penicillinase, an enzyme naturally produced by some bacteria that neutralized the effect of penicillin. In 1945, Alexander Fleming warned of the danger of antibiotic resistance in his speech as he accepted the Nobel Prize in medicine (awarded jointly with Chain and Howard Florey). In streptomycin's early trials, satisfaction with its success was accompanied by concern. In Britain, the national Medical Research Council conducted a landmark study of streptomycin that randomized the allocation of streptomycin treatment for patients in order to create an unbiased test of its effectiveness.[51] Published in 1948, the study concluded that adults treated with streptomycin improved by 43 per cent more than patients who only took bedrest. But 20 per cent of the streptomycin cohort developed resistance to the drug after six months. Experts elsewhere observed drug resistance, too. Some doctors refused to send their patients home from hospitals with antibiotics; others refused to prescribe them altogether.

By 1960, cases of resistance were documented worldwide for the three leading anti-tuberculosis drugs: streptomycin, para-aminosalicylic acid (PAS), and isoniazid. The initial response to the problem was to prescribe the drugs in combination since bacteria that were resistant to one antibiotic were seldom resistant to two or three. Cures became more difficult to complete. Whereas streptomycin had required injections for several months, multi-drug cures often took twelve to eighteen months and caused many more side effects. PAS, for example, often caused violent nausea, and isoniazid caused gastrointestinal discomfort and rashes. After the symptoms of tuberculosis eased and patients stopped taking medicine, a few hardy bacteria often survived to multiply again. In regional populations and in individual patients, practitioners recognized the start of a biological arms race. Against each drug combination, sooner or later the evolutionary energy in many billions of bacteria produced a winning formula. The patients who were most often cured lived in countries with a solid health care infrastructure that provided consistent supplies of drugs and supervised regimens. Outside the developed world, these conditions often were not met.

In the early 1980s, and probably before, the emerging AIDS epidemic further tilted the biological scales in favor of tuberculosis. From the perspective of tuberculosis bacilli, HIV was heaven-sent: it caused no distinctive symptoms to advertise itself, only immune suppression that made its human hosts vulnerable to other diseases. Prior to the late 1970s, tools had not been developed that could identify HIV. The first warning signs came in 1982, as doctors in the United States and Haiti observed that Haitians infected with the new pathogen also suffered disproportionately from tuberculosis. Health care workers in Zaire (now the Central African Republic) noticed the same thing. It would soon be clear that tuberculosis was the most common **opportunistic infection** that resulted from HIV infection. However, through the end of the 1980s, public health agencies in most developed countries failed to respond aggressively to the emerging crisis.

Circumstances were grim where antibiotic resistance and HIV infection converged and reinforced each other. In 1990, New York City had the largest HIV-positive population in North America, and 40 per cent of the city's new tuberculosis cases displayed drug resistance. It was apparent that drug-resistant infections were passing *between* patients, not merely arising in individuals who were treated unsuccessfully.[52] The problem of drug resistance mounted as many patients of limited means found it impossible to obtain the drugs or comply with demanding treatment regimens. High levels of intravenous drug use spread infection through needles, and both federal and various state antidrug policies created concentrations of infected prison inmates by imposing mandatory sentences for drug-related crimes.

Other nations experienced a similar synergy of negative forces. For example, the collapse of the Soviet Union in the early 1990s caused social dislocation and erosion of health care services. As the twenty-first century began, intravenous drug use and high incarceration rates fanned tuberculosis transmission in the Russian Federation. Conditions were even worse in regions such as sub-Saharan Africa that had not benefited from antibiotics to the same extent as Europe and North America. As chapter 11 will discuss, sub-Saharan Africa has also encountered relatively high rates of HIV infection, which causes immune system suppression. This influenced the region's experience with tuberculosis: in South Africa, Botswana, and Zambia, HIV primed millions of people for tubercular disease, caused either by dormant infections or person-to-person transmission.

As annual rates of reported new infections climbed steeply in many countries, health experts took notice. In April 1993, the WHO declared tuberculosis a global health emergency and endorsed a more consistent global approach to the crisis. The new method was called directly observed therapy, short course (DOTS), and it combined successful aspects of tuberculosis treatment that had been tested since the 1970s. The DOTS strategy required aid groups and national governments to provide case detection with microscopy, an uninterrupted supply of drugs, and reporting systems that verified treatment results for individuals and populations. Experts devised a "short course" drug regimen of 6 to 8 months that cured most patients and enabled higher levels of compliance than longer treatments. By the end of 2002, 180 countries had adopted DOTS, enabling access to the program for an estimated 69 per cent of the world's population. More than 13 million people were treated between 1995 and 2002, with an estimated average cure rate of

82 per cent.[53] DOTS was praised as cost-effective, and the program secured the support of the World Bank, which controlled a large share of the funds available for global health programs.

As the statistics above suggest, the DOTS program helped some regions achieve notable reductions in tuberculosis rates. China, for example, pursued an energetic DOTS program that included free drugs, incentives for doctors who enrolled patients in treatment, and identity cards that tracked patients and encouraged compliance. A survey conducted in 2000 estimated that China's program had eliminated roughly 660,000 cases of tuberculosis in ten years. However, some observers also questioned whether DOTS deserved all the credit for the decline. Disparities were noted between eastern China and poorer Western regions where rates of tuberculosis remained high among rural communities and ethnic minorities.[54] In general, the success of DOTS depended upon the level of health care infrastructure that was available in a community or region. Moreover, as numerous experts pointed out, DOTS did not directly address the specific challenges posed by drug-resistant tuberculosis or HIV-related infections. Improvements to DOTS, introduced under the banner "DOTS-plus," have addressed some of the criticisms. In addition, the WHO has recommended that people living with HIV (PLHIV) be preventively given isoniazid, one of the "frontline" drugs for tuberculosis control.[55]

Conclusion

By the late twentieth century, tuberculosis control had entered an era of acronyms. In the last six decades, a vaccine (BCG), supervised antibiotic treatment (DOTS), and, most recently, isoniazid preventive therapy (IPT) have all had some positive outcomes, but their overall effect on the global burden of tuberculosis has been modest. No medical technology has controlled tuberculosis by itself. Instead, recent history confirms what social critics such as Charles Dickens recognized in the nineteenth century: tuberculosis is a social disease that reflects persistent inequalities and hardships within a nation or community.

Viewed over the long term, however, it is also clear that tuberculosis presents different problems than it did a century ago and that human actions have magnified the challenges. In the nineteenth and early twentieth centuries, tuberculosis was primarily a disease of urban poverty that accompanied growing cities and concentrations of industrial activity. Thereafter, the incidence of tuberculosis diverged to reflect the fault lines of the global economy. After World War II, human interventions created the problem of drug-resistant TB, and HIV infection greatly amplified the spread of tuberculosis, particularly in Africa. The disease still affects the urban poor disproportionately, but it now may be described as a disease of exclusion that also affects Indigenous communities, ethnic minorities, rural dwellers, intravenous drug users, and refugees from war or famine. As Salmaan Keshavjee and Paul Farmer have pointed out, only a tiny fraction of the individuals who are diagnosed with drug-resistant tuberculosis receive treatment that is considered the standard of care in the United States. Meaningful reductions in the incidence of tuberculosis will require equity in health-care delivery that goes beyond the measures that have been attempted in the last two decades.[56]

In the late nineteenth century, scientific researchers such as Robert Koch proposed germ theories as a means to explain the spread of disease. This conceptual shift did not lead immediately to numerous effective treatments. However, it motivated widespread changes to institutions and individual behavior that, alongside medical interventions, contributed to a decline of tuberculosis cases in developed countries. It appears that surveillance, isolation of the sick in sanitoria, rising living standards, and the self-control commended by the "gospel of germs" all had a role to play in the improved health outcomes that Westerners experienced in the early twentieth century. Equally significant over a longer term, the discourse concerning tuberculosis enlisted ordinary citizens in *preventive* campaigns to monitor and adjust their own behavior to promote individual and communal health. The presumption that an alignment exists between self-control, good health, and effective social membership has only strengthened with time. In the twenty-first century, as wearable (and embedded) technology has enabled individuals to monitor their own heart rate, breathing, and sleep, the ideal of self-regulated health has reached a new level of internalization.

The tightening web of social controls has also encouraged government measures that targeted immigrants, the poor, or other people whose actions or beliefs seemed outside the mainstream. In a global context, can equity in health care be achieved in ways that respect the cultures and the personal autonomy of individuals around the world?

WORKSHOP: SCIENTIFIC KNOWLEDGE
AND THE SELLING OF GERMS

In the spring of 1882, Robert Koch's Berlin lecture and subsequent article concerning tuberculosis struck a chord with scientists. Many research papers, laboratory innovations, and even the personal memoirs of other researchers attest to Koch's direct influence. However, we may also consider the broader social impact of various germ theories over a longer term. How did claims about disease-causing microbes encourage people to change their behavior? What happened when technical scientific concepts left the laboratory and lecture hall to be interpreted and adapted in nonscientific contexts?

To answer these questions, historians must turn to a different range of primary sources. For example, scholars have analyzed advertisements that "sold" ideas concerning the role of germs to consumers in the late nineteenth and early twentieth centuries. Ads often created pithy narratives that linked new explanations of the causes of disease to everyday situations. Above all, they generated interest in health-related products—mouthwash, household cleansers, or porcelain toilets—by warning about germs and proclaiming the need to destroy them.

Efforts to sell such products influenced more than hygiene; they reinforced beliefs about the natural world, notions concerning gender roles, and attitudes about social class. The latter was especially important in the United States, where rising prosperity had created a substantial middle class that could afford a range of sanitary products and home furnishings. By recommending regular use of cleansers and toiletries, the ads encouraged a disciplined, consistent attention to one's surroundings and personal habits. It was not enough merely to address imminent dangers; sanitary products were cast as proactive measures that would forestall risks for individuals and their loved ones, especially children. Discerning consumers were advised to heed medical experts and consider scientific knowledge about germs as an advance that would contribute to their safety and quality of life.

Historical research with advertisements or other mass media has clear pitfalls, especially when such works are analyzed without other types of evidence. By themselves, ads may illuminate what an advertiser wanted consumers to believe or assumed that consumers would already know. However, ads do not explain motivations or actions, nor do they reveal what individuals thought after reading them. Moreover, the concepts that appear in one type of media may be presented very differently in posters, pamphlets, or broadcasts that were designed to meet other objectives.

Evidence drawn from mass media often plays a supporting role for social historians. But this does not limit the appeal or value of these sources. For an observant researcher, they may inspire a broader analysis of an important dimension of popular culture.

"The Etiology of Tuberculosis"—Robert Koch (10 April 1882)

Koch first delivered his famous paper at a demonstration for a scientific society in Berlin. Some of the text outlined methods for staining and culturing bacteria that he displayed to the audience. However, Koch also highlighted several claims of general interest: (1) his improved staining methods enabled groundbreaking findings; (2) the "tubercle bacilli" were present in every human and animal case of the disease; (3) the bacilli were distinct, living beings that grew and reproduced in the body; (4) bacilli isolated from one animal induced tuberculosis when they were inoculated into another one; and (5) the bacilli were, in fact, the same as the "tubercle virus" that others suspected to exist. They caused tuberculosis.

Koch's demonstration was remarkable because it provided convincing evidence for these related claims. They provided a powerful explanation of the cause of tuberculosis. By implication, his argument suggested that one could avoid tuberculosis, and probably other diseases, by avoiding germs.

... If the importance of a disease for mankind is measured from the number of fatalities which are due to it, then tuberculosis must be considered much more important than those most feared infectious diseases, plague, cholera, and the like. Statistics have shown that 1/7 of all humans die of tuberculosis....

The nature of tuberculosis has been studied by many, but has led to no successful results. The staining methods which have been so useful in the demonstrations of pathogenic microorganisms have been unsuccessful here. In addition, the experiments which have been devised for the isolation and culture of the tubercle virus have also failed, so that Cohnheim has had to state in the newest edition of his lectures on general pathology, that "the direct demonstration of the tubercle virus is still an unsolved problem." [*Julius Friedrich Cohnheim (1839–1884) was a leading pathologist at the University of Leipzig.*]

In my own studies on tuberculosis, I began by using the known methods, without success. But several casual observations have induced me to forego these methods and to strike out in a new direction, which has finally led me to positive results.

The goal of the study must first be the demonstration of a foreign parasitic structure in the body which can possibly be indicted as the causal agent. This proof was possible through a certain staining procedure which has allowed the discovery of characteristic, although previously undescribed bacteria, in organs which have been altered by tuberculosis....

Because of the quite regular occurrence of the tubercle bacilli, it must seem surprising that they have never been seen before. This can be explained, however, by the fact that the bacilli are extremely small structures, are generally in such small numbers, that they would elude the most attentive observer without the use of a special staining reaction. Even when they are present in large numbers, they are generally mixed with fine granular detritus in such a way that they are completely hidden, so that even here [*i.e., at Koch's demonstration*] their discovery would be extremely difficult....

[*Koch presents criteria that, he asserts, must be fulfilled to confirm that a specific microbe causes a disease.*]

On the basis of my extensive observations, I consider it as proven that in all tuberculous conditions of man and animals there exists a characteristic bacterium which I have designated as the tubercle bacillus, which has specific properties which allow it to be distinguished from all other microorganisms. From this correlation between the presence of tuberculous conditions and bacilli, it does not necessarily follow that these phenomena are causally related. However, a high degree of probability for this causal relationship might be inferred from the observation that the bacilli are generally most frequent when the tuberculous process is developing or progressing, and that they disappear when the disease becomes quiescent.

In order to prove that tuberculosis is brought about by the growth and reproduction of the bacilli, the bacilli must be isolated from the body, and cultured so long in pure culture, that they are freed from any diseased production of the animal organism which may still be adhering to the bacilli. After this, the bacilli must bring about the transfer of the disease to other animals, and cause the same disease picture which can be brought about through the inoculation of healthy animals with naturally developing tubercle materials....

[*Koch outlines techniques for culturing bacteria. He then discusses experiments in which guinea pigs were inoculated with tubercles from various diseased animals and humans. The fact that he observed identical disease processes in each guinea pig suggests that tubercle bacilli cause diseases in different animals and different human organs. The infections that he observed were directly caused by the inoculation, not some other source.*]

Cultures of tubercle bacilli were prepared from guinea pigs which had been inoculated with tubercles from the lungs of apes, with material from the brains and lungs of humans that had died from miliary [*i.e., severe and systemic*] tuberculosis, with cheesy masses from phthisistic [*i.e., tubercular*] lungs, and with nodules from lungs and from the peritoneum
[*in the lower abdomen*] of cows affected with bovine tuberculosis. In all these cases, the disease processes occurred in exactly the same way, and the cultures of bacilli obtained from these could not be differentiated in the slightest way. In all, fifteen pure cultures were made of tubercle bacilli, four from guinea pigs infected with ape tuberculosis, four with bovine tuberculosis, and seven with human tuberculosis....

The results of a number of inoculation experiments with bacillus cultures inoculated into a large number of animals, and inoculated in different ways, all have led to the same results. Simple injections subcutaneously [*i.e., through the skin*] or into the peritoneal cavity, or into the anterior chamber of the eye, or directly into the blood stream, have all produced tuberculosis with only one exception....

All of these facts taken together lead to the conclusion that the bacilli which are present in the tuberculous substances not only accompany the tuberculous process, but are the cause of it. In the bacillus we have, therefore, the actual tubercle virus.

Formamint—*Scientific American* (1915)

Formamint was a British product that was popular in Europe as well as the United States. It combined formaldehyde with milk sugar. This ad connects germs to the increasingly common experience of crowding in urban spaces and mass transport such as streetcars and trains. It commends regular attention to oral hygiene, not only to treat illness but also as a preventive measure. The key part of the ad's composition is the artist's rendering of harmful, invisible germs that are destroyed by the product. Many ads emphasized that germs were harmful agents that could not be perceived with the naked eye. The main text of the ad follows.

Formamint—The Germ-Killing Throat Tablet

—his sore throat may be *yours* tomorrow!

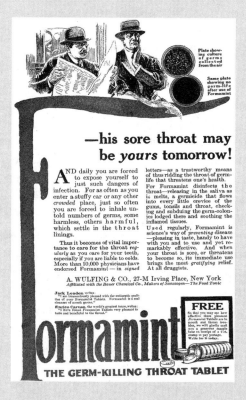

IMAGE 6.3a "Formamint—The Germ-Killing Throat Tablet"

And daily you are forced to expose yourself to just such dangers of infection. For as often as you enter a stuffy car or any other *crowded* place, just so often you are forced to inhale untold numbers of germs, some harmless, others harmful, which settle in the throat linings.

Thus it becomes of vital importance to care for the throat *regularly* as you care for your teeth, especially if you are liable to colds. More than 10,000 physicians have endorsed Formamint—in *signed* letters—as a trustworthy means of thus ridding the throat of germ-life that threatens one's health.

For Formamint disinfects the throat—releasing in the saliva as it melts, a germicide that flows into every little crevice of the gums, tonsils and throat, checking and subduing the germ-colonies lodged there and soothing the inflamed tissues.

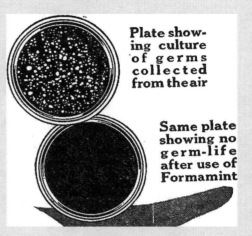

IMAGE 6.3b A depiction of "germ-life"

Used regularly, Formamint is science's way of *preventing* disease—pleasing in taste, handy to have with you and to use and yet remarkably effective. And when your throat is sore, or threatens to become so, its immediate use brings the most *gratifying* relief. At all druggists.

Lysol Disinfectant—*The Ladies' Home Journal* (1918)

Advertisers for cleansers frequently targeted literate middle- and upper-class women. They encouraged homemakers (or their servants) to attend carefully to domestic surroundings. This ad lists and visually depicts areas of the house deemed potentially unclean. It encourages persistent attention to germs—and routine use of the cleanser—as appropriate conduct. The text also creates a narrative concerning pervasive, "lurking" germs that will ambush family members at vulnerable moments to cause sickness.

Five spots where germs may lurk

Sinks, drains, toilet bowls, garbage pails, floors, corners—these are the spots where germs breed in your home. You cannot see disease germs, but that does not alter the fact that they breed by the millions and are a constant menace to health.

And so when some member of your family happens to become a trifle run-down, an excellent opening is offered for an attack of contagious sickness.

Proper disinfection kills disease germs and checks the breeding of germ life. Proper disinfection means that all places where germs might lurk or breed should be sprinkled with a solution of Lysol Disinfectant at least twice a week.

A little Lysol Disinfectant should be added to scrubbing water, too. Being a soapy substance, Lysol Disinfectant helps to clean as it disinfects. A 50¢ bottle makes 5 gallons of germ-killing solution. A 25¢ bottle makes 2 gallons.

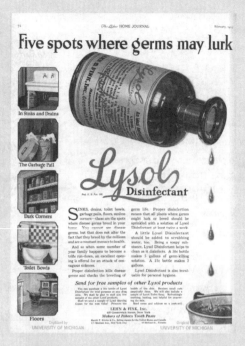

IMAGE 6.4a "Five spots where germs may lurk"

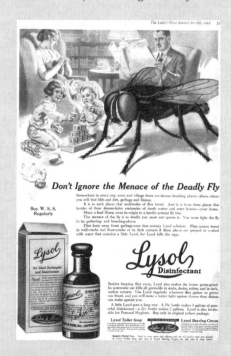

IMAGE 6.4b "Don't Ignore the Menace of the Deadly Fly"

Lysol Disinfectant is also invaluable for personal hygiene. [*Into the 1940s, some ads advertised the use of Lysol for "feminine hygiene"—to flush the vagina with a mild solution to destroy harmful bacteria and reduce odor. Similar measures performed after sex were also considered a means of birth control, a use that ads did not mention explicitly.*]

Lysol Disinfectant—*The Ladies' Home Journal* (1919)

Scientific findings concerning the spread of disease-causing agents placed a new focus on flies, mosquitoes, and lice. Advertisements introduced insights drawn from the study of malaria, typhoid, and yellow fever into everyday situations. The ads—and, in this example, an outsized fly—depicted ordinary insects as existential threats to family life and homes that should offer shelter from a dangerous world. As in other ads, the following text equates the existence of germs with the spread of disease.

Don't Ignore the Menace of the Deadly Fly

Somewhere in every city, town and village there are disease-breeding places—places where you will find filth and dirt, garbage and disease.

It is in such a place that multitudes of flies breed. And it is from these places that hordes of these disease-bearing emissaries of death scatter and enter homes—your home.

Many a fatal illness owes its origin to a hardly-noticed fly.

The menace of the fly is so deadly you must not ignore it. You must fight the fly in its gathering- and breeding-places.

Flies keep away from garbage cans that contain Lysol solution. Flies cannot breed in wall-cracks and floor-cracks or in dark corners if these places are sprayed or washed with water that contains a little Lysol, for Lysol kills the eggs.

Besides keeping flies away, Lysol also makes the home germ-proof. Its systematic use kills all germ-life in sinks, drains, toilets, and in dark, sunless corners. Use Lysol regularly wherever flies gather or germs can breed, and you will make a better fight against disease than disease can make against you.

INTERPRETING THE DOCUMENTS

1. Make a list of the attributes or qualities that Koch assigns to microbes. Do the same for the advertisements. Even when no facts are contradictory, how do the depictions differ?
2. Review the discussion of Koch in chapter 5. Upon what kind of evidence did Koch base his claims about germs? Upon what do the advertisements base their claims?
3. According to the ads, how does human behavior influence the spread of disease? What attitude toward the natural world does such advertising encourage?

MAKING CONNECTIONS

1. How does Robert Koch define disease? How does his definition differ from conceptions of disease early in the nineteenth century? In the sixteenth century?

2. Compare the physical effects of tuberculosis to those of cholera or bubonic plague. How might the different manifestations of these diseases lead to contrasting images of the sufferers and societies that these diseases influenced?

3. How do Koch's methods differ from those of John Snow and William Farr? How would you compare their roles in debate over public health measures?

For further reading: Nancy Tomes, "Epidemic Entertainments: Disease and Popular Culture in Early-Twentieth-Century America," *American Literary History* 14, no. 4 (2002): 625–52.

Notes

1. WHO, "Tuberculosis" (September 2018), https://www.who.int/news-room/fact-sheets/detail/tuberculosis.

2. Thomas R. Lerner et al., "*Mycobacterium tuberculosis* Replicates within Necrotic Human Macrophages," *Journal of Cell Biology* 216, no. 3 (2017): 583–94.

3. Iñaki Comas et al., "Out-of-Africa Migration and Neolithic Co-expansion of *Mycobacterium tuberculosis* with Modern Humans," *Nature Genetics* 45, no. 10 (2013): 1176–82; Sharon Levy, "The Evolution of Tuberculosis," *BioScience* 62, no. 7 (2012): 625–29.

4. Monica H. Green, "The Globalisations of Disease," in *Human Dispersal and Species Movement: From Prehistory to the Present*, ed. Nicole Boivin, Rémy Crassard, and Michael D. Petraglia (Cambridge: Cambridge University Press, 2017), 499–502.

5. Helen Bynum, *Spitting Blood: The History of Tuberculosis* (Oxford: Oxford University Press, 2012), 10–14.

6. My thanks to Prof. Faith Wallis for sharing an early version of her essay, "Disease 1000–1300," forthcoming in Richard Oram, Philip Slavin, and Timothy Newfield, eds, *A Handbook of Medieval Environmental History*, volume 2 (1000–1350) (Leiden: Brill, 2019).

7. Carolyn A. Day, *Consumptive Chic: A History of Beauty, Fashion and Disease* (London: Bloomsbury Publishing, 2017).

8. Francis Adams, ed. and trans., *The Extant Works of Aretæus the Cappadocian* (London, 1856), 310–12.

9. Clark Lawlor and Akihito Suzuki, "The Disease of the Self: Representing Consumption 1700–1830," *Bulletin of the History of Medicine* 74, no. 3 (2000): 467.

10. Clark Lawlor, *Consumption and Literature* (Basingstoke: Palgrave Macmillan, 2006), 140.

11. William Johnston, *The Modern Epidemic: A History of Tuberculosis in Japan* (Cambridge, MA: Harvard University Press, 1995), 130–32.

12. Karl Marx, *Capital: Critique of Political Economy*, trans. Samuel Moore and Edward Aveling (Mineola: Dover Publications, 2011), 528.

13. R.R. Trail, "Richard Morton (1637–1698)," *Medical History* 14, no. 2 (1970): 169–70.

14. Donald G. McNeil Jr, "Promising Malaria Drug Has a Striking Drawback: Blue Urine," *New York Times*, 9 February 2018.

15. Andrew Mendelsohn, "Biology, Medicine and Bacteria," *History and Philosophy of the Life Sciences* 24, no. 1 (2002): 13–15.

16. Gretchen Condran, "The Elusive Role of Scientific Medicine in Mortality Decline," *Journal of the History of Medicine and Allied Sciences* 63, no. 4 (2008): 520–22.

17. Amy Fairchild, *Science at the Borders: Immigrant Medical Inspection and the Shaping of the Modern Industrial Labor Force* (Baltimore: Johns Hopkins University Press, 2003), 100.

18. David S. Barnes, *The Making of a Social Disease: Tuberculosis in Nineteenth-Century France* (Berkeley: University of California Press, 1995), 83.

19. Bynum, *Spitting Blood*, 119.

20. Nancy Tomes, *The Gospel of Germs: Men, Women and the Microbe in American Life* (Cambridge, MA: Harvard University Press, 1999), 179–80.

21. Barbara Gutmann Rosenkrantz, "The Trouble with Bovine Tuberculosis," *Bulletin of the History of Medicine* 59, no. 2 (1985): 160.

22. Bynum, *Spitting Blood*, 170–73.

23. James Colgrove, "The McKeown Thesis: A Historical Controversy and Its Enduring Significance," *American Journal of Public Health* 92, no. 5 (2002): 725–29.

24. Cynthia Anne Connolly, "Determining Children's 'Best Interests' in the Midst of an Epidemic: A Cautionary Tale from History," in *Nursing Interventions through Time: History as Evidence*, ed. Patricia D'Antonio and Sandra B. Lewenson (New York: Springer Publishing, 2011), 20–21.

25. Michael Worboys, "Joseph Lister and the Performance of Antiseptic Surgery," *Notes & Records of the Royal Society* 67 (2013): 199–209, https://doi.org/10.1098/rsnr2013.0028.

26. S. Robert Lathan, "Caroline Hampton Halsted: The First to Use Rubber Gloves in the Operating Room," *Proceedings of the Baylor University Medical Center* 23, no. 4 (2010): 389–92.

27. Flurin Condrau, *Lungenheilanstalt und Patientenschicksal: Sozialgeschichte der Tuberkulose in Deutschland und England im späten 19. und frühen 20. Jahrhundert* [*Tuberculosis Sanatoria*

and Patient Fates: The Social History of Tuberculosis in Germany and England in the Late Nineteenth and Early Twentieth Centuries*] (Göttingen: Vandenhoeck & Ruprecht, 2000), Abb. 11, p. 58.

28. Sheila Rothman, *Living in the Shadow of Death*: *Tuberculosis and the Social Experience of Illness in American History* (Baltimore: Johns Hopkins University Press, 1995), 198.

29. Alison Bashford, *Imperial Hygiene*: *A Critical History of Colonialism, Nationalism and Public Health* (London: Palgrave Macmillan, 2004), 75.

30. Connolly, "Cautionary Tale," 26.

31. B.M.A., "Dispensary Treatment for Consumption in France," *Charity Organization Review* 21, no. 126 (1907): 321.

32. Rothman, *Shadow of Death*, 188–89.

33. "Report of the Inaugural Meeting of the Toronto Association for the Prevention ... of Tuberculosis, May 8, 1900" (Toronto, 1900), 11.

34. Graham Mooney, "The Material Consumptive: Domesticating the Tuberculosis Patient in Edwardian England," *Journal of Historical Geography* 42 (October 2013): 152–66.

35. Thomas Mann, *The Magic Mountain*, trans. H.T. Lowe-Porter (London: Penguin, 1969 [1924]), 167.

36. Quoted in Steven Cassedy, *Connected: How Trains, Genes, Pineapple Keys and a Few Disasters Transformed Americans at the Dawn of the Twentieth Century* (Stanford: Stanford University Press, 2014), 21.

37. Bashford, *Imperial Hygiene*, 77.

38. Mahito Fukada, *Kekkaku no Bunkashi* [*A Cultural History of Tuberculosis*] (Nagoya: University of Nagoya Press, 1995).

39. James Daschuk, *Clearing the Plains: Disease, Politics of Starvation, and the Loss of Aboriginal Life* (Regina: University of Regina Press, 2013), 100–103; Maureen Lux, "Perfect Subjects: Race, Tuberculosis and the Qu'Appelle BCG Vaccine Trial," *Canadian Bulletin of Medical History* 15, no. 2 (1998): 277–80.

40. Liza Piper and John Sandlos, "A Broken Frontier: Ecological Imperialism in the Canadian North," *Environmental History* 12, no. 4 (2007): 759–70.

41. Margaret W. Koenig, *Tuberculosis among the Nebraska Winnebago* (Lincoln: Nebraska State Historical Society, 1921), 43.

42. Mary Ellen Kelm, *Colonizing Bodies: Aboriginal Health and Healing in British Columbia, 1900–1950* (Vancouver: UBC Press, 2011), 57–80.

43. Joseph D. Aronson and Carroll E. Palmer, "Experience with BCG Vaccine in the Control of Tuberculosis among North American Indians," *Public Health Reports* 61, no. 23 (1946): 19.

44. Christian W. McMillen, *Discovering Tuberculosis: A Global History, 1900 to the Present* (New Haven, CT: Yale University Press, 2015), 83.

45. Christian W. McMillen and Niels Brimnes, "Medical Modernization and Medical Nationalism: Resistance to Mass Tuberculosis Vaccination in Postcolonial India, 1948–55," *Comparative Studies in Society and History* 52, no. 1 (2010): 180–209.

46. Niels Brimnes, "Another Vaccine, Another Story: BCG Vaccination against Tuberculosis in India, 1948 to 1960," *Ciência & Saúde Coletiva* 16, no. 2 (2011): 397–407.

47. Randall Packard, *White Plague, Black Labor: Tuberculosis and the Political Economy of Health and Disease in South Africa* (Berkeley: University of California Press, 1989), 291.

48. Selman Waksman, "History of the Word 'Antibiotic,'" *Journal of the History of Medicine and Allied Sciences* 28, no. 3 (1973): 284–86.

49. CDC, "Achievements in Public Health, 1900–1999: Control of Infectious Disease," *Mortality and Morbidity Weekly Report* 48, no. 29 (1999): Box 2.

50. Randall M. Packard, *A History of Global Health: Interventions in the Lives of Other Peoples* (Baltimore: Johns Hopkins University Press, 2016), 109.

51. Iain Chalmers, "Why the 1948 MRC Trial of Streptomycin Used Treatment Allocation Based on Random Numbers," *Journal of the Royal Society of Medicine* 104, no. 9 (2011): 383–86.

52. Laurie Garrett, *The Coming Plague: Newly Emerging Diseases in a World Out of Balance* (New York: Farrar, Straus and Giroux, 1994), 516–22.

53. WHO, "Global Tuberculosis Control Report 2004: Surveillance, Planning, and Financing" (Geneva: WHO, 2004), 1–2, http://apps.who.int/iris/bitstream/10665/42889/2/9241562641.pdf?ua=1.

54. S. Bertel Squire and Shenglan Tang, "How Much of China's Success in Tuberculosis Control Is Really Due to DOTS?" *The Lancet* 364 (2004): 391–92; Yan Guo and Yangmu Huang, "New Challenges for Tuberculosis Control in China," *The Lancet, Global Health* 4, no. 7 (2016): e434.

55. WHO, "The Three I's for TB/HIV: Isoniazid Preventive Therapy (IPT)" (2018), http://www.who.int/hiv/topics/tb/3is_ipt/en/.

56. Salmaan Keshavjee and Paul Farmer, "Tuberculosis, Drug Resistance and the History of Modern Medicine," *New England Journal of Medicine* 367, no. 10 (2012): 931, 935.

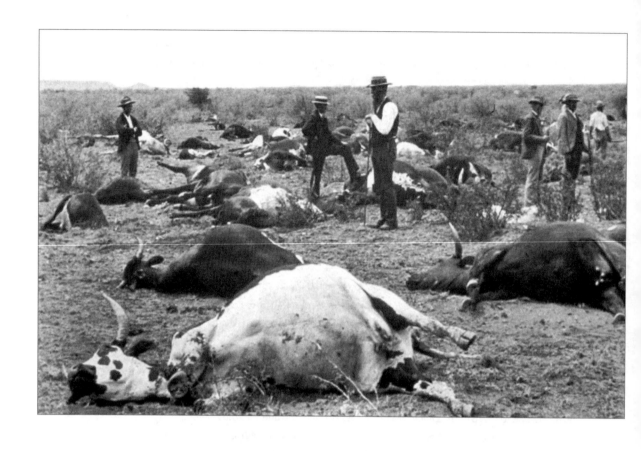

IMAGE 7.1 Rinderpest cull near Vryburg, southern Africa (ca 1896). The cattle in this picture were shot to stop the spread of rinderpest. The pandemic killed millions of wild and domesticated animals and transformed ecology in eastern and southern Africa.

RINDERPEST, IMPERIALISM, AND ECOLOGICAL UPHEAVAL

7

O n 22 December 1889, a total eclipse blotted out the sun over the Great Rift Valley in southern Uganda and Kenya. At Lake Naivasha, northwest of Nairobi, it was said that a white bull rose from the water, sniffed the cows on the shore, and sank back beneath the surface.[1] These were viewed as portents of a great mortality of beasts and humans that struck East Africa in the years that followed. Crops were ravaged by locusts and drought, but the most widespread disaster was rinderpest, a disease that destroyed vast numbers of domesticated and wild animals. The ecological and social changes were profound: in landscapes once grazed by huge herds, the advance of thornbush and tall grass created new habitats for insects and pathogens that would have sweeping consequences of their own. Across East Africa, sleeping sickness, smallpox, and other diseases killed millions of people and shredded the fabric of many communities. The Maasai herdsmen of Kenya called this era *Emutai*—a complete "finishing-off" or destruction of their herds and way of life.

The relationship between human and animal diseases is a familiar theme in the history of modern medicine. As we have seen, Edward Jenner's smallpox vaccine built on eighteenth-century observations of cowpox. Ever since, research with animals has enabled the development of other theories, vaccines, and medications. However, the *social* impact of animal diseases, including their influence on human health, merits a larger role in many historical narratives. In the Middle Ages and the early modern era, few forces disrupted rural and pastoral communities across Eurasia more deeply. As noted in chapter 1, a devastating cattle plague swept across Europe in the early fourteenth century, greatly weakening societies that would soon be struck by plague. At the end of the nineteenth century, a rinderpest panzootic in the Indian Ocean basin accompanied European attempts to seize control of Africa. For Europeans, the measure of colonialism was the acquisition of territory, labor, and raw materials. For African pastoralists, it was the loss of the animals that furnished the necessities of life.

Along with smallpox, rinderpest is (as of 2011) one of two diseases that have now been eradicated from nature by human efforts. While this was a significant public health achievement, rinderpest's broader history illustrates ecological relationships that humans only partially control (if at all). Great rinderpest panzootics involved more than animals. They took place in periods of disruption caused by climate shifts, war, or food shortage. The configuration of forces shifted over time as the scale of livestock transport and human ecological impact increased after 1850. The history of rinderpest demonstrates that we cannot understand the human disease environment without recognizing its connections to the animal one.

Etiology and Early History

Livestock epizootics have affected humans since communities first began to raise animals in large concentrations. Cattle suffer from bacterial respiratory infections such as contagious bovine pleuropneumonia—called "lung plague"—and bovine tuberculosis. The bacterium that causes the latter disease, *Mycobacterium bovis*, may also infect humans. In the early 1920s, it served as the basis for a widely used human vaccine (see chapter 6). Cattle also suffer from foot-and-mouth disease (FMD), a highly transmissible viral infection that does not infect people. (A different virus causes the hand, foot, and mouth disease that is prevalent among children in some settings.) Tropical disease researchers have been especially concerned with a variety of cattle diseases that are caused by parasitic **protozoa**. These are single-celled organisms that conventionally are distinguished from bacteria by the presence of a membrane-bound nucleus. Most protozoan infections are spread by arthropod vectors (i.e., mosquitoes, flies, and ticks). They include Texas fever and East Coast fever—both spread by ticks—and **trypanosomiasis**, a lethal infection of cloven-footed animals that is usually spread by tsetse flies. As discussed later in this chapter, some species of African trypanosomes also cause trypanosomiasis in humans. We will discuss malaria, the most widespread protozoan infection of humans, at greater length in chapter 9.

Alongside these diseases, rinderpest (named with the German term for "cattle plague") has markedly influenced European and global history. The rinderpest virus (RPV), a **morbillivirus**, was closely related to the microbes responsible for canine distemper and human measles. Unlike the viruses responsible for smallpox or yellow fever, morbilliviruses are **RNA viruses** composed of ribonucleic acid (RNA) enclosed in a protein sheath. Other RNA viruses include the causal agents of EVD, influenza, and SARS. Morbilliviruses, like other RNA viruses, mutate very quickly because the enzyme that synthesizes new molecules (called RNA polymerase) lacks a "proofreading" capacity that prevents changes as genetic material is transcribed. Morbilliviruses are highly infectious, and RPV was usually lethal. RPV affected the lining of the throat, lungs, and urogenital system of cattle and wild animals, including wildebeest, buffalo, bush pigs, and some species of antelope. In addition to dehydration and a characteristic stench, the disease caused profuse diarrhea, drooling, nasal secretions, and eye discharges that were important means of transmission. The few animals that survived rinderpest enjoyed lifelong immunity, and antibodies that passed from mothers to offspring also provided resistance for a short time. Rinderpest existed in a variety of genetic lineages that varied in virulence, but mortality often ranged upward of 80 per cent when herds were first exposed to the virus. A farming community's initial encounter with rinderpest was usually an apocalyptic event.

The overlap of rinderpest and human disease has intrigued historians of medieval Europe. Researchers once thought that rinderpest and measles had ancient origins, but recent molecular clock analyses suggest that they diverged in the Middle Ages sometime between the ninth and twelfth centuries.[2] Previously, a now-extinct morbillivirus may have caused plagues that struck both humans and animals in ways that differed from more recent epizootics. Although the disease or diseases that caused long-ago animal plagues cannot be identified with certainty, scholars have reassessed burial sites and texts from the early European Middle Ages in light of data emerging from evolutionary biology. Timothy Newfield has drawn attention to two short periods, 569–70 CE and 986–88 CE, for which some evidence suggests that a measles-rinderpest ancestor caused substantial mortality in both humans and cattle.[3] This theory is attractive but not airtight. Tools do not yet exist to harvest remnants of RNA viruses from ancient skeletons. If this becomes possible, researchers may flesh out a history of rinderpest's ancestor that combines insights from history, archaeology, and biology.

Observers commonly associated outbreaks of cattle disease with the trains of livestock that accompanied traveling armies. This dynamic may have been at work during a cattle panzootic that affected large expanses of Eurasia and reached western Europe in the early fourteenth century. Widespread cattle deaths were reported in Mongolia beginning in the late 1280s. Herds of cattle that accompanied the armies of Khan Uzbeg or other leaders of the Golden Horde potentially brought the disease from the Caspian basin or from further east across the Asian steppes.

However, the simple transfer of germs from one place to another cannot be the whole story. As noted in chapter 1, beginning in the late thirteenth century global shifts in climate created widespread ecological disturbances that affected plants and animals in numerous ways. Particularly in the years 1315–22, cold, wet weather in western Europe created conditions that aided the spread of various pathogens. Sheep suffered from scab, a severe skin disorder caused by mites; sodden fields and swollen creeks provided habitat for parasitic liver flukes that infected numerous livestock and sometimes humans. Cooler temperatures weakened livestock and made it more likely that they would be herded into enclosures where diseases would spread rapidly. A lack of good fodder in these lean years left herds malnourished and susceptible to infections. Because medieval and early modern farms used manure as fertilizer, outbreaks of cattle disease may have contributed to low crop yields for years after torrential rains destroyed arable fields.[4]

The cattle disease outbreaks began in Europe around 1310. A major epizootic apparently erupted in Bohemia around 1315 and spread across Europe to the British Isles by 1321. Again, evidence cannot confirm a diagnosis of rinderpest, but the symptoms and the spread of disease that observers described suggest that RPV played an important role, perhaps in conjunction with other pathogens. In England, where manorial records and monasteries provide some of the best evidence, the cattle and oxen mortalities in large herds reached roughly 60 per cent.[5] Small-scale farmers lost draft animals needed to sow crops and cows that provided beef and milk. Other economic trends made matters worse. A normal shortage of cattle and animal products would encourage prices to rise. In this case, however, fears of contamination meant that prices for butter, meat, and hides actually fell. A near-contemporary lyric, *Poem on the Evil Times of Edward II*, described the combined challenges of cattle death and food scarcity:

> The cattle all died quickly, and made the land all bare so fast,
> Came never a wretch into England more aghast,
> And though that mortality was stopped of beasts that bear horns,
> God sent on earth another dearth of corn....[6]

Deprivation from beef, veal, and milk products, alongside low crop yields in the mid-1310s, may have had lasting health effects for those who endured the panzootic and lived to experience the Black Death. While the precise links remain to be clarified, it seems clear that the destinies of humans and livestock were joined in this era of catastrophe.

Rinderpest in Early Modern Europe

Although European populations eventually recovered from the shocks of the fourteenth century, rural communities remained vulnerable to climate shifts that affected livestock, foodstuffs, and associated commodity markets. Intermittent cattle disease outbreaks were one ecological crisis among many in a world that most people experienced as unforgiving or capricious. While much of this history remains uncharted, the cultural repercussions of ecological crisis ranged beyond food supply, household structure, and other demographic factors. For example, scholars have drawn a suggestive link between shifts in climate and the timing of Europe's peak period of witchcraft accusations. The connection was especially strong after 1560, when temperatures again dropped and remained low for another seventy years.[7] As violent weather events destroyed crops and icy winters froze cattle, in some regions a supernatural explanation for misfortune gained currency. Numerous witchcraft trials convulsed the southern German lands, southern France, and parts of Scotland.

To be sure, the causes and consequences of witch trials ranged far beyond human relationships with crops and livestock. The central notion behind the persecutions was that the accused—often women who performed healing or cared for children and animals—had formed a pact with the devil in order to perform evil deeds. Lawyers had articulated a legal concept of the demonic pact in the late fifteenth century. Elites considered witchcraft a perverted form of religious heresy, but at the village level, where accusations took place, the conflicts usually focused around the circumstances of everyday life. The most frequent charge was "weather making," but people were also accused by their neighbors of poisoning cattle or passing diseases between cattle and humans. For example, in 1663 a woman named Tempel Anneke was burned at the stake in Braunschweig, Germany, after she confessed to several crimes that included sickening cattle in her nearby village. Allegedly, she had harmed the cows with salamanders that had come from her body after she fornicated with the devil.[8]

Such trials were often limited to one or two victims but, on occasion, widespread suffering heightened the impact of allegations that desperate people made under torture. In 1627, broadsheets among several German territories blamed witchcraft for a series of late frosts, cattle diseases, hailstorms, and epidemics. A few confessions incited a panic, and after numerous trials several thousand persons were burned as suspected witches in Würzburg, Mainz, Rhineland, and Westphalia. Ruling princes and magistrates yielded to (and at times encouraged) the justice demanded by villagers, especially in smaller polities where weak political and judicial systems failed to stem a tide of popular fear.[9]

Circumstances had shifted by the early eighteenth century, when large-scale epizootics erupted among cattle during warfare conducted by large national armies. The dynamic differed little from the spread of plague, the pox, and typhus among soldiers. As military campaigns grew to involve many thousands of combatants, vast supply trains crowded livestock together and moved sick animals from one region to another. Beginning in 1709, on the heels of battles between Russian and Swedish forces in Ukraine, a disease believed to be rinderpest spread from Russia south and west into Poland and Croatia. From then on, the disease was afoot in Europe throughout the century, with major epizootics that coincided with the War of Austrian Succession (1740–48) and the Seven Years' War (1756–63).

In all, cattle disease killed an estimated 200 million animals in Europe during the eighteenth century and exerted constant pressure on animal husbandry and the agricultural economy. Within particular regions, the pattern of outbreaks had a cyclical character. An outbreak would kill a majority of the vulnerable animals in a year or two; thereafter, the few remaining animals were mostly immune and the risk of outbreak was low until more cattle were either born or imported from elsewhere.[10] In territorial states of the Holy Roman Empire and elsewhere, the steady stream of regulations concerning the livestock trade reflected a perception that crisis might break out at any moment.[11]

As discussed in chapter 1, eighteenth-century European governments attempted to use quarantine and *cordons sanitaires* to halt the spread of bubonic plague. The same was true for rinderpest, but an additional tool was also available: the slaughter of animals that were suspected of contamination. In 1713, this drastic step was commended by Bernardino Ramazzini (1633–1714), a professor in Padua (Italy) who drew comparisons between rinderpest and smallpox. His claims gained the attention of the pope's personal physician, Giovanni Maria Lancisi. As a result, cattle herds in the sizable territories controlled by the pope were freed of rinderpest in less than a year. In some cases, strong governments pursued similar policies. In 1742–43, the governor of the Dauphiné region in France ordered troops to form *cordons sanitaires* around contaminated areas, much as the region around Marseille had been isolated after the plague outbreak in 1721. States with weaker central governments, such as the Dutch Republic, found it difficult to impose extreme measures over the objections of merchants and breeders. From the late seventeenth century forward, many authorities required inspections and assessed penalties on cattle traders who did not obtain health certificates or who attempted to sell infected animals. Sites where cattle disease had been discovered were quarantined and the sale of animal products such as hides or beef were prohibited.

The implementation of such rules depended on the actions of local leaders. Some were not inclined to enforce lengthy quarantines, and smugglers found ways to evade controls. But in general, campaigns against rinderpest reflected the growing influence of government in matters of health and economy and an increased recognition that livestock health was a strategic national concern. Veterinary medicine gained some independence and stature as an intellectual discipline. After Europe's first veterinary school was founded in Lyon in 1761, England's Royal Veterinary College was established in 1791, followed by several programs in the German lands.

Despite these steps in animal science, most eighteenth-century animal care resembled the human medicine of the time. To prevent harmful miasmas, stalls were washed with vinegar or fumigated by burning sheep's dung or juniper berries. Popular tracts proposed healing recipes that included theriac (or treacle) to be prepared with honey, opium, and dozens of other ingredients. Nothing worked consistently, and the futility of such remedies provided fodder for humorists. In an anonymous poem published by the British *Gentleman's Magazine* in 1747, a farmer despaired after giving his cow a dose of his own medicine: "The bishop'[s] drink, which snatch'd me from the grave/ Giv'n to my cow, forgot its pow'r to save."[12] The analogy of rinderpest and smallpox was of particular importance because it inspired some farmers to try a type of inoculation procedure on their cattle. One common method was to soak a thread in secretions from an infected animal and then to pass the thread under another animal's skin. Another was to introduce "morbid" material from the nasal discharges of an infected animal into an incision made in another animal's dewlap (a flap of skin beneath the lower jaw).[13] Such practices became common among some English and Dutch farmers into the nineteenth century. In South Africa, Boer farmers (Africans of Dutch and French descent, more often called Afrikaners today) attempted similar procedures as well.

After 1820, steamships and then railways transformed the long-distance livestock trade and facilitated the spread of various cattle diseases. In the 1830s and 1840s, both foot-and-mouth disease and bovine pleuropneumonia circulated freely in Europe and crossed the Atlantic to herds in the eastern United States. Rinderpest broke out with renewed violence in the 1860s after a period when it had mostly been confined to Russia and parts of Austria-Hungary that imported Russian cattle. Despite urging from veterinarians, notably the English veterinary surgeon John Gamgee, most states did not act aggressively until the disease had spread widely.[14] In 1866, governments in Britain and the Netherlands (formerly the Dutch Republic) reluctantly adopted policies of quarantine and slaughter after several hundred thousand cattle had perished.[15] The Netherlands called out army and navy troops for enforcement, and farmers were reimbursed 60 per cent of the value of sick cattle and full price for other slaughtered animals.

In the late nineteenth century, rinderpest was effectively eliminated from western Europe, although the danger remained that it would be reintroduced from other regions. In part, its disappearance reflected the increased ability of officials to monitor borders, compel obedience to health standards, and rely upon trained veterinarians. But another factor was important, too: instead of live animals the international beef trade increasingly shipped meat that was cooled to temperatures that killed RPV. This shift (and the unanticipated result) was enabled in the 1880s by ships outfitted with refrigeration systems that used compressed air, ammonia, or carbonic acid. The new technology allowed frozen beef and mutton from New Zealand or Australia to arrive safely in London after a voyage of less than two months. Live animals continued to travel as well, of course, but the scale of necessary surveillance and the overall risk that disease would be reimported dropped significantly.

At the same time that rinderpest was in retreat across Europe, it spread rapidly in regions that were colonized by European soldiers, engineers, and administrators. For many inhabitants of Africa and Southeast Asia, the arrival of cattle diseases in the 1880s transformed entire landscapes and signaled a new era marked by European influence.

The Time of *Ciinna*: Cattle Disease, Social Collapse, and Colonization, 1885–1905

In November 1884, European leaders met in Berlin to lay claim to various parts of Africa. The agreements they reached, from which Africans themselves were excluded, reflected a serene confidence in the centrality of European interests and values in world affairs. The imperial ventures of this period are often viewed through a European prism. In the conventional account, European corporations and governments were motivated by increasing demand for raw materials, such as rubber and ivory, and the hope that Africans would eventually purchase the goods produced in industrialized lands. Conquests were enabled by what Daniel Headrick called the "tools of empire."[16] New weapons, such as breech-loading rifles and early machine guns, provided Europeans an overpowering military advantage. The telegraph enabled communication once conquest was achieved. Larger steamships enabled the rapid spread of goods and troops on a scale that previously was impossible.

The most visible cause of change was the opening of the Suez Canal. Completed in 1869, the new maritime artery reduced the sailing time between London and Bombay by several weeks. Europeans used the new "Highway to India" for travel in greater numbers throughout the Indian Ocean basin. Dutch and Spanish settlers sought to expand their influence on Java and the Philippine Islands, where they had established footholds in the sixteenth century. On Africa's east coast, European merchant companies established strategic outposts near the entrance to the Red Sea. In southern Africa, British colonists and soldiers jockeyed for position among older settlements of Boers and African polities that included the Zulu, Basuto, and Xhosa peoples. The discovery of large diamond deposits and then gold in the African interior created an insatiable demand for laborers to excavate mines and search for precious stones by hand.

But other important dimensions of the African colonial encounters were beyond European intention and control. This era was marked by profound ecological upheaval, driven by weather, war, and the unforeseen impact of transplanted plants and animals. A series of El Niño events—caused by warming in the eastern tropical Pacific Ocean—reduced the strength of seasonal rains in 1876–79, 1889–91, and 1896–1902. These caused lengthy droughts and crop failures; the latter were aggravated by growing global markets for foodstuffs, such as rice, that encouraged the transport of food to the wealthiest buyers rather than the hungriest regions. There were epidemics, too. In the 1890s, bubonic plague began a global tour that resulted in millions of deaths in India alone, and waves of cholera struck South Asian islands and numerous port cities in the late 1880s and again around 1900.

Rinderpest's spread in the Indian Ocean basin was fueled by the increased tempo of trade and colonial contact. By the mid-nineteenth century the disease was already **enzootic** in much of British India. There it caused an estimated 200,000 cattle deaths per year; some of the highest losses coincided with Britain's outbreak in 1865–67. The disease was also known in Egypt, where an outbreak was apparently touched off in 1841 by Russian cattle that arrived with a British army. While some evidence suggests that rinderpest may have then spread south by the 1870s, most scholars accept that Italian forces introduced the disease to East Africa during an effort to establish an Eritrean colony in 1885–87.[17] Soon after the Suez Canal opened, the Italian Rubattino Navigation Company founded a coaling station at Assab, a desert coastal town. In 1885, Italian troops landed to extend control over a strip of neighboring territory, including the port of Massawa that formerly was controlled by Egypt. The Italians imported some cattle from Naples, including some originally from India, and thereafter rinderpest spread into eastern Africa by the end of 1886 or early 1887.

Rinderpest was only one of several challenges that overwhelmed East Africa during the late 1880s and early 1890s. Before its arrival, herds suffered from bovine pleuropneumonia and East Coast fever. Droughts caused widespread crop failures after 1885. In a region already under stress, rinderpest struck a hammer blow. Many families saw their herds decimated in just a few days. Dry conditions forced domestic and wild animals to converge on scarce water sources, which contributed to the spread of human diseases as well as animal ones. As many communities completely collapsed, millions of people died in the regions that would become Ethiopia, southern Sudan, and Kenya.

Some of the most moving testimony about the pandemic's course in 1891 was later recorded in oral narrations by members of the Borana Oromo tribe of southern Ethiopia.[18] They referred to that year as *ciinna*, a time when everything came to an end and the world was turned upside down. In the Borana's recollections, cattle died in droves, emitting a putrid stench, and the carcasses were consumed by black flies so numerous that they filled the air with the hum of vibrating wings. The disappearance of entire herds erased wealth and social class, reducing everyone to the same level of poverty and desperation. People ate boiled animal skins, dug up the few remaining plants, and picked through animal dung to glean undigested seeds. For many narrators, the most telling sign of distress was the behavior of wild animals (*gorjam*). Since many game animals died from rinderpest, starving hyenas and other predators attacked humans so weakened by starvation that they were helpless. Smallpox followed on the heels of rinderpest to complete the devastation.[19]

The Borana narratives also testify to human tenacity and resilience. Communities adopted novel trading and agricultural strategies and reconstituted families that had dispersed during the struggle to survive. However, in many regions rinderpest combined with other forces to dissolve traditional patterns of social organization and to accelerate colonial control over land and labor. Colonial measures to stop rinderpest had some effect, at least in southern Africa, but resettlement policies also worsened some aspects of the general ecological crisis. The following sections will consider how events unfolded in parts of Africa and elsewhere in the Indian Ocean basin.

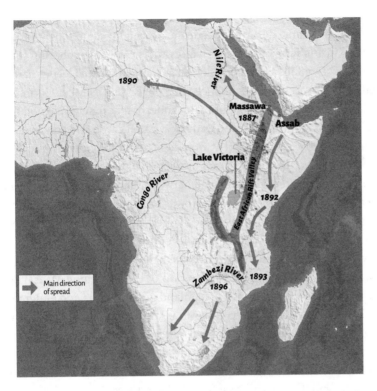

MAP 7.1 Rinderpest in Africa, 1888–1898. Rinderpest spread rapidly among the mobile pastoral peoples of East Africa for several years. Although its advance was halted at the Zambezi River for months, it also spread through southern Africa after the spring of 1896.

Social Disruption and Environmental Upheaval

In the early 1890s, Europeans in East Africa initially were concentrated near the coast and had only a modest presence inland. As British commercial interests expanded into the interior, the Imperial East Africa Company attempted to construct a railway between the coast and Lake Victoria. By 1895 the company had failed, and it ceded direct control to the British government over protectorates that formed the bases of Kenya and Uganda. Immediately to the south, Germany created the colony of Tanganyika, which, along with the coastal state of Zanzibar, eventually became the nation of Tanzania.

Among the tribes affected by the European arrivals were Maasai herders whose savannahs and highlands straddled the regions claimed by Britain and Germany. Rinderpest arrived in 1891 and almost completely wiped out their herds.

Numerous Maasai became destitute practically overnight; some sought protection in adoption or kinship with other tribes while others raided neighboring communities for cattle.[20] By 1896, a contingent of Maasai under a ritual leader named Olanana entered into an informal alliance with the British. Neither Germans nor British in East Africa paid much attention to rinderpest at first. Some noted that the disease killed wild animals as well as domesticated cattle and concluded that it was a distinctively African scourge that would not affect imported livestock.

By the early 1900s, the Maasai faced profound challenges and the British hand had strengthened. Tensions emerged between Olanana's faction and communities led by Senteu, another leader who was based in northern Tanganyika. As the British presence increased, a labor force largely imported from India completed the railway. Outbreaks of East Coast fever prompted European settlers to push for access to "clean" areas that were considered free of the scourge. Eventually, British troops forced roughly 20,000 of the remaining Maasai and their cattle to vacate the most desirable highland grazing areas and emigrate south. The Maasai were pushed into environments that they found less bountiful, and they were denied the flexibility to move with their herds to ecological niches that met their cattle's changing needs. Decades later, African elders insisted that the British had told them "*Shomo Ngatet mikiwa ol-tikana*," which means "Go to the south and may malaria/East Coast fever kill you there."[21]

As rinderpest moved further south, it crossed the Zambezi River in the spring of 1896 and reached southern African colonies that were controlled by Britain but inhabited primarily by Boers and African tribes. When infected trek oxen collapsed on the road, transport riders forsook the carcasses and their loads to local thieves. In the Protectorate of Bechuanaland, the traditional home of the pastoralist Tswana people, steep cattle losses followed a drought and a wave of crop-eating locusts the previous year. British governors were already in the process of imposing a land ownership scheme that assigned migrating herders to reserves and limited their access to watering holes and rivers. Africans, understandably, suspected that Europeans sought to benefit from rinderpest, or even that Europeans were poisoning cattle to remove African claims to the land. In fact, there is little doubt that colonial authorities disproportionately imposed culling of herds and other protective measures on Africans. Only African travellers, for example, were expected to undergo "dipping"—immersion in liquid disinfectant at checkpoints—and then to wait until they were dry before continuing on. Both Boer and Tswana cattle owners resented British efforts to build fences and quarantine herds, since measures that concentrated cattle herds in small areas made them vulnerable to infection. Gary Marquardt has recently suggested that social tensions and changing pastoral management practices probably contributed to the swift diffusion of disease.[22]

Historians have considered how rinderpest influenced several rebellions against European rule that coincided with the pestilence's arrival in southern Africa. On the border of the British Cape Colony and Basutoland, fencing operations and recruitment of border guards apparently aroused the suspicion of young Mosutu warriors. Charles van Onselen suggested that their leader, Makhaola, used the political tensions created by rinderpest to mobilize his kinsmen to resist British rule.[23] Elsewhere, spiritual leaders—in ways that resembled the response of some European clergy to cholera—suggested that the disease was a divine punishment intended to prompt religious and social renewal among Africans. While such responses may have had revolutionary implications, more recent scholars have suggested that most indigenous Africans, as opposed to their chiefs, pursued other concerns. As Phuthego Molosiwa has explored, the collapse of cattle populations created both a subsistence crisis and profound social disruption.[24] Since men were expected to provide cattle as a bride price, couples postponed or refrained from marriage. Food shortages upended conventional family roles. Men who had been accustomed to field work or hunting now joined women and children as foragers of wild plants, worms, and insects. As deeply rooted customs of food sharing became harder to honor, food preparation and mealtimes became more secretive activities.

From the colonizers' point of view, rinderpest and famine offered incentive for men to take jobs digging in mines, laying railway ties or stringing telegraph wire. Numerous African men did participate in an emerging economy for migrant workers. However, to the colonizers' frustration, many men did not consider work for wages to be meaningful employment, and they abandoned their jobs to assist with crops or other food-related tasks with their families. The colonial myth of the "lazy African" had less to do with work ethic than with competing values, survival imperatives, and the reluctance of Africans to give up traditional life patterns for those imposed by newcomers.

A British officer in East Africa, Frederick Lugard, famously observed in 1893 that rinderpest "in some respects has favored our enterprise. Powerful and warlike as the pastoral tribes are, their pride has been humbled and our progress facilitated by this awful visitation. The advent of the white man had not else been so peaceful."[25] This may have been true where armed conflict between Europeans and Africans was concerned. However, rinderpest and other ecological forces wrought violent change throughout Africa and Southeast Asia that far exceeded the impact of any battle.

Ecological Transformations

In Africa, rinderpest not only posed a new disease challenge, it aggravated an ancient one: the burden of several diseases known collectively as trypanosomiasis. The diseases result from infection with several species of African trypanosomes, single-celled protozoan parasites that mature in tsetse flies. Trypanosomes are transmitted by blood-feeding flies to various cloven-footed grazing animals and also humans. Although Human African Trypanosomiasis (HAT) no longer ranks with malaria or AIDS as a cause of mortality, tens of thousands of Africans die from sleeping sickness annually and roughly 70 million people live in regions that remain at risk.[26]

There are several species and subspecies of African trypanosomes; their interactions with various hosts have evolved over millions of years and we may never fully understand their impact upon early human history. Trypanosomal infections certainly affected cattle and sheep from the time that these domesticated animals were introduced to Africa. It is possible that mosquitoes that harbored malaria-causing parasites targeted humans, in part, because trypanosomes reduced the susceptible populations of large mammals.[27] In the absence of large herds, humans became the preferred host. We will return to this issue in chapter 9. Here, the historical relationship between trypanosomiasis and rinderpest allows us to consider one set of human and ecological interactions in slightly greater detail.

The various protozoa that cause sleeping sickness are subspecies of *Trypanosoma brucei*. They are named for a Scottish researcher, David Bruce, who first observed trypanosomes in 1895 and then, in 1903, demonstrated that tsetse flies transmitted the protozoa to humans. One key aspect of trypanosomal infection is the differential susceptibility of various mammals. Native African species such as antelope and bush pigs may host trypanosomes but seldom develop serious disease. Domesticated livestock such as cattle, which were introduced to Africa roughly 10,000 years ago, are more vulnerable. Their infections, called *nagana*, cause fever, anemia, and cachexia (wasting). Disease usually ends in death. *T. brucei* subspecies also vary in their human impact. *T. brucei brucei* only infects grazing animals; *T. brucei rhodesiense* mostly does as well, but in certain circumstances this subspecies may also cause virulent human outbreaks of sleeping sickness. *T. brucei gambiense* primarily infects humans—and is by far the most frequent cause of human disease—but other animals can maintain reservoirs of infection.

The parasites that cause HAT primarily circulate in the bloodstream and initially cause fever, joint pain, and swollen lymph nodes. Left untreated, however, they enter the central nervous system and other organs to cause extreme lethargy and sleep disruption. Infection with *T. brucei rhodesiense* commonly ends in death after two to three months, while the hosts of *T. brucei gambiense* may endure chronic weakness for two to three years before death. Treatment for sleeping sickness remains very difficult. Several drugs are used for chemotherapy. Some medicines are effective only in early stages of infection, while others are highly toxic or hard to administer.[28]

Trypanosomal infections of humans were a serious challenge long before the arrival of rinderpest. Although relatively little is known about the prevalence of sleeping sickness before the mid-nineteenth century, West African slave traders were on the lookout for it at least a century earlier and rejected slaves with telltale symptoms. Outbreaks were recorded on the West African coast in the 1860s and thereafter the disease spread, causing high mortality throughout equatorial Africa over the next several decades. Around 1890, the arrival of European cattle and their diseases upset the balance of trypanosomes, flies, wildlife, and domesticated herds in central and East Africa. In southern Uganda near the northern shores of Lake Victoria, rinderpest decimated animal populations. Large tracts of land, once grazed by thousands of cattle and cleared by shepherds, developed thickets of thornbush and other vegetation that offered congenial tsetse fly habitat. As populations of native wildlife recovered, trypanosomiasis flared with a vengeance once cattle stocks were replenished in the later 1890s.

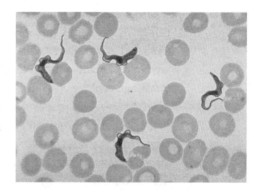

IMAGE 7.2 Trypanosomes. This photomicrograph depicts a human blood smear with *Trypanosoma brucei* parasites magnified 1,000x. Similar to malarial protozoa, African trypanosomes have a complex life cycle with stages in both insects and mammals. Humans are the main host of *T. brucei gambiense*.

Swift human mortality in the Ugandan protectorate suggests that the more virulent *T. brucei rhodesiense* protozoa were involved. One analysis has proposed that this epidemic was caused by parasites that reached new areas when cattle were imported to replace devastated herds.[29] Many factors caused local variation in the overall picture, but estimates of annual mortality in Uganda between 1900 and 1904 range upward from 200,000 people. A desperate colonial government forced thousands of people to resettle miles away from the shore of Lake Victoria. This initially failed to stop the epidemic, and the high population densities in resettlement communities also increased many Ugandans' susceptibility to smallpox and other diseases. Sleeping sickness also spread south along the shores of Lake Tanganyika.[30] By 1920, deaths from the disease in sub-Saharan Africa numbered at least 1 million.

Because of rinderpest, human diseases, and forced migrations, many savannahs in East and central Africa were almost completely emptied of people and livestock. Government intervention further tipped the scale against attempts to reclaim land for grazing or cultivation. European newcomers viewed the bushlands, which recently had been pastures for livestock, as remnants of a primordial African wilderness. As Fred Pearce has suggested, the experience of colonists, tourists, and sportsmen gave rise to a Western notion of an unchanging "wild" Africa that required protection from the forces of modernization. Colonists passed laws and eventually established wilderness preserves, such as the Serengeti in northern Tanzania, to protect large game. Such policies mostly ignored the roles in grassland ecology of wildlife, cattle, and environmental forces such as fire. Instead, wildlife preserves provided an enduring haven for tsetse flies and their hosts.[31]

In Southeast Asia, rinderpest had a similar impact on animals, food procurement, and the human disease landscape. After 1850, periodic rinderpest outbreaks erupted among cattle passing through markets in Hong Kong (1860), Calcutta and its surroundings (1864), Shanghai (1872), and Singapore (1874). Rinderpest may have been present in Java (then ruled by the Netherlands) beginning in the 1860s, but an especially severe outbreak began in 1879. As the cattle mortality mounted, veterinarians from the Netherlands imposed quarantines, oversaw the building of fences guarded by soldiers, and ordered the destruction of numerous cattle herds. It is unlikely that these measures did much good. In four years, an estimated 220,000 animals died and the disease established a lasting presence on the neighboring island of Sumatra.[32]

Conditions were even worse in the Philippine Islands, where violent revolt against Spanish colonizers and the incursion of American forces magnified the ecological stresses of colonization. Prior to the late nineteenth century, cattle imports to the Philippines were relatively modest. Meat was not an important part of the Filipino diet, and the water buffaloes (called *carabaos*) that were raised in the islands were used chiefly to plow rice fields. The arrival of many foreign workers in the 1870s, which included large numbers of Chinese as well as Spaniards, led to an increase of thousands of animals imported for beef. Rinderpest arrived in the mid-1880s, with shipments of either cattle or sheep. A substantial outbreak in

1886–87 was followed by a general epidemic a decade later that coincided with an uprising led by Andrés Bonifacio (1863–1897) in August 1896.

As the Filipino revolution stalled, the arrival of US naval troops in May 1898 further clouded the political picture. As noted in chapter 4, the United States attacked Spanish territories in the Caribbean and the Pacific after an explosion on the battleship *Maine* in the harbor at Havana, Cuba. American forces destroyed Spanish ships in the Philippines and occupied the capital city, Manila. Filipino patriots declared a new republic but the United States refused to recognize their independence. A second battle for Manila between Americans and Filipinos began in early February 1899. US forces prevailed and the Philippines were declared a US territory in summer 1902, although guerrilla resistance continued for another decade.

During this turbulent period, outbreaks of rinderpest contributed to overlapping subsistence and disease crises among Filipino communities. US military practices of requisitioning some *carabaos* and killing others exacerbated the problem, as did the flight of Filipinos away from destroyed villages and zones of colonial influence or conflict. Although statistics do not provide a full picture, a census that the US military conducted of most of the islands in 1903 estimated that roughly 630,000 cattle died in 1902 alone.[33] On Luzon, the most populous island, whole regions faced cattle depopulation. Without plow animals, many rice fields were left untended for years. As the food supply and economy of rice-producing areas collapsed, families dug up roots and tubers for survival. Neglected farmland turned into a wilderness of standing water and uncontrolled vegetation. This created an ideal habitat for *Anopheles* mosquitoes that carried malaria, and hungry female mosquitoes with no cattle to feed upon greatly increased human exposure to infection. The 1903 US census tallied 211,993 deaths from malaria; actual mortality was undoubtedly higher for that year and fatalities were probably at the same level for several years afterward. In addition to outbreaks of typhoid, smallpox, and tuberculosis, a wave of cholera also killed an estimated 200,000 inhabitants in 1902–1903.[34]

In Southeast Asia, as in Africa, human and ecological forces worked in tandem to disrupt food and water supplies, uproot communities, introduce new pathogens, and increase the influence of old ones. In the late 1890s, Africa's "continental cattle plague" also provided a focal point for an international scientific elite that harnessed investigations of disease and hygiene to the interests of expanding colonial empires.[35]

The Legacy of Tropical Medicine

As discussed in chapter 4, after 1875 the emerging discipline of tropical medicine influenced European and American strategies in the Caribbean and Latin America. In Africa, too, a small network of specialists—mostly students of the new research institutes in London, Liverpool, Paris, and Berlin—viewed tropical disease research as an arena of competition and collaboration. As Thaddeus Sunseri has noted, the rapid advance of germ theory encouraged a "culture of experimentation" among European and American scientists who attempted numerous experiments with animals and humans that involved blood transfusions and vaccine preparations.[36] There were other concerned parties on the ground as well. European governments and colonial corporations viewed Africa's beasts—and its humans—as a source of economic profit, and this sensibility influenced the response to rinderpest and other diseases. Local farmers and veterinarians, especially in southern Africa, contributed expertise and sometimes contradicted the opinions of European visitors. African communities often resisted European efforts at control or attempted to migrate beyond the sphere of European influence.

In the fall of 1896, the British Cape Colony government invited Robert Koch to tackle the rinderpest challenge. Although he was Europe's leading microbiologist, Koch had been wounded by his failure with tuberculin (see chapter 6). His divorce and remarriage to a much younger woman scandalized associates and reinforced his status as an outsider. Koch's first voyage to sub-Saharan Africa began a period in which he largely forsook the European research milieu to become a globetrotting consultant in public health. He was eager for new discoveries. In Africa, he wrote to a colleague, "the streets are still paved with the gold of science."[37] As researchers had discovered, the transmission of tropical diseases among insect vectors and mammalian hosts raised many fascinating questions. Moreover, Koch had become increasingly interested in the spread of pathogens among populations as opposed to the effects of microbes on individuals. Ever since his work on anthrax, Koch had perceived the value of animal models for human medicine, and he welcomed the prospect of research involving large numbers of cattle.

Koch arrived in December 1896 and set up an isolated compound, financed by the De Beers diamond company, near the large mine at Kimberley.[38] Like other researchers in southern Africa, Koch was influenced by Emil Behring's recent success using inoculation with blood serum to induce immunity to diphtheria (see chapter 6). His own experiments had an element of trial and error. Koch first attempted to use contaminated material taken from goats and sheep to create a weak form of rinderpest that could serve as a basis for a vaccine. After mixed results, he switched strategies and inoculated healthy animals with bile (or gall) taken from animals that had recovered from rinderpest. In March 1897, Koch claimed success for his treatment and forecast an end to the rinderpest epidemic. He then departed for India and left controversy in his wake. Koch's sponsors in the Cape Colony supported the bile treatment. Others argued that Koch's claims were exaggerated and that he had taken ideas from local experts without acknowledging them. That same year, two scientists who lived in Africa, Arnold Theiler (1867–1936) and Herbert Watkins-Pitchford (1868–1951), proposed a vaccination procedure that combined blood from an infected animal with serum from one that had recovered. This method proved safer than Koch's, and it was later refined by two scientists from the Pasteur Institute, Jules Bordet (1870–1961) and Jean Danysz (1860–1928). Thousands of southern African cattle received vaccines in the late 1890s, but rinderpest still destroyed about half the cattle population and at least that proportion of susceptible wildlife.

Koch made several more trips to Africa and to Pacific islands where he explored the epidemiology of cattle and human diseases, including Texas fever, malaria, nagana, and sleeping sickness. With British assistance, in May 1906 Koch established a compound on the Ssese Islands of Lake Victoria on the border of the Ugandan protectorate.[39] Removed from critics (and ethical safeguards), Koch experimented on sleeping sickness patients with doses of **atoxyl**, an arsenic compound that British researchers had studied as a treatment for animal trypanosomal infections. In humans, atoxyl had drawbacks. It sometimes damaged the optic nerve and caused partial or total blindness, and the drug's effects on symptoms did not continue after treatment stopped. But atoxyl also reduced the level of protozoa in peripheral blood vessels and thus prevented feeding mosquitoes from ingesting the parasites and spreading them. This was not very helpful for individual patients, but atoxyl did reduce the spread of sleeping sickness within a population.

Although this phase of Koch's research is less well known than his earlier work, its impact was considerable in both Western nations and their colonies. Koch concluded from his experiences that parasites might live in an animal for an extended time, either before or after obvious symptoms of disease appeared. (Other scientists had noted this dynamic before—Pasteur, for example, had noted that some chickens who survived fowl cholera still excreted virulent bacteria.) Koch's research further consolidated the concept of animals—or humans—that

More Than Guinea Pigs: Animal Testing in Vaccine Development

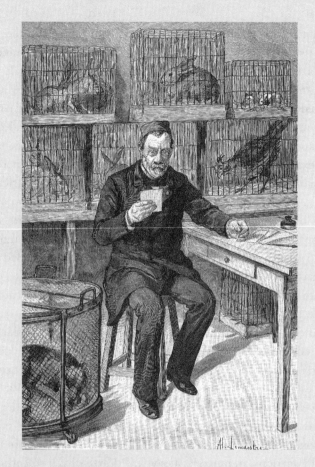

IMAGE 7.3 Louis Pasteur with animals. This drawing from 1893 appeared in a children's magazine published in Paris. It was recognized that animal experiments were essential for vaccine research.

Scientists have not made every medical advance by themselves. Experiments with animals have enabled critical progress in vaccine development, and such tests remain important in some areas of research.

Animal experimentation and dissection have a long history. In antiquity, a Hippocratic author described experiments with pigs, and Galen's writings on anatomy demonstrated familiarity with the internal organs of dogs and apes. However, animal experiments did not become controversial until the mid-nineteenth century, when many investigators in Europe and Britain staged invasive procedures on live animals—vivisection—to explore topics such as nerve function or the effects of injected chemicals.

Many scientists, notably the esteemed naturalist Charles Darwin (1809–1882), argued for restraint, and some rejected animal testing altogether. Britain's Parliament ordered minimal restrictions in the Cruelty to Animals Act (1876) and anticruelty advocates enjoyed some public support. However, prevailing sentiments shifted after 1890 when researchers discovered that blood serum from immunized animals could cure diphtheria. Live horses provided the large quantities of blood that the procedure required. The success of diphtheria antitoxin and the perceived value of other animal tests effectively muted the antivivisection movement.

In the twentieth century, scientists relied on "animal models" to study the transmission of pathogens and to develop vaccines. These studies were especially important for viral infections such as influenza because the pathogens could not be cultured (and, at first, could not even be seen). Various criteria determined the choice of animal. In the 1930s and 1940s, researchers turned to ferrets to model the spread of influenza. Ferrets were inexpensive and easy to handle but, most importantly, ferret flu symptoms resemble human ones—they sneeze the way that humans do. Researchers cultivated viral strains in many generations of mice to keep them alive, and they also used mice to conduct studies of antibodies. In the mid-1930s, a team led by Joseph Stokes (1896–1972) sacrificed more than 11,000 mice to prepare for a human clinical trial.

Experiments with primates pose thorny ethical issues, but in some instances scientists have found them indispensable. For example, humans are the only natural host for polioviruses, and primates were the sole nonhuman alternative for some essential research. In the 1910s, researchers at the Rockefeller Institute conducted studies with rhesus monkeys. Several decades later, a team led by Jonas Salk (1914–1995) at the University of Pittsburgh used 15,000 monkeys in a massive study of poliovirus typing. Policy makers and the American public accepted the need for animal testing when children's lives were at stake. Research with primates continues today (on a smaller scale) with investigations of simian immunodeficiency virus (SIV) strains, which are closely related to human immunodeficiency virus (HIV) strains.

In recent years, some advocates for animals have pressed for a complete end to animal testing. On balance, scientists have not agreed with this position, but the long-running debate concerning animal welfare has had important results. Responsible researchers now acknowledge an ethical obligation to limit animal testing and to treat animals in their care as humanely as possible. Most importantly, researchers are obliged to weigh the harm caused to animals against the value of the potential findings. In some cases, innovations in method now allow them to substitute laboratory tests in place of experiments with animals.

Studies conducted with some animals may directly benefit others. For example, researchers have turned their attention to influenza strains that infect birds. A vaccine for avian flu will benefit many millions of birds and humans alike.

were in a "carrier state" and might spread pathogens to others even when they appeared healthy themselves. Applied to Europe, this insight influenced control measures for diseases such as typhoid and legitimated bacteriological screening to confirm that individuals harbored no dangerous germs. As Christoph Gradmann has put it, the concept of a carrier state "facilitated a conception of infected individuals as a threat to society that needed to be dealt with through isolation and control."[40] Moreover, Koch's approach, labeled by one historian as "test and treat," prioritized the effort to stop the spread of disease in populations over the cure of individual patients.[41] Government officials increasingly viewed the health of human bodies as a collective resource to be fostered for economic or political benefit.

Notions that were related to the carrier state concept also influenced US administrators in the Philippines, who now accepted that microbes were a primary cause of disease. In the wake of war, many Filipinos faced deprivation and appeared weakened and susceptible to illness. Blood analyses seemed to indicate high levels of malaria and infection with other "animal parasites." Similar to colonial agents in Panama, who sought to segregate local workforces from immigrants (see chapter 4), US medical authorities warned against Filipinos who might act as physical reservoirs for tropical disease. These officials thought the danger was heightened because of lax sanitary habits among the locals. "The natives do not keep their hands clean, although it is said their bodies are washed daily," noted one surgeon. He concluded, "at all events, they are not microscopically clean."[42] Concepts of racial hierarchy persisted, even as the focus of the colonists' concerns shifted from unhealthy tropical environments to the biological and cultural characteristics of Indigenous peoples. Evidence drawn from microscopy served to explain the causes of infection but it also could be used to reinforce longstanding stereotypes.

In Africa, a focus on the health of populations reinforced the treatment of Africans as a collective workforce or economic commodity rather than as individuals.[43] European overlords pursued similar objectives as they combated sleeping sickness and other diseases, although their tactics varied. British officials, as we have seen, resettled Ugandans away from Lake Victoria and also attempted to clear bush and drain swamps where tsetse flies would breed. Where resettlement was not permanent, the results were shortlived. Nonetheless, British Uganda's estimated annual mortality rate from sleeping sickness dropped from roughly 200,000 between 1900 and 1904 to less than 25,000 between 1905 and 1909.[44] Whereas the British attempted to limit human contact with disease-spreading mosquitoes, French doctors tried a different approach in French Equatorial Africa and in Cameroon, a territory that Germany ceded to France after World War I. In regions where thick jungle made bush clearance impossible, French practitioners trained their sights on the pathogens in infected individuals. After 1917, the effort was led by Eugène Jamot (1879–1937), who organized mobile teams that walked to remote jungle villages to perform diagnoses and inject drugs. Armed with microscopes and syringes, the feats of Jamot's squads were astonishing: in just one year, 1928, they detected more than 54,000 cases of sleeping sickness and treated them with atoxyl or tryparsamide, another arsenic compound.[45] For millions of inhabitants of central and West Africa, colonial medicine meant a line of villagers that ended with a jab in the shoulder, hip, or buttock.

What were the consequences of the sweeping European campaigns? From the Europeans' perspective, the goal was to shield colonial agents from disease and safeguard workers who provided rubber, metals, palm oil, and other natural resources. Certainly, many thousands of African lives were spared, and in areas where sleeping sickness was rampant whole villages were saved.[46] However, the measures taken to diminish the impact of some diseases contributed to the spread of others. Millions of injections were performed with syringes that retained small amounts of blood. In the jungle, equipment was not always sterilized before reuse. There is considerable evidence that blood-borne pathogens, especially hepatitis C, were transmitted by campaigns against sleeping sickness, malaria, and syphilis. Blood in a contaminated syringe may have transmitted another pathogen that caused obvious symptoms only years later—HIV. We will consider this at greater length in chapter 11.

Because numerous animals harbor trypanosomes, the eradication of sleeping sickness has proven impossible even in this century. The account of rinderpest, however, has a more definitive conclusion. Koch was overconfident in 1897 when he predicted imminent eradication, but scientists, public health officials, and cattle owners have made this vision real in the last twenty years.

Rinderpest Eradication

Rinderpest remained a global threat in the early twentieth century. In August 1920, a herd of infected zebu cattle shipping from India to Brazil stopped over at the port of Antwerp (Belgium) and crossed paths with cattle bound for European destinations. Various outbreaks were stamped out in a few months, but the crisis led French officials to convene an international conference on animal diseases. In 1924, the World Organization for Animal Health (known by the French acronym OIE) began formal international collaboration and soon developed health and safety standards for the trade in land animals. OIE remains a leading international body that, since 2001, has also adopted animal welfare as a key priority.

Like other viruses, RPV could not be observed directly before the invention of electron microscopes in the early 1930s. In the meantime, however, vaccine researchers attenuated virulent material by passaging it through numerous generations of animals. In the 1920s, at a British research institute in Izatnagar, India, J.T. Edwards passaged bovine RPV through goats to create a vaccine that did not require serum. This vaccine could be freeze-dried and was easy to distribute. A Korean researcher, Junji Nakamura (1903–1975), followed a similar procedure using rabbits. Nakamura's "lapinized vaccine" was not only used in Mongolia and China, it was eventually sent to Kenya. In the 1940s and 1950s, French Equatorial Africa, China, and India conducted campaigns that vaccinated more than 100 million cattle, and the annual number of reported rinderpest cases dropped tenfold.

The steep climb to full eradication required more than scientific innovation.[47] Improvements to the vaccine incorporated techniques from polio researchers, who had pioneered the use of tissue cultures to grow numerous viral strains for testing. In Kenya, a team led by English veterinary scientist Walter Plowright (1923–2010) used calf kidney tissue to develop a rinderpest vaccine that conferred lifelong immunity for all types of cattle. Under the aegis of a multinational effort called Joint Project 15, individual African countries continued to make headway with vaccination. In 1979, only Sudan reported new infections. But funding and surveillance efforts lapsed, and it later became clear that rinderpest had circulated undetected among wild animals and herding communities in both East and West Africa. In the early 1980s, outbreaks originating in Nigeria and Sudan swept across the middle of the continent and killed several million animals.

In 1994, the United Nations Food and Agriculture Organization (UN-FAO) established the Global Rinderpest Eradication Programme (GREP) to oversee a comprehensive global strategy. Decision makers increasingly relied upon computer modeling to focus vaccination strategies. The campaign also benefited from a new heat-resistant vaccine, introduced in 1990, that could be stored without refrigeration for thirty days. Without the need for a "cold chain" provided by coolers or refrigerated trucks, it was possible to deliver vaccines to herders in the most remote regions in Africa. As with smallpox eradication, the participation of local partners was a final, essential ingredient for success; the training of numerous community-based workers empowered individual livestock owners to ensure the safety of their own herds. At the turn of the twenty-first century, East Africa was the last known reservoir of rinderpest. After an unconfirmed outbreak in southern Sudan in 2000, active surveillance confirmed that the virus did not circulate there after 2001, and another small outbreak in Kenya was also stopped. By June 2011, both the OIE and the UN-FAO had declared rinderpest eradicated from nature.

Conclusion

Because human measles closely resembles rinderpest, could its eradication be next? There are signs that this is possible. Measles was declared eliminated from the United States in 2000, and in September 2016 the PAHO verified that endemic measles transmission had been eliminated throughout the Americas. On the other hand, that same year measles also caused 90,000 deaths worldwide. In Europe, a resurgence of the disease began in 2017 and more than 40,000 cases and 39 deaths were reported in the first six months of 2018. Reimportation to the Americas remains a constant possibility.[48] An outbreak that began in December 2014 at a Disneyland park in California resulted in nearly 150 cases scattered across seven US states, Mexico, and Canada.[49] In April 2019, officials in New York City ordered mandatory vaccinations in some neighborhoods after nearly 300 cases were reported in the borough of Brooklyn.[50] Like rinderpest, measles is highly contagious. In order for a community to attain the widespread protection that is conferred by herd immunity, over 90 per cent of the population must acquire immunity from previous exposure or (ideally) through vaccination. In a globally connected world, in which well over 100 million children are born each year, only full eradication can remove the need for continued global surveillance and vaccination.

Where animal diseases are concerned, surveillance strategies that were pioneered to stop rinderpest are useful against new threats. The dangers now include bovine spongiform encephalitis (BSE), a lethal infection of the central nervous system that was first identified in 1986. Humans who eat contaminated nerve tissue may ingest the causal agent—a misfolded protein called a prion—and develop **Creutzfeldt-Jacob disease** (although this condition may have other causes as well). Particularly between the late 1980s and early 2000s, disease-causing prions spread when cattle were fed infected meat and bone meal that were the by-products of industrial slaughter. Fears of BSE led to tighter regulations and damaged the international market in cattle products for years. As with rinderpest, the enforcement of new rules intended to stop disease reflected the counterpoint of economic and public health objectives.

To date, total human deaths related to BSE apparently number only in the hundreds, but the disease demonstrates how pathogenic material might spread beyond agricultural settings. The likelihood of such events has increased because of industrial farming practices. Since the 1960s, livestock farming of poultry, pigs, cattle, and fish has greatly increased in intensity, meaning that animals are raised in crowded facilities that contain hundreds of thousands or even millions of animals. This vastly multiplies the biological exchanges among animals, their body wastes, and fluids, which then necessitates the widespread use of antibiotics in animal feed. This, in turn, increases the risk that a pathogen will emerge that can infect humans or—perhaps more likely—that genetic material from agriculture will transfer into a human pathogen to make it more virulent or difficult to treat. As the next chapter will discuss more fully, influenza further illustrates the potential for cross-relationships among human and animal pathogens.

Intensive animal farming is a recent development in a longer story: in the modern era, human societies have vastly increased both the number of domesticated animals and the ecological impact of livestock farming and transport. In the fourteenth century, the impact of a cattle plague (probably rinderpest) was greatly aggravated by ecological disruption caused by climate shifts. Environmental factors also played a significant role later on, but from the eighteenth century forward the scope of rinderpest outbreaks increasingly reflected the impact of human forces, particularly an increased scale of warfare, imperialism, and cattle movement. Once steamships enabled the global transport of infected cattle,

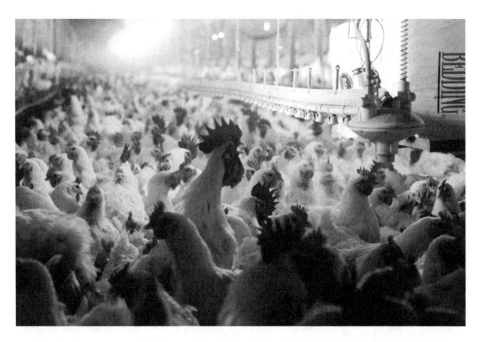

IMAGE 7.4 A commercial chicken production house. In 2011, this facility near Myerstown, Pennsylvania, warehoused 17,000 poultry that produced roughly 2.5 million chicks. In such facilities, packed living conditions require the use of antibiotics in feed to prevent disease. This contributes to the emergence of new strains of avian influenza and other pathogens.

rinderpest fundamentally shifted the balance of microbes, mammals, and insects across Africa and Southeast Asia. Diseases not only weakened African societies as Europeans extended their influence, they also shaped African land use and labor patterns through the twentieth century.

In the early twentieth century rinderpest epidemics tended to exaggerate an already widening gap between Western countries that had only recently eliminated the disease and nations in Africa and Southeast Asia that were experiencing it for the first time. In 1918–19, successive waves of influenza had the opposite effect, at least superficially. Emerging on the heels of World War I, the influenza pandemic has a claim—perhaps a singular one—to be an experience truly shared by the vast majority of humanity.

WORKSHOP: RINDERPEST AND COLONIAL TENSIONS IN SOUTHERN AFRICA

The history of colonization might seem grounded in the basic divide between new arrivals and traditional inhabitants, colonizers and colonized. In fact, the relationships and conflicts in colonial settings are seldom so simple. Often, the historian's first task is to unravel the divisions *within* large groups that might at first appear to be cohesive. This is certainly true when we consider the diverse responses to rinderpest in southern Africa. The ecological catastrophe exacerbated numerous social tensions across the spectrum of colonial societies.

The following excerpts discuss events that took place in 1896 on the boundary of several political entities: the Bechuanaland Crown Colony, which only months before had been annexed by British authorities to join the Cape Colony to the south; the Transvaal South African Republic; and the Orange Free State. The latter states were ruled by colonists of Dutch origin (the Boers) whose ancestors had arrived in the seventeenth century. The region was also populated by Bantu-speaking Tswana peoples who were native to southern Africa.

While these groups all viewed each other with suspicion, the rinderpest crisis pitted British government officials against livestock owners in every camp. British veterinary surgeons sought to stamp out the disease by building fences, patrolling borders, and shooting cattle that were diseased or exposed to infection. Both Boer and British farmers often opposed these measures, and they collaborated in border actions to protect their herds or thwart the eradication campaign. Many farmers believed that inoculations would protect their herds. In the Bechuana lands, tribespeople viewed the actions of all white South Africans with suspicion and perceived fence-building as a potential prelude to further British annexation. Tswana communities were themselves often divided along a generational line, as younger men supported more aggressive responses to the government measures than their elders.

The following observations of two veterinary surgeons represent the view of a beleaguered scientific elite that faced resistance on all sides. The texts come from a book-length collection of veterinary reports that were forwarded by the Cape Colony governor to the British Houses of Parliament. The surgeons record events before Robert Koch's arrival (in December 1896) and the systematic development of several inoculation procedures. The authors do not believe that any of the inoculations performed by farmers on their own were effective.

"Mr. Soga's Report"—Jotello Festiri Soga (1897)

Jotello Soga was an unusual man. His mother (Janet Burnside) was Scottish, and his father (Tiyo Soga) was the first black South African ordained as a minister in the United Presbyterian Church. His father's social status provided Soga with opportunities that were rarely available

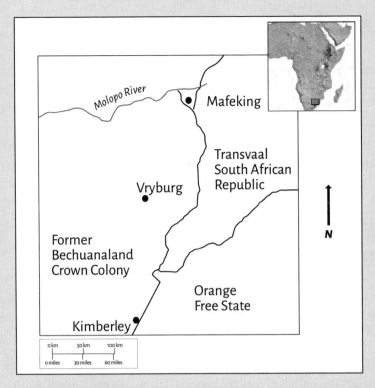

MAP 7.2 Southern Africa, 1896. In spring 1896, veterinary officials hoped to contain rinderpest north of the Molopo River (in southern Bechuanaland north of Vryburg). This effort failed and the disease soon spread throughout southern Africa.

to a man of mixed heritage. After attending veterinary school in Scotland, in 1889 Soga became Second Assistant Veterinary Surgeon to the British Cape of Good Hope colony.

Soga submitted his report to the Cape Town Chief Veterinary Surgeon. He describes events soon after rinderpest crossed the Molopo River. As a trained practitioner of elite status, Soga approaches rinderpest and Tswana South Africans in a manner consistent with white European colonial administrators. He has some training in bacteriology and he hopes for an expert scientific solution that will supersede the uninformed attempts at inoculation by local farmers. His remarks, although measured, nonetheless reveal that rinderpest is spreading like an uncontrolled wildfire.

On the 26th of March, by special dispatch, I was summoned to Mafeking, there to await your arrival anent [*i.e., for reason of*] the disease Rinderpest, which was then causing such consternation in the Protectorate. A short *resumé* of this awful scourge will be sufficient, with a few important facts....

On the 15th [*15 April 1896*] an outbreak, supposed to be Rinderpest, was reported from Sunnyside [*about 6 kilometers northeast of Mafeking*] by a native named Wellem to Mr. R. Cowan, manager.... As this was really the first authentic outbreak in Bechuanaland, it might be interesting to give in detail a result of this and other outbreaks, behind the first line of defense— "the Ramathlabama Molopo line." [*This refers to the region south of the Molopo River.*]

Europeans, farmers, and natives could not at first grasp the seriousness of the situation, owing to the salient fact that no sooner had the disease made its appearance in a herd reported by the vigilant police, than one of your staff was, within the shortest notice, on the spot; the verdict being given for destruction, was carried out immediately. Under these circumstances very few had seen the virulent effect of Rinderpest until too late. To myself, had we had thorough cooperation of the European and Native, very little destruction of stock [*cattle*] would needs have taken place....

[*At Sunnyside*] [w]ithin three weeks there was not the semblance of a case of Rinderpest. Careful burial of all infected and killed, also disinfection of people who visited the place was carried out. A strong guard of police, under Sergt. Nelson, was placed around the infected spot. The suspected eight kraals adjoining [*i.e., nearby animal enclosures*] were carefully supervised.

I may here state that many of the low Vaalpense [*poor families subjected to harsh treatment by other Indigenous groups*] had brought their pots to partake of the already dead cattle; these [*people*], fortunately, had not yet left. These I had dipped [*i.e., bathed in disinfectant fluid*], hands and utensils washed in Jeyes' [*disinfectant*] fluid, yet no outbreak occurred. These people were a great source of the spread of Rinderpest, their wandering habits, mostly by night, was a cause of great trouble. Human vultures in the extreme, and they would do anything for meat, a strange magnetism guiding them to infected or dead cattle. These are poor people, or, as I might term them, *slaves*, which they virtually are, among the Baralongs, caused us much anxiety. Moreover, it is a scandalous shame that slavery should exist in our midst....

[*Soga then records his actions at another farmstead less than three weeks later.*] 4th May—It was reported to me that suspected cases were seen at the junction of the Setlagoli and Molopo Rivers [*about 40 kilometers northwest of Mafeking*], a native Roukoquarrie and also Abram, being the afflicted. On my arrival, eighty (80) were dead in the kraal, and one hundred sixty-odd sick outside, the police meantime guarding them. Out of 342 head [*of cattle*] Roukoquarrie had nine (9) remaining, of which five (5) again were shot by the police.... [W]e had occasion to use very severe measures with the Vaalpense, threatening the same with bastinado [*hitting the soles of their feet*], and, I can assure you, sir, it was effective. We burned and buried pounds and pounds of biltong [*i.e., cured meat. Officials feared it was produced from infected cattle*], which might have infected the farms further south....

[*Soga then claims that an Indigenous chief brought contaminated livestock into a Bechuanaland reserve across the border from the Transvaal South African Republic.*]

About the middle of August was our most eventful time in Bechuanaland; a perfect influx of contamination came from the Transvaal side, introduced, in the first instance, by the natives of the Setlagoli Reserve. The chief Moshet, for certain reasons, fled into Setlagoli with a good following, leaving a good quantity of stock in the Transvaal meanwhile. Seeing that all communication (by means of wire fence was to prevent his cattle coming in), was likely to be cut off, and disease being prevalent in the Transvaal, slipped his cattle into the reserve ... setting the whole native reserve alight. So much so that with astounding rapidity, before we could check the spread, the whole reserve was alight, and past redemption as regards shooting.... Out of computed 20,000 head of cattle, something like 500 remain....

[*Soga reiterates his belief that inoculation and disinfectant chemicals are not effective, and efforts to rely on them have hampered efforts to stamp out the disease.*]

Inoculation and drenching [*dipping in disinfectant*] has been a curse; instead of retarding the disease, it has spread it.... Our only means up to the present, until science gives us a thorough preventive, is to destroy the disease by shooting and clear belts [*i.e., regions free of rinderpest*], when starvation, for want of a host or habitat, Rinderpest will die out. Clear proof we have that the organism does not last very long on the veldt. This is an important point; but how long it may remain in salted cattle [*cured meat or salted hides*] is not yet determined, until such time that science can assure us that a solution of these facts is accomplished, it is our bounden duty to retard the progress of Rinderpest by natural means, which as other countries have already proved effectual.

Fatalism seems to be the order of the day with many [*other people*]; what a childish, churlish idea. Surely this should not be the principle of an enlightened people. To this I attribute, in great measure, the cause of the failure of the prevention of the spread of Rinderpest in Bechuanaland—a want [*i.e., lack*] of co-operation.

"Resolutions Passed at Rinderpest Conference" (1897)

This excerpt was written by either Chief Surgeon Duncan Hutcheon or his First Assistant John Borthwick. On 30 August–1 September, authorities from several South African states agreed to a rinderpest strategy: culling of infected herds and the construction of lengthy wire fences to be patrolled by police. The excerpts from the following October indicate the vigorous popular resistance to the eradication plan.

On the 3rd idem [*3 October 1896*] I left Vryburg by the early morning train for Dry Harts, being accompanied by Captain Fuller and Mr. Piers, private secretary to Mr. Faure, to carry out the regulations on certain farms, the owners of which had reported to the Commission that the disease had appeared amongst their cattle, but that they would not allow them to be shot. We met Mr. Theron, the Field-Cornet at Dry Harts Station, and proceeded in company to the farms in question. We met with considerable opposition from these men, and some of them danced round us with loaded guns, and threatened us with all sorts of terrible consequences if we touched their cattle, but by exercising a firm and patient attitude we succeeded in overcoming their active opposition, but the temper of the people was such that it was evident to me that we could not continue the stamping-out policy in that district with any hope of success. An exaggerated belief in the benefit of inoculation had by this time got such a hold on the Transvaal farmers [*i.e., farmers in the neighboring Transvaal South African Republic*], that they gave their friends on the Colonial side their active sympathy against the shooting of their cattle, and doubtless encouraged them to bring their cattle into the Transvaal, in order to avoid their destruction, as four of our farmers rushed over the line in one night with their cattle. Another farmer, who attempted to take his cattle through by raising the [*wire*] fence bodily, was caught in the act by the police, and, therefore, did not succeed, much to my annoyance, as his cattle were already affected, and had to be shot. I am of the opinion that he afterwards considered himself lucky, as his son, who was one of those that got through, lost nearly the whole of his herd. I returned to Vryburg late on the 5th idem....

[*The surgeon describes his defense of livestock culls at a community meeting in Vryburg. In the face of unified opposition, the culling policy is abandoned in the district around the town.*]

On Monday, October 12, a semi-public meeting was held at the Rinderpest Committee-room at Vryburg. A large majority of those present had come to protest against the continuance of the policy of attempting to stamp out rinderpest by the slaughter of infected herds. I endeavored to reason with them, and tried to explain to them what the result of their opposition would be as compared to the benefit of the action of the Government, but they were—with a few exceptions, principally merchants—quite against any further slaughter, being determined to inoculate their cattle, as exaggerated reports of the preventive effects of this operation were at that time being widely circulated. I was very reluctant to abandon the policy that I had all along advocated so strongly, but I had come to realize a fortnight previous [*i.e., two weeks earlier*] that the farmers would not consent much longer to its continuance, and although I felt very sorry for the farmers who were so misled by glowing reports, I could hardly blame them for opposing a policy which hitherto had failed to stamp out the disease. But this was due mainly to the prolonged drought and scarcity of water which necessitated the constant movement of cattle throughout the district.... It was therefore practically decided at that meeting, that the policy of attempting to stamp out the disease in the Vryburg district should be abandoned. After the meeting, I left the same evening by train for Kimberley to attend a meeting of farmers held at Klein Karreepan.

INTERPRETING THE DOCUMENTS

1. Why did many cattle owners believe that inoculation would protect their cattle?
2. Across southern (and eastern) Africa few written sources or oral transcriptions record the firsthand perspective of Africans. What do you think were the main objectives of the tribespeople that Soga describes? What did the cattle represent in tribal society?
3. How do you think the rinderpest pandemic influenced administrative efforts to establish British rule in the Cape Colony and elsewhere in southern Africa?

MAKING CONNECTIONS

1. Compare the social tensions during the rinderpest outbreak to the social unrest during Europe's urban cholera outbreaks (chapter 5) and the Indian response to British anti-plague measures (chapter 1). What were the similarities and differences?
2. Compare the popular attitude toward expert authority (in this case veterinarians) with public health officials in Europe. Do doctors and veterinarians face similar challenges?

For further reading: Pule Phoofolo, "Face to Face with Famine: The BaSotho and the Rinderpest, 1897–99," *Journal of Southern African Studies* 29, no. 2 (2003): 503–27.

Notes

1. Richard Waller, "Emutai: Crisis and Response in Maasailand, 1883–1902," in *The Ecology of Survival: Case Studies from Northeast African History*, ed. Douglas H. Johnson and David M. Anderson (London: Lester Crook Academic Publishing, 1988), 75.
2. Y. Furuse et al., "Origin of Measles Virus: Divergence from Rinderpest Virus between the 11th and 12th Centuries," *Virology Journal* 7 (March 2010): 52–56. A time frame of the late-ninth to the tenth century is proposed in Joel O. Wertheim and Sergei L. Kosakovsky Pond, "Purifying Selection Can Obscure the Ancient Age of Viral Lineages," *Molecular Biology and Evolution* 28, no. 12 (2011): 3362–63.
3. Timothy P. Newfield, "Human-Bovine Plagues in the Early Middle Ages," *Journal of Interdisciplinary History* 46, no. 1 (2015): 1–38.

4. Philip Slavin, "The Great Bovine Pestilence and Its Economic and Social Consequences in England and Wales," *Economic History Review* 65, no. 4 (2012): 1239–66.

5. Philip Slavin, "Flogging a Dead Cow: Coping with Animal Panzootic on the Eve of the Black Death," in *Crisis in Economic and Social History: A Comparative Perspective*, ed. A. T. Brown, Andy Burn, and Rob Doherty (Woodbridge: Boydell Press, 2015), 120.

6. Quoted in Timothy P. Newfield, "A Cattle Panzootic in Early Fourteenth-Century Europe," *Agricultural History Review* 57, no. 2 (2009): 166.

7. Wolfgang Behringer, "Climate Change and Witch-Hunting: The Impact of the Little Ice Age on Mentalities," *Climatic Change* 43, no. 1 (1999): 335–51. Behringer asserts that "witchcraft was the unique crime of the Little Ice Age," 346.

8. Peter A. Morton, ed., and Barbara Dähms, trans., *The Trial of Tempel Anneke* (Toronto: University of Toronto Press, 2017), 85.

9. Behringer, "Witch-Hunting," 345. See also Clive A. Spinage, *Cattle Plague: A History* (New York: Plenum Publishers, 2003), 334–35.

10. Peter A. Koolmees, "Epizootic Diseases in the Netherlands, 1713–2002," in *Healing the Herds: Disease, Livestock Economies and the Globalization of Veterinary Medicine*, ed. Karen Brown and Daniel Guilfoyle (Athens, OH: Ohio University Press, 2010), 19–41.

11. Dominik Hünniger, "Policing Epizootics: Legislation and Administration during Outbreaks of Cattle Plague in Eighteenth-Century Northern Germany as Continuous Crisis Management," in Brown and Guilfoyle, *Healing the Herds*, 76–91.

12. Spinage, *Cattle Plague*, 365.

13. C. Huygelen, "The Immunization of Cattle against Rinderpest in Eighteenth-Century Europe," *Medical History* 41, no. 2 (1997): 182–96.

14. Mark Harrison, *Contagion: How Commerce Has Spread Disease* (New Haven, CT: Yale University Press, 2012), 213–20.

15. Spinage, *Cattle Plague,* 181; Koolmees, "Netherlands," 26–27.

16. Daniel R. Headrick, *The Tools of Empire: Technology and European Imperialism in the Nineteeth Century* (Oxford: Oxford University Press, 1981). Headrick surveys health, medicine, and imperialism in *Power over Peoples: Technology, Environments and Western Imperialism, 1400 to the Present* (Princeton: Princeton University Press, 2010), 226–50.

17. Richard Pankhurst, "The Great Ethiopian Famine of 1888–1892: A New Assessment," *Journal of the History of Medicine and Allied Sciences* 21, no. 2 (1966): 100– 02. Clive A. Spinage, *African Ecology: Benchmarks and Historical Perspectives* (Berlin: Springer-Verlag, 2012), 1057–59, presents the Egyptian hypothesis.

18. Waktole Tiki and Gufu Oba, "Ciinna—The Borana Oromo Narration of the 1890s Great Rinderpest Epizootic in North Eastern Africa," *Journal of Eastern African Studies* 3, no. 3 (2009): 479–508.

19. Richard Pankhurst, "The Great Ethiopian Famine of 1888–1892: A New Assessment: Part 2," *Journal of the History of Medicine and Allied Sciences* 21, no. 3 (1966): 271–94.

20. Richard Waller, "The Maasai and the British 1895–1905: Origins of an Alliance," *Journal of African History* 17, no. 4 (1976): 529–53.

21. Quoted in Lotte Hughes, "'They Give Me Fever': East Coast Fever and Other Environmental Impacts of the Maasai Move," in Brown and Gilfoyle, *Healing the Herds*, 152.

22. Gary Marquardt, "Building a Perfect Pest: Environment, People, Conflict and the Creation of a Rinderpest Epizootic in Southern Africa," *Journal of Southern Africa Studies* 43, no. 2 (2017): 349–63.

23. C. van Onselen, "Reactions to Rinderpest in Southern Africa, 1896–97," *Journal of African History* 13, no. 3 (1972): 473–88.

24. Phuthego P. Molosiwa, "White Man's Disease, Black Man's Peril?: Rinderpest and Famine in the Eastern Bechuanaland Protectorate at the End of the 19th Century," *New Contree*, no. 71 (December 2014): 1–24.

25. Quoted in Fred Pearce, "Inventing Africa," *New Scientist* 167, no. 2251 (2000): 32.

26. Peter Babokhov et al., "A Current Analysis of Chemotherapy Strategies for the Treatment of Human African Trypanosomiasis," *Pathogens and Global Health* 107, no. 5 (2013): 242.

27. James L.A. Webb Jr, *Humanity's Burden: A Global History of Malaria* (Cambridge: Cambridge University Press, 2009), 37–39.

28. Geoff Hide, "History of Sleeping Sickness in East Africa," *Clinical Microbiology Reviews* 12, no. 1 (1999): 112–14.

29. E.M. Fèvre et al., "Reanalyzing the 1900–1920 Sleeping Sickness Epidemic in Uganda," *Emerging Infectious Diseases* 10, no. 4 (2004): 570–72.

30. Maryinez Lyons, *The Colonial Disease: A Social History of Sleeping Sickness in Northern Zaire, 1900–1940* (Cambridge: Cambridge University Press, 2002), 68–73.

31. Pearce, "Inventing Africa," 33.

32. Spinage, *Cattle Plague*, 487.

33. Arleigh Ross D. Dela Cruz, "Epizootics and the Colonial Legacies of the United States in Philippine Veterinary Science," *International Review of Environmental History* 2 (2016): 150.

34. Ken De Bevoise, *Agents of Apocalypse: Epidemic Disease in the Colonial Philippines* (Princeton: Princeton University Press, 1995), 163.

35. Deborah J. Neill, *Networks in Tropical Medicine: Internationalism, Colonialism, and the Rise of a Medical Specialty, 1890–1930* (Stanford: Stanford University Press, 2012), 205–206.

36. Thaddeus Sunseri, "Blood Trials: Transfusions, Injections, and Experiments in Africa, 1890–1920," *Journal of the History of Medicine and Allied Sciences* 71, no. 3 (2016): 319.

37. Quoted in Christoph Gradmann, "Robert Koch and the Invention of the Carrier State: Tropical Medicine, Veterinary Infections and Epidemiology around 1900," *Studies in History and Philosophy of Biological and Biomedical Sciences* 41, no. 3 (2010): 235.

38. Facil Tesfaye, "Medical Expeditions and *Scramble for Africa*: Robert Koch in Africa, 1896–1907" (PhD diss., McGill University, 2013), 64–83.

39. Wolfgang U. Eckart, "The Colony as Laboratory: German Sleeping Sickness Campaigns in German East Africa and in Togo, 1900–1914," *History and Philosophy of the Life Sciences* 24, no. 1 (2002): 69–78.

40. Gradmann, "Robert Koch," 238.

41. Guillaume Lachenal, "A Genealogy of Treatment as Prevention: The Colonial Invention of Treatment as Prevention (TASP)," in *Global Health in Africa: Historical Perspectives on Disease Control*, ed. Tamara Giles-Vernick and James L.A. Webb Jr (Athens, OH: Ohio University Press, 2013), 75.

42. Quoted in Warwick Anderson, *Colonial Pathologies: American Tropical Medicine, Race, and Hygiene in the Philippines* (Durham, NC: Duke University Press, 2006), 59.

43. Megan Vaughan, *Curing Their Ills: Colonial Power and African Illness* (Cambridge, MA: Polity Press, 2004), 202.

44. Daniel R. Headrick, "Sleeping Sickness Epidemics and Colonial Responses in East and Central Africa," *PLOS Neglected Tropical Diseases* 8, no. 4 (2014): e27772.

45. Jacques Pepin, *The Origins of AIDS* (Cambridge: Cambridge University Press, 2011), 177.

46. Pepin, *Origins of AIDS*, 124.

47. Amanda Kay McVety, *The Rinderpest Campaigns: A Virus, Its Vaccines, and Global Development in the Twentieth Century* (Cambridge: Cambridge University Press, 2018), 121–63.

48. WHO Measles Factsheet (2017), http://www.who.int/mediacentre/factsheets/fs286/en/; W.Y. Leong, "Measles Cases Hit Record High in Europe in 2018," *Journal of Travel Medicine* 25, no. 1 (2018), https://doi.org/10.1093/jtm/tay080.

49. Jennifer Zipprich, "Measles Outbreak—California, December 2014–February 2015," *Morbidity and Mortality Weekly Report* (*MMWR*) 64, no. 6 (2015): 153–54.

50. Tyler Pager and Jeffery C. Mays, "Measles Outbreak: New York Declares Measles Emergency, Requiring Vaccination in Parts of Brooklyn," *New York Times*, 9 April 2019, https://www.nytimes.com/2019/04/09/nyregion/measles-vaccination-williamsburg.html.

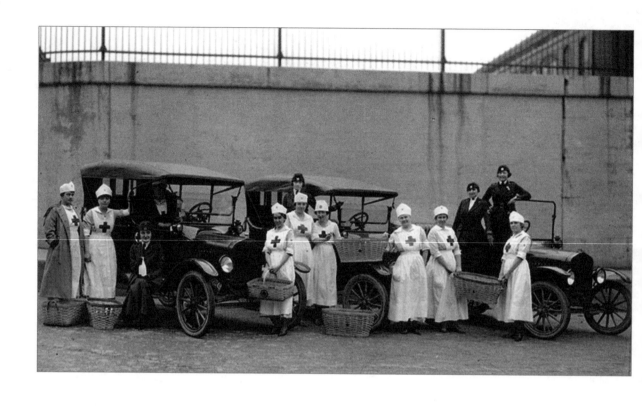

IMAGE 8.1 The Detroit Red Cross Corps. During the global pandemic of 1918–19, female nursing corps were instrumental in the response against flu. Medicines were ineffective, and good nursing care was the only real treatment.

INFLUENZA 1918—ONE
PANDEMIC, MANY EXPERIENCES

8

n Katherine Anne Porter's short novel, *Pale Horse, Pale Rider* (1939), a young woman named Miranda tumbles into delirium during a life-and-death struggle with influenza:

> Silenced she sank easily through deeps under deeps of darkness until she lay like a stone at the farthest bottom of life, knowing herself to be blind, deaf, speechless, no longer aware of the members of her own body, entirely withdrawn from all human concerns, yet alive with a peculiar lucidity and coherence; all notions of the mind, the reasonable inquiries of doubt, all ties of blood and the desires of the heart, dissolved and fell away from her, and there remained of her only a minute fiercely burning particle of being that knew itself alone.... This fiery motionless particle set itself unaided to resist destruction, to survive and be in its own madness of being, motiveless and planless beyond that one essential end. Trust me, the hard unwinking angry point of light said. Trust me, I stay.[1]

Miranda's illness mirrored Porter's own, which the author experienced in October 1918 while living in Denver, Colorado, and writing for the *Rocky Mountain News*. Porter survived influenza; a young soldier who befriended and nursed her did not. Of her brush with death Porter later noted: "It just simply divided my life, cut across it like that. So that everything before that was just getting ready, and after that I was in some strange way altered, ready. It took me a long time to go out and live in the world again."[2]

For millions of people, the great influenza pandemic that struck in the fall of 1918 was a turning point even more profound than the "Great War" that it accompanied. To a degree, the two crises were inseparable. Movements of troops propelled the pandemic that, in turn, sapped the strength of combatants in the war's final European battles before the armistice on 11 November. However, the pandemic also spanned the globe from South Africa, to the furthest reaches of the Canadian Arctic, to remote Pacific islands that faced some of the highest mortality of all. Between one-quarter and one-half of the globe's human inhabitants experienced symptoms of influenza; at least 50 million deaths over just eighteen months have been attributed to its effects, including roughly 675,000 in the United States and 50,000 in Canada. Healthy young adults experienced unusually high mortality. Pandemics caused by smallpox, bubonic plague, or cholera may once have killed a higher proportion of certain populations, but no other disease has ever dealt a blow more concentrated and widespread than influenza in 1918 and 1919. Initial attempts to create vaccines were unsuccessful, and biomedical treatments of the time were also of little use. The best defense against the flu was effective nursing care.

If any event in history might be claimed as a common human experience, surely this pandemic would be it—and yet, as historians investigate the impact of influenza in 1918–19, its unity dissolves into a mosaic of contrasting experiences, ideas, and actions. The pandemic raises basic questions that, in different ways, concern both historians and health advocates: what is a "global event," and how can we describe the interaction of local circumstances with forces that influence the whole world?[3]

Etiology and Early History

Influenza has many guises and moves swiftly. Researchers distinguish several virus types—A, B, and C—according to their protein structures (a fourth influenza type only affects cattle). A-type influenza, the main culprit for human illness, has evolved in tandem with birds. Waterfowl are its most common natural reservoir, but the virus may also be hosted by domesticated poultry and numerous mammals including bats, horses, swine, and humans. Swine may host both avian and human types of influenza. Accordingly, swine are considered a "mixing bowl" where new flu strains may emerge. In the human body, these variants may be poorly recognized by the immunity that individuals have previously acquired. Influenza typically incubates for roughly two days before symptoms develop, but hosts may be able to infect others even sooner. With modern transport, influenza can spread across an entire continent or even the globe within weeks.

Influenza A's many subtypes are named according to combinations of two surface proteins: spike-shaped hemagglutinin (HA or H) and mushroom-shaped neuraminidase (NA or N). So far, eighteen subtypes of hemagglutinin (H1–18) and eleven subtypes of neuraminidase (N1–11) have been identified. Thus, numerous protein combinations are possible, although only a few influenza subtypes have been associated with human disease. That is just on the microbe's surface—within its protein envelope, each influenza A virus has eight genetic segments of RNA that can be exchanged with other influenza viruses. The precise composition of circulating viruses changes rapidly because mutation of the surface proteins, especially HA, occurs frequently. This process, called **antigenic drift**, helps the virus evade a host's immune response. Less often, viruses undergo **antigenic shift** in one of two ways: either an entire virus jumps from one kind of host to another, or an animal and human virus exchange genetic material (a process called reassortment) in ways that also affect the surface proteins. Variation in the virus influences its tropism—its adaptation to particular cells and tissues—which helps determine how readily the virus will spread from one respiratory tract to another.

In addition to the influenza virus's capacity for rapid change, many environmental factors influence its transmission. In temperate regions, a high incidence during wintry "flu seasons" has been noted for centuries. Low relative humidity and temperatures of ~5 degrees Celsius (~40 degrees Fahrenheit) are especially conducive to the airborne spread of the microbe between hosts.[4] The precise reasons for this relationship are difficult to explain; conditions among microbes, water droplets, and animals apparently all have parts to play. It may be that the virus itself is more stable at low temperatures, or that hosts shed viruses more readily in cooler conditions. The virus usually spreads between hosts that are only a few feet apart, but low relative humidity encourages small moisture droplets that can carry it further. One study of influenza in a subarctic climate has further suggested that sudden drops in temperature and humidity increase the risk of transmission, perhaps because of the impact of weather changes upon respiratory tracts.[5] Although influenza regularly causes several million severe illnesses and roughly 300,000–600,000 deaths each year, much remains unknown about the dynamics of transmission among humans or between animals and humans.[6] Not surprisingly, investigators have focused on the origin of the 1918 influenza, its distinctive symptoms, and why it was so widespread and lethal among people in the prime of life (see figure 8.1).

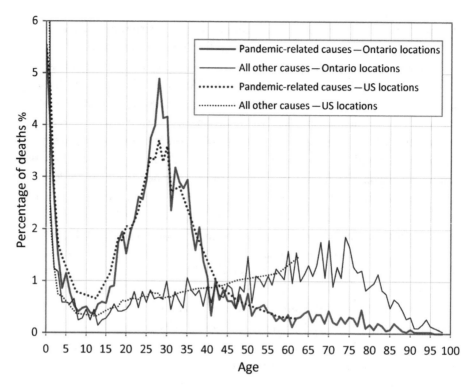

FIGURE 8.1 Mortality and age in North America, September–December 1918. This graph illustrates the disproportionate death from pandemic-related causes that took place among young adults in the United States and the Canadian province of Ontario. For example, nearly 5 per cent of all flu-related deaths in Ontario were among people aged 28. By contrast, people aged 60 in Ontario only accounted for ~0.3 per cent of flu-related deaths. The pandemic caused a much higher death rate for individuals in their twenties and thirties than all other causes of death combined. Flu-related mortality in the United States followed an identical profile. Source: Alain Gagnon et al., "Age-Specific Mortality during the 1918 Influenza Pandemic: Unravelling the Mystery of High Young Adult Mortality," *PLOS One* 8, no. 8 (2013): e69586.

The long detective story began in 1918 when US Army clinicians harvested tissue from victims and preserved the samples in paraffin wax. In the early 1930s, researchers isolated human and swine influenza viruses and eventually harvested genetic material from Arctic gravesites that were encased in permafrost after 1918–19. In the 1990s, PCR sequencing techniques allowed researchers to knit RNA fragments together, map an entire genome, and identify the cause of the 1918 pandemic as influenza A, subtype H1N1. Thereafter, a clone of this virus was recreated and used in animal tests. Researchers believe that pandemic H1N1 originated in horses or birds. It was entirely novel to humans in 1918, or shortly before, and evolved along the way so that at least two different H1N1 virus strains circulated during the pandemic. It remains unclear how pigs or other mammals might have functioned as intermediate hosts.[7]

What have researchers learned about the physical effects of the deadliest flu? Analysis of tissue samples preserved from the fall of 1918 suggest that two overlapping patterns accounted for the extremely high mortality.[8] In most cases, an aggressive bacterial infection accompanied the virus and caused pneumonia that destroyed the lungs. Less frequently, in perhaps 10–15 per cent of cases, the disease caused individuals to accumulate liquid in their lung tissues. A terrifying death ensued as they drowned in bodily fluids and their faces turned an ashen-blue or purple color from lack of oxygen. The underlying question of what caused these symptoms has been a focus of recent investigation.

Influenza's most common symptoms—fever, sore throat, body aches and fatigue, and inflamed mucous membranes—do not readily distinguish it from other diseases that are described in historical accounts. Influenza may have belonged among the fevers noted by the Hippocratic writers, Galen, and other theorists, but its ancient role remains obscure. Although scholars are reasonably confident that influenza pandemics have recurred since the early sixteenth century, analysis of the era before the nineteenth century is mostly educated guesswork.[9] With regard to the past 150 years, research suggests that influenza pandemics often have been followed by periods of high mortality from respiratory disease. It may be that widespread influenza outbreaks initiate "pandemic eras" in which a heightened incidence of other ailments fall in influenza's train.

It is, therefore, not surprising that many observers did not readily separate influenza from other maladies until the late nineteenth century. As discussed in chapter 5, by the 1830s industrial forces had begun to increase the size of cities and hasten the arrival of cholera and other epidemic diseases by railway and steamship. After 1847, working in London's General Registry Office, statistician William Farr began to distinguish influenza-attributable deaths and assign values of excess mortality to assess the impact of various epidemics. Alongside his contributions to the debate over cholera and "zymotic diseases," Farr's methodical approach did much to define influenza as a discrete disease. To a few of Farr's contemporaries, such as the Irish hospital physician Robert Graves (1796–1853), it became apparent that influenza killed more people than cholera, in part because influenza struck people who already suffered from bronchitis, asthma, or tuberculosis. However, most practitioners were less precise than Farr and Graves or failed to recognize the outbreaks of severe influenza that probably took place throughout Europe in 1847 and 1857.

Birth Year,
Immunity, and
the Future of Flu

For more than a century, influenza viruses have been a riddle: why does flu seem worse in some years than others? What factors determine which people will suffer the worst effects from the flu?

Until recently, investigators of the 1918–19 pandemic explored these questions by focusing on flu-related mortality in various age groups. Mortality during the pandemic was remarkably high among people in their twenties and thirties. Accordingly, researchers considered what characteristics were shared by people in this age group that would make them susceptible to severe symptoms. A leading hypothesis was that they experienced an immune system overreaction: signaling proteins, known as cytokines, essentially went haywire and summoned massive amounts of immune cells that clogged the lungs. In essence, healthy young adults were vulnerable because of the (destructive) strength of their body's immune response.

In 2016, a research team conducted a study to answer a new question: did an individual's first exposure to influenza influence how the immune system responded to influenza viruses later in life? The crux of the study concerned "H"s: the eighteen subtypes of hemagglutinin proteins in different human and avian influenza viruses (see figure 8.2). Researchers have established that viruses fall into two groups according to the amino acids that make up the proteins. Group 1 viruses include H1 and H2 seasonal strains and H5 avian strains; Group 2 viruses include seasonal H3 strains and H7 avian strains.

The team hypothesized that individuals would develop immune resistance to the first influenza virus they encountered as children and other viruses in the same group. Individuals would also be more susceptible to viruses in the other group. Moreover, this "imprinting" of the immune system would last their entire lives. Thus, immunities of different age cohorts would be matched or mismatched against future flu strains, depending on each virus's protein structure.

The researchers tested this thesis with data from two strains of influenza that have emerged recently: H5N1, first observed in 1997, and H7N9, first observed in 2013. Both were "avian strains" of flu transmitted from birds to humans (often to poultry workers). These viruses caused few human cases of

Group 1	Group 2
H1N1 (1918)	H3N2 (1968)
H2N2 (1957)	H7N9 (2013)
H5N1 (1997)	

FIGURE 8.2 Recent influenza viruses and apparent date of emergence.

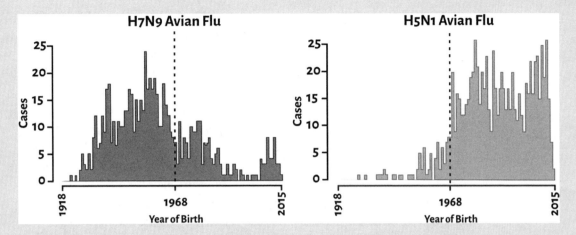

FIGURE 8.3 Birth year and influenza virus susceptibility. The two graphs suggest how the pandemic of H3N2 influenced immunity patterns against two strains of avian flu. For children born after 1968, exposure to H3N2 strengthened immunities to Group 2 viruses, including H7N9. That cohort also displayed less resistance to H5N1, a strain that is in Group 1. Source: Katelyn M. Gostic et al., "Potent Protection against H5N1 and H7N9 Influenza via Childhood Hemagglutinin Imprinting," *Nature* 354, no. 6313 (2016): Fig. 2.

disease worldwide, but the illnesses were severe and resulted in very high mortality. H5N1's protein makeup placed it in Group 1 and H7N9's composition placed it in Group 2. For the years 1997–2015, the team analyzed roughly 1,500 reported cases of severe illness caused by these strains (see figure 8.3). With various factors taken into account, the data indicated that people born before 1968 were highly susceptible to H7N9 and relatively resistant to H5N1. For people born after 1968, the situation was reversed: H5N1 caused serious illness while H7N9 did not.

Why would 1968 be a turning point for human immunities to influenza? In that year, a worldwide pandemic of the H3N2 "Hong Kong flu"—a Group 2 virus—began a period in which the global circulation of Group 1 viruses was less dominant. Thus, the first influenza exposure for children born after 1968 was more often to a Group 2 virus. Accordingly, they developed immunities to other Group 2 viruses (including H7N9), while children born before 1968 had developed immunities to Group 1 viruses (including H5N1). The mismatch of acquired immunity with a flu strain made individuals more vulnerable to severe illness.

In short, the findings suggest that a person's age is not the most important factor that determines their resistance to various influenza viruses. Instead, *initial childhood exposure* markedly influences how a person's body reacts to influenza thereafter. This research offers a new explanation for the extraordinary mortality from H1N1 in 1918–19: a different kind of influenza virus imprinted the immune systems of the hardest-hit cohort when its members were young children in the 1880s and early 1890s.

Beyond history, will this research affect vaccine development and the shots people receive? In the future, it may be possible for individuals to select a flu shot that strengthens immunity in areas that require support. Work in this area will assist prediction and public health strategies, particularly when a new pandemic influenza strain emerges. Influenza is still a puzzle with missing pieces and there is much to learn about how the first exposure to a pathogen shapes immunity for a lifetime.[10]

Quite different was the emergence, several decades later, of the "Russian flu" in 1889. While influenza would cause much higher mortality in 1918, this pandemic forced a reckoning of its own: at least a million people died worldwide as waves of infection circled the globe several times between the fall of 1889 and the winter of early 1894. This flu arrived in an era marked by new technologies that were rapidly knitting together large parts of the world. By 1890, more than 120,000 miles of railroad enabled swift transport across Russia and western Europe, and North American rail networks were of comparable scale. The rapid movement of people was matched by an increasingly rapid flow of information. In 1851, the first telegraph cable had been laid between Calais (France) and Dover (England) to link London and other key cities of northern Europe. Fifteen years later, a permanent telegraph line was laid across the Atlantic and networks of cable crisscrossed Europe and North America. The Russian flu was the first pandemic that could be tracked by millions of people more or less in real time.

Some observers certainly associated the pandemic with the increased scale and speed of human travel. However, the growing awareness of global interconnectedness also encouraged new environmental explanations. In an article that American newspapers reprinted widely, Philadelphia physician Roberts Bartholow (1831–1904) attempted to combine germ theory with a "seed and soil" analogy that was akin to the approach of Max von Pettenkofer. Although Bartholow attributed individual cases of influenza to "some micro-organism or its ova" that irritated mucous membranes and bronchial surfaces, he also considered broader factors that enabled its spread and produced what he called a "systemic poisoning."[11] Minor epidemics, he thought, did not develop "sufficient momentum" to venture beyond regions with a certain soil and climate. Bartholow concluded that the great epidemics must be related to enormous global disturbances that were caused by "the sun with its photosphere and magnetic storms."

Spurred by the new bacteriology, many European researchers also hunted for a microbial culprit. The most likely candidate, a bacterium, was put forth by the scientist with the best pedigree: Richard Pfeiffer (1858–1945), a protégé and the son-in-law of the august Robert Koch. Other researchers soon confirmed that Pfeiffer's bacillus—called *Bacillus influenzae*—appeared in great quantities in the sputum of infected individuals. The bacillus failed to cause flu when it was inoculated into various mammals and, therefore, it did not fulfill Koch's postulates that were thought to prove conclusively that a pathogen caused disease (see chapter 5). But observers were prepared to overlook this fact. Cartoons depicted influenza as a beastly, impish little "microbe of the sneeze."[12]

It was this pandemic, rather than the "Spanish flu" three decades later, that propelled the notion of a disease-causing microbe into wide circulation. As discussed in chapter 6, the discourse concerning tuberculosis provided another avenue for "germ talk" and associated products and practices to enter the lives of Westerners. None of this was of any immediate use in 1918; germ theories had little to offer for effective treatment or prevention. And when influenza struck again, it seemed to be everywhere at once.

Influenza in 1918–1919

Since 1927, when Edwin Oakes Jordan (1866–1936) first reviewed the epidemiology of the pandemic, researchers have suggested several possible sites of origin.[13] Many scholars have pointed to the US state of Kansas. In February 1918, a major influenza outbreak at the Fort Riley military base was preceded by unusually violent cases in nearby Haskell County. Soldiers from the base soon circulated throughout the United States and overseas. A second theory focuses attention on an earlier outbreak at Étaples, France, where a disease called "purulent bronchitis" was noted in December 1916. At this hub of the French war effort, soldiers came and went by the tens of thousands and lived in close proximity to large numbers of chickens and pigs that were raised to feed them. A third hypothesis points to a mysterious outbreak of respiratory disease in the Shanxi province of northern China. In spring 1918, thousands of Chinese workers bound for France arrived at a port near Victoria, on Canada's Vancouver Island, where hundreds fell ill and were placed in medical care. Reports of severe pulmonary disease followed these conscripts across Canada and to labor camps in France. The origin debate lingers, but the fact that various scenarios are plausible carries a lesson of its own. As John Barry has noted, the potential for a US origin of the pandemic "warns investigators where to look for a new virus. They must look everywhere."[14]

The overall profile of the pandemic is most often described as three waves that coursed around the globe, beginning in early 1918. Unlike the 1889 pandemic, which reappeared annually over several winter seasons, the phases that began in 1918 occurred in relatively swift succession. At first, in late winter and spring 1918, the outbreaks were episodic and dispersed. H1N1 influenza may have circulated at this time, but no samples have been analyzed to confirm it. In late August, a well-defined second phase began with nearly simultaneous outbreaks in ports on three continents: Freetown, Sierra Leone; Brest, France;

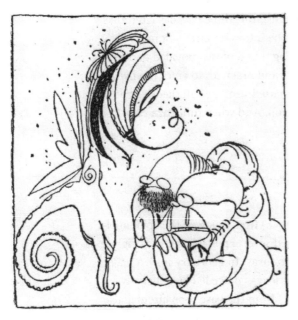

IMAGE 8.2 "The Biologists—'Come on, precious! ... Tell us who you are!'" This cartoon by Lluis Bagaria first appeared in the Spanish newspaper *El Sol* in May 1918. Researchers kneel beseechingly before influenza, depicted as a strange chimera. Its causes remained mysterious since microscopes of the time did not enable observers to identify the virus.

and Boston, Massachusetts and a nearby military staging area named Camp Devens. Very few locations were left untouched. The great majority of victims sickened and died between the end of August and November 1918. The mortality rate for the infected was extraordinary; in a typical year influenza causes case mortality of roughly 0.1 per cent, but in 1918 the rate exceeded 2.5 per cent, at least twenty-five times higher.[15] A third phase began early in 1919, and lingered in some places until early 1920, but caused fewer deaths. None of the waves originated in Spain; the moniker "Spanish flu" reflected the willingness of this nation's newspapers to report the disease's impact because it was not a combatant in World War I.

In many regions, especially where wartime personnel were on the move, influenza spread rapidly along railways and steamship routes, and it fanned out into countrysides from urban centers. In the United States, the pandemic moved west from the eastern seaboard, north from the Gulf of Mexico up the Mississippi River, and inland from west-coast ports. In Canada, it has been suggested that infection spread from the United States, not among troops returning from Europe, and that soldiers spread the disease as they traveled west to join a trans-Siberian expeditionary force.[16] Regardless, the main paths of diffusion were shipping routes down the St Lawrence Seaway and west via the Canadian Pacific Railway. Elsewhere, newly completed rail systems in central and southern Africa and steamships in the Congo River basin provided conduits for the movement of disease. Railroads in India and rivers in China also served as transmission routes.[17] Most developed nations reported overall mortality rates between 4 and 10 people per 1,000 and seemingly faced a similar level of impact from the pandemic. One comparison may illustrate: the United States, Japan, and New

Zealand differed dramatically in population—with 105 million, 57 million, and 1 million inhabitants, respectively—but their reported overall mortality rates were similar (for the US, the rate was 6.4 per 1,000; for Japan, 4.5 per 1,000; and for New Zealand, 5.8 per 1,000). Reports from western European nations, even the main combatants Germany and France, reflect a comparable experience.

However, the consistent picture offered by such numbers is deceptive. For much of the world, the available records permit only cautious generalizations. Nonetheless, it is clear that non-Western nations often (but not always) faced substantially higher mortality than Western ones, and the way that influenza interacted with other forces varied considerably from place to place. In Iran, for example, Amir Afkhami has estimated that at least 8 per cent (80 per 1,000) of the total population died of influenza-related causes. Here the impact of influenza was exacerbated by famine, high rates of malaria and hookworm (caused by parasites that live in the small intestine), and perhaps also by high levels of opium use.[18] In Tanzania, which had been controlled by Germany, influenza struck a population that was destabilized by intermittent fighting and stripped of food and livestock by both German and British forces. James Ellison suggests that some communities lost 10 per cent of their inhabitants, mostly young adults, between October and December 1918. Overall, the pandemic was probably the worst short-term demographic crisis in southern Africa's recorded history.[19] In contrast, the sparse evidence available for China suggests that its inhabitants experienced relatively low mortality outside of principal port cities. Unlike Japan and the island of Taiwan under Japanese control, China's lack of railway and steamship travel slowed influenza's progress across the country.[20] India faced the greatest mortality of any nation; estimates of the total influenza mortality in the subcontinent range upward from 17 million people.

As these brief examples indicate, at the level of large populations there was no typical encounter with pandemic influenza. Likewise, the pandemic's impact varied *within* communities as well. While a single chapter cannot address this topic fully, the following sections explore factors that helped create diverse landscapes of disease.

Influenza in War

The impact of influenza in warfare prior to the fall of 1918 is difficult to assess. Its common, nonlethal symptoms often were not viewed as a distinct threat that merited comment. During most conflicts, there were worse diseases to worry about. In Eurasia, bubonic plague accompanied the movements of armies throughout the early modern period. Large assemblies of troops and animals contaminated water supplies and caused outbreaks of typhoid, dysentery, and cholera. In tropical regions, yellow fever and malaria influenced the course of many military campaigns. Over the long term, the cluster of maladies known as typhus has perhaps done the most to obscure influenza's wartime impact from view. Various forms of typhus are caused by bacteria that are spread by bites and discharges from their hosts—lice, fleas, and ticks that live on humans. Often lethal, typhus causes rashes, but also very high fever and severe body aches. A typhus outbreak may have hastened the disintegration of Napoleon's *Grand Armée* during its disastrous invasion of Russia in 1812–13. Although some of the causal microbes were identified by 1914, typhus killed millions of people in central and Southeast Asia during the world wars and the aftermath of the Russian Revolution (1917). In all likelihood, typhus has overshadowed various maladies that share some of its symptoms.[21]

Many of these diseases played a significant role in the first years of World War I. In 1918, however, influenza's devastating impact was distinct and terrifying. In the battlefields of France, trench combat placed millions of exhausted young men at close quarters where they could easily transmit infection. What made the conflict particularly advantageous for the influenza virus, however, was the evacuation of sick soldiers to hospitals and the frequent rotation of combatants on and off the front line. Both patterns were a godsend for pathogens in search of new hosts: hospitals concentrated men in closely spaced beds, and the supply of vulnerable hosts at the front was constantly replenished. Soldiers waiting for deployment in barracks or crowded into trains were probably at greatest risk of infection. The British Expeditionary Force reported 313,000 cases of influenza in 1918, although the actual tally was probably higher, and the French army reported more than 400,000 cases between May 1918 and April 1919. Because the United States did not field a large army until September 1918, its war experience more or less coincided with the peak of the pandemic. Tens of thousands of soldiers fell ill in camps before their departure. In France, Americans showed up and got sick: US troops hospitalized for influenza—around 340,000—exceeded the number of battle casualties by 50 per cent. Fortunately for them, however, the Germans were sick, too; their army documented more than 700,000 cases of the disease.[22]

Although influenza did not determine the outcome of World War I, the disease certainly affected how warfare was conducted. German general Erich Ludendorff famously acknowledged the severity of its impact; it is possible that the initial influenza outbreaks in spring 1918 interfered with the German army's ability to mount an offensive. In September 1918, millions of soldiers participated in two major campaigns, St Mihiel (14–16 September) and Meuse-Argonne (26 September–11 November). As thousands of troops sickened, casualties reduced fighting strength and created logistics challenges as medical personnel hastened to the front and thousands of men were shuttled back and forth. Beyond the actual battlefield, war conditions increased the incidence of lethal influenza for noncombatants. In Paris, which provided supplies for the front, deaths caused by influenza in young women dramatically outnumbered those of young men. Patrick Zylberman has suggested that young women in "front-line cities," such as Paris or Nancy, lived disproportionately in cramped conditions and faced malnutrition and disease as they worked as servants or replacement factory workers.[23] Throughout the combat zones, the combined impact of war and disease ranged beyond the soldiers.

Influenza and "Home Fronts"

Some scholars have emphasized that social inequality shaped the course of the pandemic in nations that did not face battles on home soil. This focus is a recent trend. Until the 2000s, most historians assented to Alfred Crosby's view that, although cramped housing facilitated the spread of disease, "by and large the rich died as readily as the poor."[24] Certainly, in the pandemic's immediate aftermath, the scale of suffering encouraged many observers to proclaim its universal impact. A mournful commentary in the London *Times* was typical: "[Influenza] came and went, a hurricane across the green fields of life, sweeping away our youth in the hundreds of thousands and leaving a toll of sickness and infirmity which will not be reckoned in this generation."[25]

However, when local statistics are available they often tell a different story. Already in 1931, an analyst for the US Public Health Service, Edgar Sydenstricker (1881–1936), focused on class distinctions in an analysis of data from ten cities around the country. After accounting for sex, age, and ethnic background, Sydenstricker concluded that "the lower the economic level the higher was the attack rate" for influenza; moreover, the mortality rate in "very poor" households approached three times the rate of households with a status of "well-to-do" or "moderate."[26] Although influenza spread in both rich and poor *communities*, its effects were more severe in disadvantaged *households*. Sydenstricker's analysis had its limits. His chief interest lay with industrial working families, which led him to ignore factors such as the social subordination of African American farmworkers in the South.[27] His data also did not explain the reason for the correlations he found. Were feeble people, who were more vulnerable to disease, also less capable of earning a good living? Did working or living conditions among the poor increase their chance of infection, or were there differences in health care between rich and poor? Numerous conditions were at play, Sydenstricker conceded, but he rejected the claim that influenza was an entirely "democratic" pestilence.

Overall, it seems clear, as Howard Phillips and David Killingray have suggested, that "the poor, and those living in overcrowded and insanitary conditions, were more likely to catch and to die from the virus."[28] For example, Esyllt Jones's study of Winnipeg suggests that death was concentrated in a poor northern district inhabited by Jewish and Slavic immigrants whose dwellings were segregated from better-off Anglo-Canadians. The socio-economic disparity did not merely cause more deaths—Jones claims that Winnipeg's experience with influenza galvanized social protest that took the form of a general workers' strike in May 1919.[29] In Europe, an investigation of neighborhoods in Kristiania, Norway (now Oslo), identified correlations related to the income status of neighborhoods and the size of dwellings. Individuals who lived in one-room apartments faced influenza mortality that was 50 per cent higher than those who lived in four to six room apartments. Collectively, the inhabitants of Kristiania's most impoverished parishes (i.e., districts) experienced mortality that was almost 50 per cent higher than mortality in the wealthiest district.[30] However, not all local studies have drawn precisely the same conclusion. In a detailed analysis of the town of Christchurch, New Zealand, Geoffrey Rice determined that well-paid professionals were less likely to fall ill than skilled and semiskilled workers, and that lower-quality housing and sanitation seemed to correlate with illness.[31] But Rice also considered these facts to be less important than the high mortality among parents with young children and the potential for the disease to strike everyone. In the face of such a widespread event, every community—and perhaps every historian—can offer a different narrative.

Indigenous Experiences

Around the world during the influenza pandemic, Indigenous communities suffered disproportionately compared to other groups. Where statistics are available, the contrast is stark. The estimated mortality among Indigenous Canadians was 37.7 per 1,000, compared with 6.1 per 1,000 for the entire country. In some provinces, such as British Columbia, the death rate among Indigenous people was even higher. In New Zealand, the death rate for Maori was estimated at 43.3 per 1,000, more than seven times the rate among people of European descent.[32]

At the time, Western observers attributed high Indigenous mortality to inherited "racial" characteristics or innate weakness. As discussed in chapter 3, a version of this claim persisted among historians who suggested that genetic traits, or at least a lack of genetic diversity among Indigenous peoples, explained uniformly high death rates when diseases struck. But for influenza, as for most other diseases, no relevant genetic differences have been isolated at the level of populations. Attention now focuses on the complex suite of immune characteristics that can vary among families and even among individuals. Certainly, some Indigenous communities existed in relative isolation and therefore experienced few opportunities for individuals to acquire immunities. In 1918, this was especially true for the inhabitants of previously remote Pacific islands. Before the arrival of steamships on their shores in the 1830s, these small societies were protected by distance and travel times that exceeded the duration of infections such as influenza or measles. Even in the later nineteenth century, the isolation was self-reinforcing, as brushes with various diseases encouraged Indigenous communities to avoid the sick. In 1918, however, individual and communal defenses broke down unless extraordinary measures were taken.

The experience of inhabitants on the Samoan Islands provides an especially dramatic example of the differential impact of disease among Indigenous communities. In the early twentieth century, control over this South Pacific archipelago was divided between Germany and the United States. In 1914, as World War I began, Britain launched a blockade of Germany's ports and prevented its navy from reaching the South Pacific colonies. Pacific nations rushed to fill the breach, and forces from New Zealand assumed control over German (or Western) Samoa in August. A few years later, the Samoan experience of pandemic influenza diverged along political lines. In Western Samoa (on the island of Upolu), the ship *Talune* arrived from Auckland, New Zealand, on 7 November 1918 with infected passengers and crew aboard. No precautions were taken and influenza began a violent rampage that killed more than 7,500 people (about 20 per cent of the island's population) in less than two months. Forty miles distant, on the American-controlled island of Tutuila, officials recognized the danger of influenza at the outset. Arrivals were quarantined, and, as conditions in Western Samoa became known, its ships were refused entry altogether. Quarantine was maintained until mid-1920, apparently with the enthusiastic support of the populace, and the island did not record a single influenza death.

We might conclude from Samoa's experience that exposure to the influenza virus was the most important (or perhaps the only) variable that determined the fate of Indigenous peoples. However, other factors were also important, as illustrated by the contrasting experiences of two Canadian communities in the Lake Winnipeg region, Norway House and Fisher River. In the late nineteenth century, Indigenous inhabitants of the area had responded in different ways to the growing impact of European immigrants and the diminishing supply of fur-bearing animals that supported a trapping economy. Indigenous individuals based at Norway House in the summer continued to work traplines in the winter and were forced to travel hundreds of miles in cold weather. At Fisher River, former traders and trappers worked at a saw mill, performed wage labor, and kept livestock. These activities kept them sedentary year-round. In 1918–19, an estimated 18 per cent of the individuals connected to Norway House died from influenza. Mortality was concentrated in able-bodied adults (ages 21–65) and in select families that experienced more than one death. The outbreak began in December, when many families were trapping in snowy forests, far beyond the reach of any assistance when they fell ill. Circumstances differed in Fisher River, where 13 per cent of the inhabitants died and 80 per cent of the deceased were twenty years of age or younger. The available records do not afford a complete picture, but Karen Slonim suggests that children and young adults in Fisher River experienced other respiratory diseases, such as tuberculosis, that aggravated the influenza-related mortality.[33] Overall, communal supports enabled Fisher River to withstand the pandemic more effectively than Norway House's isolated trappers, but the sedentary context also increased the risks from other concurring diseases. In these communities, as elsewhere, generalizations about an "Indigenous experience" of influenza have only limited value.

Influenza and Medical Practitioners

As the analyses of Fisher River and Norway House suggest, sustained and attentive care contributed to reduced mortality and greater communal resilience.
Although many trained doctors and nurses labored heroically during the pandemic, their efforts yielded very different results.

In some respects, elite medical researchers experienced the least success and
greatest frustration during the pandemic. Since the 1880s, the exploration of
vaccines, treatments, and disease-causing pathogens had advanced by leaps and
bounds. In the United States, the Johns Hopkins University in Baltimore had
created a leading center for medical research. Then, in October 1918, several
Hopkins experts witnessed the horrific outbreak at Camp Devens and left
stunned and disturbed. In the following year, antiserums and vaccines were
tested in haphazard fashion by various research groups. At first, many preparations were derived from Pfeiffer's *B. influenzae* bacterium. When mounting
evidence suggested that *B. influenzae* was, in fact, a "secondary invader" rather
than the causal pathogen, more vaccines targeted secondary infections such as
pneumonia rather than influenza itself. As the scientific disarray became
apparent, the American Public Health Association (APHA) produced a set of
standards to be met by vaccine trials to ensure the quality of data. One key
criterion was a control group; vaccine tests should pair vaccinated subjects with
an equivalent nonvaccinated group that had identical exposure to the disease in
question. This initiative contributed significantly to the consistency and quality
of medical research in the coming decades but it did not pay immediate divi-
dends. Although the pandemic of 1918–19 did little over the long term to
diminish popular esteem for medical science, disease experts were humbled by
failure.

The pandemic offered other lessons to those who tended the sick. Doctors,
like medical researchers, grappled with the realization that they could offer no
cure for influenza. The tangible measures that contributed to a patient's
well-being—blankets, clean sheets and clothes, essential food and water—fell
within the purview of nurses. When people fell ill by the hundreds, effective
nursing frequently made the difference between communities that remained
intact and ones that collapsed. Nancy Bristow has suggested that this created a
distinctively gendered response among caregivers. Nurses shared the male
physicians' feelings of dread but were also more likely to associate their work
with positive accomplishments and satisfaction. On occasion, the service of

nurses was celebrated, as in this passage from a *Literary Digest* article in 1919: "In the fight against influenza ... devoted women have served in the front ranks and many of them, uninspired by the interest and honor that helped the dough-boy act the hero, have gone down to death, if not unwept, at least unsung."[34]

Such references to women in the "front ranks" made a superficial comparison between female nurses and male soldiers. Ultimately, however, both observers and nurses themselves described their contribution in ways that emphasized their role as selfless caregivers and model women. While some trained nurses drew attention to the skill and training their profession required, on balance the discourse about nursing during and after the pandemic reinforced conventional gender roles more than it challenged them.

The Influenza Pandemic's Legacy

How may we characterize the impact of a war that took many lives and a pandemic that took even more? A few studies have attempted pieces of a narrative concerning demographic shifts of the era. In combatant countries, there were fewer marriages and relatively more single young females immediately after the war. However, as Elizabeth Roberts has pointed out, these women did not necessarily enjoy better employment opportunities. Instead, many were displaced from their wartime jobs by men who returned home.[35] Andrew Noymer and Michel Garenne have further suggested that mortality in World War I and from influenza both struck young males disproportionately but, thereafter, male life expectancy increased because the survivors were less vulnerable to tuberculosis, kidney disease, and heart disease.[36] In general, however, there is no accounting for the children, fathers, mothers, siblings, and spouses who disappeared in such great numbers over such a short time. As Terence Ranger has suggested, this may be the province of poets and novelists, who can extract meaning from a compressed episode in ways that transcend a historical narrative of events, causes, and effects.[37]

We are on slightly firmer ground when we consider the legacy of the influenza virus itself. Jeffery Taubenberger and David Morens have named the 1918 influenza the "mother of all pandemics" because influenza A pandemics thereafter have been caused by descendants of the H1N1 influenza that circulated in

1918–19.[38] After 1920, H1N1 influenza settled into a more conventional pattern of annual seasonal recurrence, and its impact lessened after the early 1950s. In 1957, a virus emerged that contained key genes from the 1918 virus but also incorporated two different surface proteins, H2 and N2. This virus caused mortality similar to 1889 but then settled into a seasonal pattern as well. In 1968, the "Hong Kong flu" (H3N2) replaced H2N2 in another pandemic event. Although widespread, this strain had relatively mild effects, perhaps because the "N" (neuraminidase) remained unchanged and antibodies that had accumulated in the world's population helped to reduce the duration and severity of illness.

In 1977, a strain of H1N1 influenza suddenly re-emerged. Analysis soon revealed that the virus's genetic composition was almost identical to samples that were collected in Scandinavia during the 1950s. The most likely scenario—a troubling one—is that human action reactivated the pathogen through a laboratory accident, a vaccine trial that went awry, or an intentional release as a biological weapon. H1N1 influenza has continued to circulate, and fortunately has not had the devastating impact of its ancestor in 1918–19. However, the likelihood that scientists revived a potential threat has sparked debate concerning biosafety standards and the appropriate scope of viral research programs. Investigators now have the means not only to release old pathogens but also to recreate or adapt them. The possible benefits of such research—for example, to develop a vaccine that is more effective than the current ones—must be weighed against risks that are perceived differently by various research communities.[39]

In addition to H1N1 "legacy viruses," other threats arise from pathogens that are endemic among animals and may infect humans as well. In January 1976, an alarming outbreak of swine influenza at Fort Dix, a US military base in New Jersey, sickened thirteen people and caused one death. While the infection did not spread, it prompted a hasty vaccination program that reached 40 million Americans before it was halted at the end of the year. WHO officials faced a similar alarm in the spring of 2009 when a human virus was identified that combined genetic material from two pre-existing swine viruses. As discussed earlier in this chapter, novel avian strains of influenza are also worrisome. In 1997, human cases of H5N1 "bird flu" were documented for the first time in Hong Kong. Between 2003 and 2009, H5N1 became rampant among birds, and the WHO reported 468 confirmed human cases and 282 deaths, a sobering case fatality rate of 60 per cent. While human cases have diminished since then, experts have feared that the virus could evolve into a form that would spread rapidly among humans. In 2013, H5N1 was joined by H7N9. This strain, which also circulates in poultry, has only resulted in approximately 1,500 reported human cases, but among them it has caused an extraordinary case fatality rate of about 30 per cent.

As noted in chapter 7, the shift to intensive animal farming in recent decades has vastly increased the potential for pathogens to evolve and circulate among birds, mammals, and humans. The World Organization for Animal Health (OIE) has developed guidelines for the reporting of animal disease, standards for their diagnosis and control, and other regulations to assure sanitary safety in the international animal trade. But risks persist, including the exposure of domesticated birds to infected wild birds, possible contamination of drinking water, and the continued circulation of swine flu in regions where bird flu is also common.[40] In 2015, a highly pathogenic virus strain entered the United States from Canada and infected 40 million birds on nearly 100 commercial poultry farms in Minnesota and Iowa. The virus spread among several wild bird species as well. Such episodes are damaging economically—the poultry were culled at a cost of more than $1 billion—and raise fears of an uncontrolled pandemic that would spread far beyond farm settings.

Human activity in the lab and on the farm has magnified the risk of a future influenza pandemic. What about efforts to develop preventive vaccines or therapy? In 1918, medicine was impotent, but researchers began to make meaningful strides after a human influenza virus was isolated with an electron microscope in 1933. Several years later, Rockefeller Foundation researchers Thomas Magill (1903–1999) and Thomas Francis (1900–1969) observed the antigenic variation among influenza A viruses. Vaccine trials soon commenced in the United States, and, as with other disease control measures, the desire to protect troops in World War II spurred further research in the 1940s. A vaccine using inactivated, or "killed," virus was introduced in 1943; fertilized chicken eggs were used to culture the needed virus after it was shown that the virus grew readily in them. Eggs are still commonly used to grow the virus used in vaccines today. A hope that researchers could develop one vaccine to provide lasting protection against various influenza strains has not been fulfilled. Instead, flu vaccines are now designed each year, one for the northern

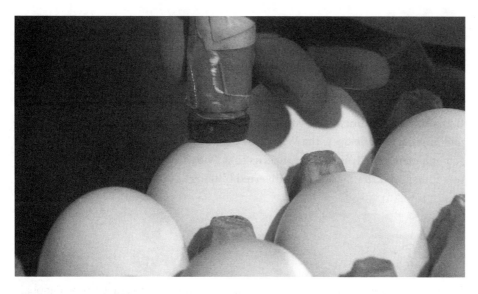

IMAGE 8.3 Culturing flu samples. A CDC scientist punctures holes in embryonated chicken eggs. A syringe will be inserted into the holes to inject viral material into a cavity where it will grow. The procedure yields large quantities of viral material for laboratory tests.

hemisphere and one for the southern hemisphere, based on data collected from monitoring stations in more than 100 countries. The high rate of antigenic drift means that the viral strains that are used to construct the vaccine may not precisely match the influenza in circulation at a given time. Data concerning vaccinations vary from country to country, but less than half of the inhabitants of Western nations receive seasonal flu shots, and elsewhere vaccination rates are even lower.[41]

In the last several decades, anti-flu medications have also been developed, but their role in the broader social response to pandemics has become controversial. While drugs such as amantadine were introduced in the late 1960s, influenza treatment entered a new phase in 1999 when the drug zanamivir (sold under the name Relenza) became available. This drug and oseltamivir (sold as Tamiflu) are **neuraminidase inhibitors**. They work by blocking the action of neuraminidase proteins, thus preventing the release of a virus's progeny from an infected cell. In the 2000s, nations that included Canada and the United States began to stockpile millions of medication doses as part of their pandemic response strategies, and in 2010 the WHO added oseltamivir to its core list of medicines that were essential for a basic health-care system. However, a growing body of evidence indicated that these NA inhibitors had modest effects: while they might reduce the duration and severity of symptoms for some people, no research about individuals or populations suggested that NA inhibitors affected transmission of influenza or hospital admissions, or reduced the likelihood of pneumonia. In June 2017, the WHO downgraded oseltamivir to the status of a "complementary" drug, amid concerns that evidence for the drug's usefulness was flimsy, and that nations had diverted billions of dollars from more useful health investments.

Conclusion

Despite many advances—in vaccines, treatment, animal care practices, and global surveillance—nothing can remove the likely prospect of another influenza pandemic. However, the popular perception of influenza remains in flux. It is a familiar seasonal burden and a looming global threat; a historical artifact and a current concern. Most often, the discourse around influenza focuses not on a potential pandemic but, rather, on its current impact among vulnerable groups (such as the elderly) and the effectiveness of vaccines for "this year's flu." Since hundreds of thousands of people die from influenza annually, routine preventive efforts compete for attention with the known but unpredictable risk of a true global crisis. When we consider pandemic influenza through the prism of biology, we may understand it as the product of "A" influenza viral subtypes. But the many manifestations of disease present distinct social and medical challenges. There is no single influenza.

As one pair of researchers recently noted, "The challenge for us humans is to learn as much about influenza viruses as they have already learned about us."[42] Efforts are focused on the development of vaccines that are effective against a broad range of influenza viruses. In the meantime, the combination of modern surveillance, current vaccines, and medicines that counter both viruses and secondary infections will reduce the impact of another pandemic in developed countries. Just as in 1918, however, disparities in access to medical and nursing care pose a challenge for the global response to a pandemic.

In *America's Forgotten Pandemic*, Alfred Crosby asked why the United States seemed so eager to leave the influenza of 1918–19 behind. The war, of course, prevented officials in many countries from commenting openly about its impact. And influenza came and went so swiftly that most institutions had no chance to react; its sudden stroke defied a measured response, just as its symptoms defied treatment. Crosby found that only in individual accounts, the kind that appear in intimate letters or oral histories, did the pandemic's deep impact become apparent.[43] As recent historians have shown, even in 1918 there was no single influenza. However, many factors that were relevant a century ago remain important as we consider the prospect of a future pandemic.

This chapter began with one literary meditation and will end with another. To British author Virginia Woolf, the muted literary response to influenza reflected an impoverishment of the English language in its response to disease. "The merest schoolgirl, when she falls in love, has Shakespeare or Keats to speak her mind for her," Woolf wrote in 1926, "but let a sufferer try to describe a pain in his head to a doctor and language at once runs dry." (Although we recall that Shakespeare barbed his plays with allusions to the pox, and Keats earned notice as a consumptive aesthete as well as a poet.) No stranger herself to severe bouts of flu and other diseases, Woolf thought that illness belonged alongside love or death as a great literary theme. Nonetheless, she conceded that "the public would say that a novel devoted to influenza lacked plot—they would complain that there was no love in it...." Woolf thought that influenza was an experience easily recognized, but difficult for a writer to mine for universal meaning: "his own suffering serves but to wake memories in his friends' minds of *their* influenzas, *their* aches and pains which went unwept last February."[44] The idea of "influenza" held more than one potential story, and the swift, terrible pandemic of 1918–19 receded before the disease's more common, mundane presence.

Pandemic flu carried no lessons about the differences between societies or environments. In contrast, as the twentieth century progressed, "tropical" diseases such as malaria signified an increasing gap between nations that still confronted them and others that did not. This was especially true after World War II, as pesticides and other tools helped Europe and North America eliminate malaria. Elsewhere, public health interventions encountered greater difficulty, and the measures themselves often created new challenges for the inhabitants of Africa and Southeast Asia.

WORKSHOP: COMING TO GRIPS WITH "LA GRIPPE" IN NEWSPAPERS AND LETTERS

Newspaper articles are an abundant and fascinating historical source for events related to World War I. However, they must be read with care: their audience, point of view, objectives, and main claims are all open to discussion. This is true even for short articles that ostensibly present "objective" information such as names and dates. Comparison with other source material reveals how print media interpret events by including or emphasizing some ideas and omitting others.

The first two written documents describe conditions at Camp Devens, a staging area where American soldiers assembled before shipping out to France. Thirty-five miles north of Boston, Massachusetts, Devens was an encampment of roughly 2,000 hectares (7.7 square miles). Although its medical facilities and staff were well regarded, in late September Devens was overwhelmed by influenza. Doctors called it "the grip" or "la grippe," the French term for the flu. Reports of the crisis often distinguished between cases of influenza and deaths caused by "pneumonia," the most obvious secondary symptom of infection.

"3000 Have Influenza at Devens"—*Boston Post* (17 September 1918)

12 New Wards Opened at Hospital; Room for 1500 More

CAMP DEVENS, Sept. 16—The second week of Spanish grip started today with 3000 patients at the base hospital. The twelve new wards built some time ago were opened to accommodate cases, and there is room for 1500 more cases. To date there is not a single death which can positively be traced to influenza.

RECEIVING BEST CARE—The base hospital area is closed to civilians, although it is not quarantined and a guard is posted to stop civilian pedestrians and autoists from entering without permission. There is no quarantine and men in uniform are allowed to pass freely. The quartermaster supply wagon brought a quantity of straw to fill bed sacks and iron cots to equip those of the new wards which have as yet been unoccupied.

Soldiers are "throwing off" the disease without having to go to the hospital. One colonel overcame it with his vigorous resistance.

Major-General McCain visited the base hospital and was satisfied that the men were receiving the best of care. In the sunshine today scores of patients lay on cots on the ward porches tucked in snugly under wool blankets.

Deaths from Pneumonia—Pneumonia caused the death today of Private George Sprague, I Company, 7th Infantry, son of Mrs. Phellan Sprague of Harrington, Me, and of Private Mellen Adams, H Company, 42nd Infantry, son of Mrs. Effie Adams, Belgrade Me. Private William Hebenstruit, H Company, 73rd Infantry, son of Mrs. Selma Hebenstruit, Worcester, died in convulsions. An examination is expected to determine the cause. Private Earl E. York, 44th Company Depot Brigade, Wells Beach Me. died from reaction following an operation.

The general staff school opened this morning with lectures by Major Day, British general staff representative and Major Bellot, the French senior instructor. It is planned to have two batteries of artillery on hand Wednesday to demonstrate how a barrage is laid down. A war strength battalion is being formed to work out problems in field tactics on the Still river combat range. Sessions of the school will be on Mondays, Wednesdays and Fridays and will be closed to visitors.

"Letter from Camp Devens, Mass."—Roy Grist (29 September 1918)
Grist was a physician at Devens who wrote to a friend during the peak of the epidemic. Almost two weeks after the newspaper article above, Grist presents a very different view of conditions at the camp.

Camp Devens, Mass.
Surgical Ward No. 16
29 September 1918

My dear Burt ...

Camp Devens is near Boston, and has about 50,000 men, or did have before this epidemic broke loose. It also has the base hospital for the Division of the Northeast. This epidemic started about four weeks ago, and has developed so rapidly that the camp is demoralized and all ordinary work is held up till it has passed. All assemblages of soldiers taboo. These men start with what appears to be an attack of la grippe or influenza, and when brought to the hospital they very rapidly develop the most viscous type of pneumonia that has ever been seen. Two hours after admission they have the mahogany spots over the cheek bones, and a few hours later you can begin to see the cyanosis [*literally,"turning blue": a sign of lack of oxygen*] extending from their ears and spreading all over the face, until it is hard to distinguish the colored men from the white. It is only a matter of a few hours then until death comes, and it is simply a struggle for air until they suffocate. It is horrible. One can stand it to see one, two or twenty men die, but to see these poor devils dropping like flies sort of gets on your nerves. We have been averaging about 100 deaths per day, and still keeping it up. There is no doubt in my mind that there is a new mixed infection here, but what I don't know....

We have lost an outrageous number of nurses and doctors, and the little town of Ayer is a sight. It takes special trains to carry away the dead. For several days there were no coffins and the bodies piled up something fierce, we used to go down to the morgue (which is just back of my ward) and look at the boys laid out in long rows. It beats any sight they ever had in France after a battle. An extra-long barracks has been vacated for the use of the morgue, and it would make any man sit up and take notice to walk down the long lines of dead soldiers all dressed up and laid out in double rows. We have no relief here; you get up in the morning at 5:30 and work steady till about 9:30 p.m., sleep, then go at it again. Some of the men of course have been here all the time, and they are tired....

I don't wish you any hard luck Old Man, but do wish you were here for a while at least. It's more comfortable when one has a friend about. The men here are all good fellows, but I get so damned sick o' pneumonia that when I eat I want to find some fellow who will not "talk shop" but there ain't none, no how. We eat it, sleep it, and dream it, to say nothing of breathing it 16 hours a day. I would be very grateful indeed it you would drop me a line or two once in a while, and I will promise you that if you ever get into a fix like this, I will do the same for you....

Good-by old Pal, "God be with you till we meet again"

Keep the Bowells open, Roy

"Showing the Courage of Soldiers"—*New York Times* (5 November 1918)
On the day this newspaper editorial was published, the news from Europe was the surrender of Austria and the re-entry of the Serbian army into the capital city, Belgrade. Predicting the imminent end of the pandemic, the article emphasizes the unity of the war effort at home and abroad.

Perhaps the most notable peculiarity of the influenza epidemic is the fact that it has been attended by no trace of panic or even of excitement.... There has been no bitterness of criticism aimed in any direction, though there has been some excuse for it, and those who escaped the disease have gone about their daily affairs steadily and hopefully, taking what precautions they could and following the good advice they received to the best of their ability. Now the scourge is disappearing—has "burned itself out" as epidemics always do, even when there is no interference with them—and in a few days we can confidently expect to see the end of the new cases and the deaths....

We have all learned to think more or less constantly in terms other than those of individual interest and safety, and death itself has become so familiar as to lose something of its grimness and more of its importance. Courage has become a common possession, and fear, when it exists, is less often expressed than ever before.

Probably the general feeling was that the danger here should be borne as bravely as the risks that are endured by our fighting men abroad. At any rate, the danger has been met and conquered, and now we are caring for the wounded just as they do in France after a big encounter with the Germans.

"Letter to the Editor"—G.R., *American Journal of Nursing* (December 1918)
The pandemic was equally severe in rural areas not directly involved in the war. In such places, which might be quite distant from a hospital, inhabitants relied on a patchwork of services that were often staffed by trained volunteers. These included local Red Cross chapters. While the Red Cross was a national organization, its ability to organize domestic relief for influenza

varied with the personnel and resources that were available. To the frustration of local nurses, many chapters prioritized the needs of the war effort above those of civilians.

This challenge and the stress of rural nursing in a time of crisis are illustrated by this letter from a North Dakota nurse (identified only as "G.R.") who wrote to her colleagues in a professional journal.

Dear Editor:

It might be interesting to you to know how a little village on the prairie of North Dakota met the Spanish influenza. We were caught wholly unprepared, as far as organization went. Our Red Cross Chapter received working orders in time, but these were disregarded by the chairman, a man of much red tape, and not at all capable of meeting any emergency with which he was not familiar. Therefore the Red Cross Chapter offered no cooperation....

My husband, a doctor, took me out one Sunday morning to "do something," as he expressed it. I found, lying on a sanitary cot, with a horse-hide robe for a mattress, four completely-dressed little children, from two to six years old, with temperatures ranging from 102° to 105°,—the boy with croup struggling for breath, and kicking the little brother at the other end of the cot, in the chin, with a new pair of shoes. They were so toxic as not to notice anything. A baby four months old, in a buggy, was defending itself from the flies and coughing, getting what solace it could from a dry bottle. In the next room lay the very delirious mother.... You can imagine the agony of soul I went through as the things which could be done in a half-way equipped place passed in review before my mind. Many times, in our county alone, these same conditions are multiplied, often with the exception of money....

The doctor [*a practitioner other than her husband*] said that we must have a hospital and that I must start it.... With the help of friends we got together beds, and enough equipment from the drug store and doctor's office, to receive our mother of nine, who was on the way in, and her three babies, the fourth was deemed not sick enough to bother about. Also the man, father of five, and a child whose days were numbered. The wildness and confusion of that first night were awful. The willing but untrained help, who left the bedside of the delirious upon any sign on their part of wishing to get up, the kind attendant whose sole concern was the croupy boy, the smoky furnace, and the multitudinous orders, and no one but myself capable of carrying them out,—are pictures that my seven years' hospital experience cannot equal ...

The only suggestion I can make is that the Home Defense nurses should be safeguarded with stricter regulations and more supervision, so that their fullest activities need not be interfered with by some chapter head who has no vision of a nurse's usefulness or of her wish to serve her country, and who can now block the nursing activities of a whole county as far as the Red Cross is concerned.... I want our nurses across [*with the troops in Europe*] to know that we at home are trying to do our part, even though it is not being talked about.

INTERPRETING THE DOCUMENTS

1. The newspaper articles are not signed. What point of view do they represent? How do the personal letters differ from them? What conclusion do you draw concerning the value of each type of source for understanding larger social or occupational groups?

2. How does the tone of Grist's letter differ from the *Boston Post* article? The documents were written two weeks apart—does this help to account for the contrast, or do you think other factors are more important? What research could you do to find out?

3. What logistical challenges did the North Dakota nurse face during the pandemic? How do you think she would react to the *New York Times* commentary?

4. How do the conditions the nurse describes compare to the accounts at Camp Devens? Do you think doctors and nurses experienced their service during the pandemic differently?

MAKING CONNECTIONS

1. For decades, influenza in 1918–19 was considered a "forgotten pandemic" because relatively little was said about it publicly at the time or for years afterward. Why do you think the pandemic received relatively little attention?

2. By 1918, various "germ theory" ideas were starting to circulate among medical professionals and a broader public. Do you think such concepts influenced the practice of medicine or public health efforts to combat influenza? How would you compare the response to the influenza pandemic with measures taken against tuberculosis?

For further reading: Alfred Crosby, "An Inquiry into the Peculiarities of Human Memory," Chapter 15 in *America's Forgotten Pandemic* (Cambridge: Cambridge University Press, 2003), 311–28.

Notes

1. Katherine Anne Porter, *Pale Horse, Pale Rider: Three Short Novels by Katherine Anne Porter* (New York: Random House, 1936), 252–53.

2. Quoted in Joan Givner, *Katherine Anne Porter: A Life* (Athens, GA: University of Georgia Press, 1991), 126.

3. The framing of this problem is influenced by Robert Peckham, *Epidemics in Modern Asia* (Cambridge: Cambridge University Press, 2016), 15.

4. Anice C. Lowen and John Steel, "Roles of Humidity and Temperature in Shaping Influenza Seasonality," *Journal of Virology* 88, no. 14 (2014): 7692.

5. Kari Jaakkola et al., "Decline in Temperature and Humidity Increases the Occurrence of Influenza in Cold Climate," *Environmental Health* 13, no. 22 (2014): 5.

6. CDC, "Seasonal Flu Estimate Increases Worldwide" (December 2017), https://www.cdc.gov /media/releases/2017/p1213-flu-death-estimate.html.

7. David M. Morens and Anthony S. Fauci, "The 1918 Influenza Pandemic: Insights for the 21st Century," *Journal of Infectious Diseases* 195 (April 2007): 1018–19.

8. Morens and Fauci, "1918 Influenza Pandemic," 1020–22.

9. J.K. Taubenberger and D.M. Morens, "Pandemic Influenza—Including a Risk Assessment of H5N1," *Review of Science and Technology* 28, no. 1 (2009): 2–3.

10. David M. Morens and Jeffery K. Taubenberger, "1918 Influenza: A Puzzle with Missing Pieces," *Emerging Infectious Diseases* 18, no. 12 (2012): 332–35.

9. David M. Morens and Jeffery K. Taubenberger, "1918 Influenza: A Puzzle with Missing Pieces," *Emerging Infectious Diseases* 18, no. 12 (2012): 332–35.

11. Roberts Bartholow, "The Causes and Treatment of Influenza," *Cincinnati Lancet-Clinic* 63, no. 1 (1890): 21–22.

12. Mark Honigsbaum, *A History of the Great Influenza Pandemics: Death, Panic and Hysteria, 1830–1920* (London: I.B. Tauris & Co, 2014), 75.

13. Mark Osborne Humphries, "Paths of Infection: The First World War and the Origins of the 1918 Influenza Pandemic," *War in History* 21, no. 1 (2013): 55–81.

14. John Barry, *The Great Influenza* (New York: Viking Press, 2004), 456.

15. Jeffery K. Taubenberger, "Genetic Characterization of the 1918 'Spanish' Influenza Virus," in *The Spanish Influenza Pandemic of 1918–19*, ed. Howard Phillips and David Killingray (New York: Routledge, 2003), 40.

16. Mark Humphries, "The Horror at Home: The Canadian Military and the 'Great' Influenza Pandemic of 1918," *Journal of the Canadian Historical Association* 16, no. 1 (2005): 235–59.

17. K. David Patterson and Gerald F. Pyle, "The Geography and Mortality of the 1918 Influenza Pandemic," *Bulletin of the History of Medicine* 65, no. 1 (1991): 10–11.

18. Amir Afkhami, "Compromised Constitutions: The Iranian Experience with the 1918 Influenza Pandemic," *Bulletin of the History of Medicine* 77, no. 3 (2003): 367–92.

19. James Ellison, "'A Fierce Hunger'—Tracing Impacts of the 1918–19 Influenza Epidemic in Southwest Tanzania," in Phillips and Killingray, *Spanish Influenza Pandemic*, 224.

20. Wataru Iijima, "Spanish Influenza in China, 1918–1920: A Preliminary Probe," in Phillips and Killingray, *Spanish Influenza Pandemic*, 101–109.

21. Typhus merits greater attention than it receives in this book. A classic account is Hans Zinsser, *Rats, Lice and History* (Boston: Little Brown & Co., 1935). The role of typhus in Nazi ideology and practice is discussed at length in Paul Weindling, *Epidemics and Genocide in Eastern Europe, 1890–1945* (Oxford: Oxford University Press, 2000); and in Naomi Baumslag, *Murderous Medicine: Nazi Doctors, Human Experimentation and Typhus* (Westport, CT: Praeger Publishing, 2005).

22. Statistics cited in Carol R. Byerly, *Fever of War: The Influenza Epidemic in the U.S. Army during World War I* (New York: New York University Press, 2005), 107; and Patrick Zylberman, "A Holocaust in a Holocaust: The Great War and the 1918 'Spanish' Influenza Epidemic in France," in Phillips and Killingray, *Spanish Influenza Pandemic*, 192.

23. Zylberman, "Holocaust," 198–201.

24. Alfred Crosby, *America's Forgotten Pandemic: The Influenza of 1918* (Cambridge: Cambridge University Press, 2003), 227–28.

25. Quoted in Christian McMillen, *Pandemics: A Very Short Introduction* (Oxford: Oxford University Press, 2016), 99.

26. Edgar Sydenstricker, "The Incidence of Influenza among Persons of Different Economic Status during the Epidemic of 1918," *Public Health Reports* 46, no. 4 (1931): 154–69. Quotes and data from 155 and Table III, 159.

27. Harry Marks, "Epidemiologists Explain Pellagra: Gender, Race and Political Economy in the Work of Edgar Sydenstricker," *Journal of the History of Medicine and Allied Sciences* 58, no. 1 (2003): 50–55.

28. Howard Phillips and David Killingray, "Introduction," in *Spanish Influenza Pandemic*, 9.

29. Esyllt Jones, *Influenza 1918: Disease, Death, and Struggle in Winnipeg* (Toronto: University of Toronto Press, 2007).

30. Svenn-Erik Mamelund, "A Socially Neutral Disease? Individual Social Class, Household Wealth and Mortality from Spanish Influenza in Two Socially Contrasting Parishes in Kristiania 1918–19," *Social Science and Medicine* 62 (2006): 923–40.

31. Geoffrey Rice, *Black November: The 1918 Influenza Pandemic in New Zealand*, 2nd ed. (Christchurch: Canterbury University Press, 2005).

32. Rice, *Black November*, 159; Karen Slonim, "Beyond Biology: Understanding the Social Impact of Infectious Disease in Two Aboriginal Communities," in *Epidemic Encounters: Influenza, Society, and Culture in Canada, 1918–20*, ed. Magda Fahrni and Esyllt W. Jones (Vancouver: UBC Press, 2012), 119; Mary Ellen Kelm, "British Columbia First Nations and the Influenza Pandemic of 1918–19," *BC Studies* no. 122 (Summer 1999): 25.

33. Slonim, "Beyond Biology," 114–41.

34. Nancy K. Bristow, "'You Can't Do Anything for Influenza': Doctors, Nurses and the Power of Gender during the Influenza Pandemic in the United States," in Phillips and Killingray, *Spanish Influenza Pandemic*, 58–70.

35. Elizabeth Roberts, *Women's Work: 1840–1940* (Basingstoke: Macmillan, 1988).

36. Andrew Noymer and Michel Garenne, "Long-Term Effects of the 1918 'Spanish' Influenza Epidemic on Sex Differential of Mortality in the USA," in Phillips and Killingray, *Spanish Influenza Pandemic*, 202–19.

37. Terence Ranger, "A Historian's Foreword," in Phillips and Killingray, *Spanish Influenza Pandemic*, xx.

38. Jeffery K. Taubenberger and David M. Morens, "1918 Influenza: The Mother of All Pandemics," *Emerging Infectious Diseases* 12, no. 1 (2006): 15–22.

39. Michelle Rozo and Gigi Kwik Gronvall, "The Reemergent 1977 H1N1 Strain and the Gain of Function Debate," *mBio* 6, no. 4 (2015): e01013–15, https://doi.org/10.1128/mBio.01013-15.

40. S.L. Knobler, A. Mack, A. Mahmoud, and S.M. Lemon, eds, *The Threat of Pandemic Influenza: Are We Ready? Workshop Summary* (Washington, DC: National Academies Press, 2005).

41. European Centre for Disease Prevention and Control (ECDC), *Seasonal Influenza Vaccination in Europe* (Stockholm: ECDC, 2017), https://ecdc.europa.eu/en/publications-data/seasonal-influenza-vaccination-europe-vaccination-recommendations-and-coverage-2007-2015.

42. Morens and Fauci, "Insights for the 21st Century," 1026.

43. Crosby, *Forgotten Pandemic*, 323.

44. Virginia Woolf, "On Being Ill," (New York: Paris Press, 2002 [1926]), 18–19.

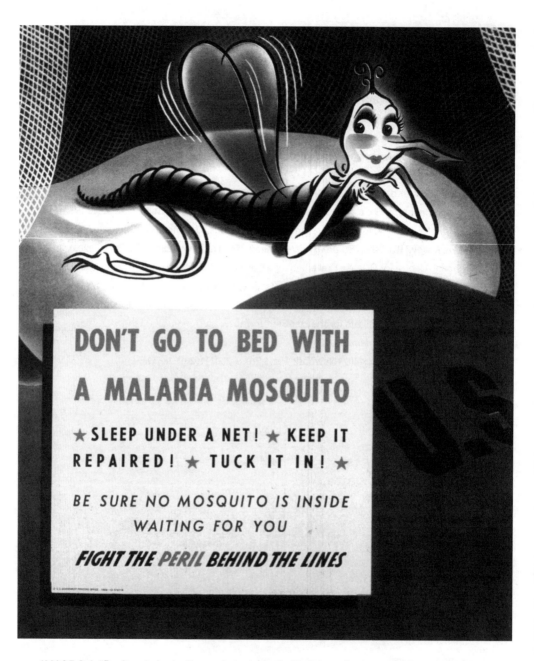

IMAGE 9.1 "Don't go to bed with a malaria mosquito." In this poster from 1943, a coquettish *Anopheles* mosquito offered US soldiers a friendly reminder to avoid unnecessary mosquito exposure at bedtime. The feminine reference, aimed at an audience of young men, played on the fact that only female *Anopheles* mosquitoes feed on human blood.

MALARIA AND MODERN LANDSCAPES

n 1946, an outbreak of malaria struck the Kipsigis reservation in the north-western region of Britain's Kenya Colony. Officials in the national medical office resolved to stamp it out by warding off mosquitoes that spread the disease. Medical officers fanned out across the countryside with canisters of pesticide to spray in dwellings. A preliminary goal of the mission was to convince tribal peoples that the chemicals were harmless. In a staged scene that was captured on film, an audience of skeptical villagers watches one British officer point a long wand at a bowl of porridge on the ground and drench it with a white powder—the chemical pesticide DDT. Another officer picks up the bowl from the ground, dips a spoon, and starts to eat.

What do we make of such a spectacle? A viewer today, who is alert to the danger of swallowing chemicals, might sympathize with the puzzled Kenyans. To the officials, however, lives were at stake and they needed to demonstrate that DDT was harmless. The pesticide had just helped win a world war. Jungles around the planet had been sprayed with it; hundreds of thousands of soldiers and millions of civilians had used it or similar chemicals to fumigate their clothes and their bodies. DDT caused no apparent damage to human health; it seemed obvious that exposure even to substantial amounts of the pesticide was preferable to the immediate, deadly threat of malaria, yellow fever, or sleeping sickness. Years later, malariologist P.C.C. Garnham (1901–1994) recalled that malaria deaths among the Kipsigis in the DDT-treated zone were less than one-tenth the toll in the untreated control area.[1]

For health workers who waged war against mosquitoes, the risks of pesticide use were more than acceptable, even when DDT's harmful effects became more apparent in the later 1940s and 1950s. Those without similar experiences, however, could be persuaded by other arguments. And many, indeed, were swayed by Rachel Carson's epochal work, *Silent Spring* (1962), that sounded an alarm about the dangers of human impact on the natural world. Carson (1907–1964) acknowledged the danger of insect-borne disease, but she suggested that indiscriminate use of pesticides actually made the problem worse—and destroyed the most effective tool humans had by causing insects to develop resistance. More than any other single work, Carson's book highlighted the concerns of a new environmental movement. The policy changes that *Silent Spring* inspired in the United States, and their ripple effects around the world, have caused bitter controversy ever since.

Human interventions have transformed not only malaria control but also the disease itself. Since antiquity, malaria has often sprouted in manufactured landscapes. Land-use strategies, particularly those related to dams, drainage, and irrigation, have deeply influenced patterns of incidence. In more recent times, parasites have developed resistance to antimicrobial chemicals, and mosquitoes have developed resistance to pesticides. Both shifts have created more dilemmas for the control of this deadly scourge. As the worldwide impact of technology upon ecosystems expanded in the mid-twentieth century, debate over malaria control became part of an ideological struggle over the human relationship to nature in the modern world.

Etiology

Malaria's complexity is humbling. "Everything about malaria," observed researcher Lewis Hackett (1884–1962), "is so moulded and altered by local conditions that it becomes a thousand different diseases and epidemiological puzzles. Like chess, it is played with a few pieces but is capable of an infinite variety of situations."[2] Hackett wrote this in 1937, when isolated cases of malaria were still diagnosed in the United States and many people still remembered their own bout with the disease. Eight decades later, malaria has all but vanished from North America, but worldwide more than 200 million people suffer from it annually. An estimated 435,000 people died from malaria-related illness in 2017.[3] Experts remain confounded by some questions that Hackett faced in the 1930s and they also confront challenges that emerged only after World War II.

Similar to the trypanosomes that cause sleeping sickness, the malaria pathogens are classified as protozoa. Malarial protozoa are grouped in the genus *Plasmodium*. Just as trypanosomes are hosted by both mammals and tsetse flies, malarial protozoa live part of their lives in mosquitoes and part in other animal hosts. Between thirty and forty different mosquito species in the genus *Anopheles* host malarial parasites in tropical, subtropical, and temperate environments.[4] These insects prefer different habitats, vary in their behavior, and transmit parasites with varying degrees of efficiency. All of these factors have influenced the success of modern anti-mosquito campaigns. In Africa and elsewhere, the *A. gambiae* mosquito has been recognized as an efficient transmitter of malarial parasites, in part because of its preference for human blood. In North America, attention often focuses on *A. quadrimaculatus*, which favors coastal lowlands but has spread elsewhere, while *A. atroparvus* has inhabited parts of Europe and Britain.

Borne aloft by insects, more than 200 species of *Plasmodium* parasites affect a range of birds, bats, lizards, primates, and mammals. Only five species of the protozoa are known to infect humans (which is quite enough). As currently understood, three of the *Plasmodia* species, *P. ovale*, *P. malariae*, and *P. knowlesi*, have had modest historical impact because of their relatively mild symptoms or limited geographic range. We shall focus primarily on the two remaining species, the more widespread *P. vivax* and the more lethal *P. falciparum*.

All five malaria-causing plasmodia have a complex life cycle (see figure 9.1) that includes stages of both sexual and asexual reproduction. Several stages of the cycle take place in the mosquito's midgut, where gametocytes develop into male and female gametes that fuse together. This union eventually creates thousands of offspring (sporozoites) that travel to the mosquito's salivary glands. As they feed, female mosquitoes inject sporozoites into the bloodstreams of various hosts. Within the secondary (or intermediate) animal host, more changes take place. The sporozoites travel to the liver and by asexual reproduction produce merozoites that re-enter the bloodstream, penetrate red blood cells, and replicate within them. Eventually, merozoites erupt from the blood cells in a remarkable, synchronized burst that releases a new cohort of parasites. The cycle recommences when some of these merozoites differentiate into gametocyte forms that circulate in the bloodstream until they are ingested by another feeding mosquito. The most frequent symptoms of malarial infection—fever spikes, weakness, and anemia—are principally related to the bursting of red blood cells at intervals of either 48 or 72 hours. Researchers have not determined how or why the parasites synchronize

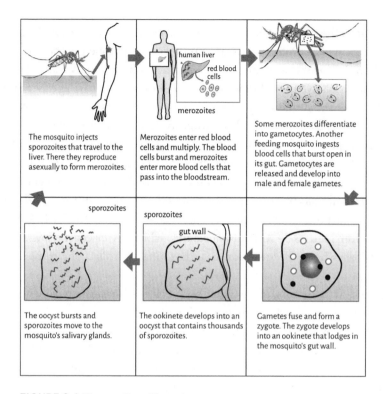

The mosquito injects sporozoites that travel to the liver. There they reproduce asexually to form merozoites.

Merozoites enter red blood cells and multiply. The blood cells burst and merozoites enter more blood cells that pass into the bloodstream.

Some merozoites differentiate into gametocytes. Another feeding mosquito ingests blood cells that burst open in its gut. Gametocytes are released and develop into male and female gametes.

The oocyst bursts and sporozoites move to the mosquito's salivary glands.

The ookinete develops into an oocyst that contains thousands of sporozoites.

Gametes fuse and form a zygote. The zygote develops into an ookinete that lodges in the mosquito's gut wall.

FIGURE 9.1 Plasmodium life cycle.

their emergence from cells; the behavior may reflect adaptation by the parasites, some aspect of host animal physiology, or a combination of both. An enlarged spleen is also characteristic of malarial infections. References to this symptom in ancient writings are often taken as an indication of malaria's presence.

Broadly speaking, this outline applies to all of the malaria-causing parasites, but the differences between them also have important consequences.[5] *P. vivax* parasites (and *P. ovale*, too) have a dormant stage in the liver as "hypnozoites" that can last for months or years before new waves issue forth to cause a relapse. Although fatigue and anemia may worsen after relapses, *P. vivax* malaria is seldom lethal in otherwise healthy people. *P. falciparum*, in contrast, has no dormant phase but produces severe anemia and may cause cerebral malaria that results in blindness, brain damage, or death. The mortality caused by malaria or malaria-related conditions has varied widely, but mortality from untreated *P. vivax* is thought to be in the range of 1–2 per cent of cases, while for *P. falciparum* it is on the order of 20 per cent. The two also have different geographic ranges that vary with climate. *P. falciparum* parasites cannot reproduce in temperatures lower than 19 degrees Celsius (~66 degrees Fahrenheit). Its presence in more temperate regions is, therefore, sporadic and often limited to summer months. The hardier *P. vivax* can survive at lower temperatures. This characteristic, as well as its ability to remain dormant, has enabled its spread among smaller populations and in a wider range than *P. falciparum*. Malarial infections may be passed from mother to child *in utero*; however, pregnant women with acquired immunity to *P. falciparum* malaria may also transfer protection that lasts for several months in newborns.

This last point brings us to the factors that influence when and how severely a person may experience malaria and its relapses. The picture is not a forgiving one. Individuals who contract malaria once may contract it again; infection with one type of malaria does not affect susceptibility to other types; and, worst of all, it is possible to suffer multiple types of malarial infection at once. In regions where one form of malaria is widespread, individuals acquire a degree of immunity after repeated infections, although young children run a high risk of severe complications. Immunity disappears when people leave the endemic region or the sources of infection are removed. Accordingly, virulent outbreaks of malaria have tended to flare up where it is intermittent, either at the edge of tropical zones that host *Anopheles* mosquitoes or in temperate regions where mosquitoes appear only in warmer weather. Since the later twentieth century, a similar dynamic has hampered public health measures that temporarily reduce malaria's burden on a population. If sources of infection return—when mosquito populations rebound after pesticide use, for example—then malaria may strike a population that has been deprived of its accumulated immunities. Interventions that reduce the risk of infection (but do not remove it completely) will, in many cases, merely delay a child's first episode of malaria.[6] There is another new problem: AIDS-related immune suppression has heightened the impact of malaria in parts of Africa and elsewhere.

Malaria has shaped human existence from the earliest times. Recent consideration of its imprint in the human genome, in tandem with other evidence, has yielded new claims about the forces that influenced early human societies. Since visions of a primitive Africa have deeply influenced perceptions of disease—and provided a foil for a Western-led modernity—recent scholarly advances in our understanding of ancient Africa offer insight into humanity's long experience with malaria.

Malaria, the Ancient Disease

Accounts of ancient history often describe the great advance of sedentary agriculture in Eurasia, built around seed planting and domesticated animals, beginning around 10,000 years ago in sites that included Mesopotamia. In this account, "crowd diseases" such as smallpox and measles originated in sites of concentrated human-animal habitation, eventually providing Europeans with some immunological advantages when they encountered less sedentary peoples in Africa and the Americas. Earlier chapters in this book indicate that recent genomics research has questioned some aspects of this narrative. The origins of smallpox date well before the emergence of agriculture, and humans may have introduced cows to the pathogen that became bovine tuberculosis. The history of malaria, too, beckons toward a more complex history of social development that relates to humanity's early African home.

Some evidence stems from genetic analysis of *Plasmodium* pathogens and their human hosts. For millions of years, *P. vivax* and *P. falciparum* evolved separately. While this much is agreed upon, debate persists over how each co-evolved with primate hosts in the distant past approximately 100,000 years ago. A common ancestor of modern *P. vivax* parasites infected early humans—whether in Africa or Southeast Asia is unclear—and, at some point, a random genetic mutation occurred that offered protection to *P. vivax* infection. The "Duffy mutation," which is carried today by about 97 per cent of central and West African populations, modifies a receptor on the surface of red blood molecules to block invasion by the *P. vivax* parasite. As a result, the Africans of these regions are often immune to the type of malaria that is most widespread around the world.

When and how did this mutation take hold? Some researchers point to recent archaeological findings for clues. It is now believed that tropical Africans conducted seasonal fishing expeditions with bone tools beginning as early as 90,000 years ago. James Webb has argued that seasonal settlements in malaria-prone areas would have produced infant mortality and gradual evolutionary pressure that favored carriers of the Duffy mutation.[7] While other researchers believe the mutation may have spread later and faster, this hypothesis combines different types of evidence in a compelling fashion.

The early evolution of *P. falciparum* raises another intriguing hypothesis. While its evolutionary trail reaches back into African apes and humanoids millions of years ago, some genetic evidence points to an increase in human *P. falciparum* infections 10,000–15,000 years ago in West Africa. Around that time, communities of seasonal migrants practiced a form of yam **paracultivation** that involved burying a wild yam head after the rest of the tuber was harvested. A reliance on yams offered tradeoffs. The tuber itself contains chemicals that inhibit the growth of malarial parasites and may have helped some individuals resist malarial disease. On the other hand, families that spent time at the rainforest's edge were constantly bitten by *Anopheles* mosquitoes. As discussed in the chapter on rinderpest, the presence of trypanosomes that killed livestock also restricted the number of large animals that diverted mosquitoes from humans. Under these circumstances, many infants probably contracted malaria and died, but the surviving inhabitants enjoyed enhanced resistance to malaria if they stayed in the local environment. Over thousands of years, paracultivation encouraged the development of more permanent settlements at the edges of rainforests.[8]

Scholars of early African societies emphasize that the exploitation of wild yams developed independently (and earlier) than seed-based agricultural practices.[9] This challenges an assumption that early Africans relied on agricultural techniques imported from elsewhere and offers insight into the demographic history of central Africa. In this region, the village-dwellers were the ancestors of Bantu-speaking peoples. The immunological advantages reaped by communities that cultivated yams, and eventually bananas and plantains, may have enabled successive waves of Bantu-speaking migrants to replace hunter-gatherers.

It may also have been in this environment that a *P. falciparum*-related genetic trait took hold: the sickle-cell gene, which is expressed by a mutated red blood cell molecule. This genetic trait, one of several that influence susceptibility to *P. falciparum*, is widespread in two different forms across central and West Africa, particularly in the Zaire basin and the Niger River delta. A child who inherits the sickle-cell gene from one parent has a vastly reduced risk of death from *P. falciparum* compared with those who do not have the trait. However, children who inherit the trait from both parents develop abnormal hemoglobin that causes blood cells to become stiff and sickle-shaped. Such cells die more quickly than normal red blood cells, and the resulting anemia causes premature death. Despite this fact, the sickle-cell trait has persisted because of the protection from malaria enjoyed by those with one normal gene and one sickle-cell gene.

For this distant history, our backward gaze necessarily relies upon modern scientific tools and inferences. Beginning in the first millennium BCE, however, we encounter malaria—or a range of diseases that probably included it—throughout Eurasia in writings that sought to insert "fevers" into meaningful patterns. Ancient texts not only demonstrate malaria's significance for classical societies, they illuminate a basic narrative about disease and environment that decisively influenced European medical thought for more than 2,000 years.

Roman Fevers and Their Legacy

Ancient Roman ideas about fevers—caused by diseases that certainly included malaria—influenced later Europeans who venerated classical civilizations. Rome's imperial expansion probably created conditions that fostered malaria's spread. Large-scale building projects caused deforestation and water runoff that expanded mosquito-friendly swamps; a steady influx of slaves and other adult immigrants ensured the presence of a susceptible population. The Pontine Marshes to the city's southeast, still a prime source of malaria in the early twentieth century, were already considered unhealthy by the ancient Romans. Wealthy inhabitants of the city, including Cicero (106–43 BCE) and Livy (59 BCE–17 CE), contrasted Rome's low-lying valleys and the flood-prone shores of the Tiber River with the purer atmosphere in the city's famous hills. Their beliefs concerning elevation and healthy air long outlived them. "Man feels his immortality in the hills," wrote William Farr in 1852. His elevation-based explanations for cholera in London owed much to the ancients' reckoning with fever.

Rome was also the vantage point of late antiquity's famous and prolific medical theorist, Galen of Pergamum. As discussed in chapters 1 and 2, Galen's Greek writings expanded and recast the Hippocratic medical tradition that originated in the fifth century BCE. Galen emphasized the role of individual humoral imbalance and innate predisposition to disease, but he also emulated the Hippocratic focus on environment that was evidenced in texts such as *Airs, Waters, Places*. Galen attributed the origins of many maladies to poisonous miasmas or putrid exhalations that arose from sources such as warm, fetid swamps. Building on the Hippocratic tradition, Galen noted that fevers had distinctive rhythms, and he linked different types of fever to excesses in certain bodily humors. Tertian fever (every first and third day) was caused by excessive yellow bile; quartan fever (every first and fourth day) by excessive black bile; and quotidian, or daily, fever by excess phlegm. Mixed forms were also possible; Galen called the variety that he considered most dangerous "semi-tertian" (a mix of quotidian and tertian). Recent research has confirmed that malaria caused by *P. vivax*, *P. falciparum*, and *P. ovale* share a 48-hour cycle that would correspond to tertian fever, while *P. malariae* has a 72-hour cycle that would correspond to quartan fever. Of course, this modern schema only partly explains the observations of fever in earlier times. As Galen and his predecessors recognized, many factors influenced the incidence of fever, just as they do today. Ancient Romans suffered from numerous fever-causing diseases, such as typhoid and influenza, without readily distinguishing one from another.

Thereafter, malaria exerted at least a modest influence in Mediterranean Europe, and the influence of fevers, at any rate, was proverbial. For example, the twelfth-century poet Godfrey of Viterbo quipped that fevers would defend Rome even when swords could not.[10] Some evidence suggests that malaria's European range began to extend further north as far as England and Scandinavia by the sixteenth century. One possible reason for this was Europe's population growth, which gained momentum after a period of slow recovery in the wake of the Black Death. In the sixteenth and seventeenth centuries, especially in coastal regions of England, France, and the Dutch Republic, landowners constructed embankment and drainage schemes to expand farmland. Such projects created pools, lowered the elevation of some coastal lands, and altered the distribution of salt and fresh water. These environmental changes, combined with increased population mobility, ensured congenial habitats for mosquitoes and a steady supply of susceptible humans. By this time, the term "mal'aria" (literally "bad air") was in use around Venice, another malaria-prone coastal community, to refer to the incidence of intermittent fevers. Here and further south, summer temperatures probably enabled *P. falciparum* to be a seasonal infection alongside disease caused by *P. vivax* and *P. malariae*.

The malaria in northern Europe's cooler climate that was caused by the *P. vivax* parasite had effects that were milder but nonetheless crippling. Shakespeare's tragedy *Julius Caesar* (1623) linked Elizabethan England to antiquity with a dramatic depiction of the illness. In the words of Caesar's rival, Cassius, malaria reduced the mighty general to a shadow, trembling and pale with glazed eyes as he groaned for water:

> He had a fever when he was in Spain,
> And when the fit was on him I did mark [*observe*]
> How he did shake. 'Tis true, this god did shake!
> His coward lips did from their color fly [*became pale*].
> And that same eye whose bend [*gaze*] doth awe the world
> Did lose his luster. I did hear him groan,
> Aye, and that tongue of his that bade the Romans
> Mark [*heed*] him and write his speeches in their books—
> "Alas," it cried, "give me some drink, Titinius"
> As a sick girl.[11]

Although some childhood mortality may have resulted from *P. vivax* malaria, its main effect was to cause chronic malaise and exacerbate the health effects of malnutrition and other infections. In parts of southeastern England, diseases that included "marsh fever" caused horrific mortality—often 50 or 60 people per 1,000 every year—throughout the sixteenth and seventeenth centuries.[12] For impoverished peasants there was no escape. They resorted to charms, folk remedies, and, frequently, to narcotics. Inhabitants of the swampy fens in East Anglia used high levels of opium and laudanum—a mix of opium and alcohol—to ward off feverish "ague-fits" caused by malaria and probably other diseases as well. Narcotic agents were put in the local beer, and even children were dosed with poppy-head tea.

Circumstances were no better in locations such as the Dombes region of southeastern France, where hard clay soil repelled rainwater and formed surface pools that attracted mosquitoes. In 1808, an observer of peasants in this "vast marsh" described them as "old at thirty, and broken and decrepit at forty or fifty. They live out their brief, miserable existences on the edges of a tomb." The writer's explanation for the peasants' suffering came straight from Galen: "Hardly have the sun's rays penetrated their dwellings than they are trudging along the dank forests to a filthy marsh from which emanates the poisoned gas that they will once again inhale."[13] At a time when Europe's largest cities were experiencing industrial expansion, the rhythm of life and death for many rural people resembled that of the later Middle Ages. Later in the nineteenth century, mechanical pumps and other industrial tools enabled drainage projects that curbed the impact of disease-carrying mosquitoes.

At the same time, Europe's colonial ventures approached their peak expansion. Malaria's impact upon the long history of colonization was twofold. The disease helped to stymie European efforts to penetrate Africa. Elsewhere, however, malaria influenced European efforts to form societies that enacted their conception of productive agriculture. Plantations, riverside settlements, and eventually large drainage projects, irrigation, and dams all transformed colonial environments. In consequence, although malaria retreated from much of Europe during the late nineteenth century, by the early twentieth century the disease was more prevalent around the world than at any previous time in history.

Malaria, the Colonial Disease

Most scholars agree that malaria was probably absent from the Americas before the end of the fifteenth century. In prehistory, migrants across the Bering Land Bridge traversed cold climates that would have extinguished the parasites.

Likewise, small outposts of Vikings in the tenth and eleventh centuries would not have sustained chains of infection.

Beginning in the late fifteenth century, trans-Atlantic voyages brought malaria to the Americas. As discussed in chapter 4, Portuguese and Spanish arrivals in the Caribbean imposed forced-labor methods that they had pioneered further east on Madeira and Saõ Tomé. After Caribbean populations were decimated and conquests on the American mainland yielded an uneven labor supply, in the mid-sixteenth century Europeans expanded the traffic in African slaves and introduced sugar plantations to the coast of Brazil. In the early seventeenth century, English colonists arrived on the Atlantic seaboard. England's thirteen colonies included several in the southeast with fertile land, hot summers, and relatively warm weather year-round. The English began to import large numbers of African slaves to the region in the later seventeenth century. In 1655, the English also wrested control of Barbados from Spain. Remarkably, the island apparently remained free of malaria until the twentieth century, although its inhabitants had their share of experience with other diseases.

As with yellow fever and smallpox, it is impossible to disentangle the impact of malaria from the broader exchange of plants, animals, and peoples around the Atlantic basin. Throughout the Caribbean and the Americas, voluntary and forced migrants contributed to various disease landscapes in ecologically distinct regions. Portuguese and Spanish explorers emigrated from Iberian regions that had both *P. vivax* and *P. falciparum* parasites. The travelers probably introduced malaria to the islands and the mainland of Central America by the 1520s. The arrival of Africans in large numbers influenced the malarial landscape because most West African slaves carried the Duffy mutation that made them immune to *P. vivax* malaria. By 1600, *P. falciparum* malaria became established in the plantations on the northeastern coast of Brazil. It also spread northward to Central America where it tormented later European expeditions alongside yellow fever. Elsewhere in South America, mosquitoes that were adapted to various altitudes and landscapes transmitted both malarial types, although not at the same levels experienced on plantations and in coastal lowlands.

Europeans adopted the plantation complex model in the Caribbean islands, where African slaves were subjected to overwork, malnutrition, and mortality from various diseases. Most imported Africans, who already had inherited immunity to *P. vivax* malaria, also developed a degree of resistance to *P. falciparum* malaria after surviving one or more cases. Europeans were at a profound disadvantage; their usual response, which meshed with their economic interests and notions of racial hierarchy, was to consider Africans naturally suited to work in harsh tropical conditions.

In North America, it is possible that French settlers introduced malaria in the higher latitudes, but the disease broke out infrequently owing to the cool climate. Further south in the mid-Atlantic region, British immigrants, some of whom hailed from malaria-ridden areas of southeastern England, introduced *P. vivax* malaria. Early accounts of the Virginia colony, established at Jamestown in 1607, suggest that the first settlers were beset by malaria in the summer and unexpectedly cold weather in the winter. By the end of the seventeenth century, several patterns had emerged in British settlements. Northern colonies such as Massachusetts and Rhode Island suffered periodic outbreaks of *P. vivax* malaria but were too cool for *P. falciparum* to penetrate. The latter became more common as one moved south from Pennsylvania into Maryland, and then to tobacco plantations in Virginia that imported large numbers of slaves by the later seventeenth century. Still further south, plantations in coastal South Carolina concentrated on rice crops that furnished an ideal habitat for malaria-carrying mosquitoes. These plantations, the Caribbean islands, and coastal Brazil formed a single zone in which *P. falciparum* malaria predominated among populations that were primarily of West African descent.

Malaria exerted great influence on the development of the United States, particularly in periods of war. Alongside the impact of smallpox and yellow fever in this era (see chapters 3 and 4), during the American Revolution malaria hobbled British troops in 1780 and contributed to the events that led to their surrender in October 1781. Malaria also caused high morbidity and mortality during the Civil War (1860–65) as Northern and Southern armies crisscrossed the eastern United States. Into the twentieth century, malarial disease was a constant presence in southern states such as South Carolina, Georgia, Alabama, and Louisiana. In more temperate regions, it caused severe outbreaks during warmer summers up and down the entire Mississippi River Valley and further west. Over time, many people of African descent lost the Duffy mutation as more children of mixed heritage were born. Europeans and Africans eventually shared vulnerability to *P. vivax* malaria as a result of life together in the United States.

The United States and Britain's other Atlantic colonies had mostly won independence by the turn of the nineteenth century. In India, however, Britain's colonial regime continued to enact sweeping social and environmental change. Here, as well as in Africa and elsewhere in the Indian Ocean basin, the introduction of an effective remedy—quinine—worked in favor of European colonial objectives.

Quinine and Colonization

Nearly four centuries after its first known use, quinine remains in the global arsenal against malarial infections. Its natural source is bark from the cinchona tree, which is native to the foothills of the Andes Mountains in modern-day Peru, Bolivia, and Ecuador. Cinchona belonged with guaiac, tobacco, sassafras, and cacao to the trade in New World botanicals that blossomed in the later seventeenth century. Unlike many other remedies from this time, quinine's antiparasitic properties were confirmed by twentieth-century criteria and tests. Cinchona bark contains more than twenty organic compounds known as alkaloids. In addition to quinine, several others have anti-malarial properties and are also used to kill some types of bacteria, relax skeletal muscles, and reduce inflammation. Quinine works in red blood cells; researchers believe it interferes with the merozoites' ability to consume hemoglobin and neutralize heme, a by-product that is toxic to the parasite. For *P. vivax* and *P. malariae* parasites, quinine can also kill gametocytes before they are ingested by mosquitoes.

Cinchona received its European name from the wife of a Spanish viceroy, the Countess of Chinchón. Seventeenth-century writers reported that the countess was healed by the bark in 1630 after she fell sick in Lima. After 1742, the influential Swiss botanist Carl Linnaeus (1707–1778) used her name for a genus of flowering plants in his influential taxonomy of living things. However, the cinchona legend does not match other evidence about the countess's biography, and other aspects of this intriguing history remain obscure. In the 1570s, Spanish botanists described a tree bark that native Peruvians consumed to cure diarrhea, but it remains unclear how that bark (if indeed it was the same) came to be used to treat fever. In any case, letters and records from an infirmary sponsored by Jesuits in Lima indicate that, by the late 1620s, they included cinchona bark with shipments to other Jesuit institutions in the Spanish viceroyalty. In 1631, a Jesuit carried samples to Rome, and the bark was used soon thereafter to treat fever. Ground into a powder, the "Jesuits' bark" was consumed several hours before the anticipated onset of fever to relieve the worst effects of "tertians" and "quartans." Alcohol or chocolate were used to mask its bitter, astringent taste.

Cinchona rapidly earned a following in Rome and other Catholic cities. Some Protestants harbored suspicions about a Catholic—or "popish"—remedy, and uncertainty about the remedy also persisted since there was no consensus concerning dosage or method of preparation. However, cinchona made important inroads after 1670. In London, this began when a young man named Robert

Talbor announced his ability to cure fever with a secret remedy. While others had tried cinchona cures, Talbor had refined his methods in the malaria-ridden coastal district of Essex. With no medical credentials, he was spurned by England's medical elite. In this era, however, physicians increasingly were ridiculed for their attachment to ancient theories, and an adroit empiric could gain the ear of influential patrons. In 1672, Talbor was appointed Physician to the King by Charles II. After the monarch knighted him in 1678, Talbor traveled to France, where success among King Louis XIV's family and friends burnished his reputation. Talbor guarded the secret until his death in 1681; thereafter, at the king's behest, a French royal physician published a work that appeared in English as *The English Remedy: Or Talbor's Wonderful Secret for the Curing of Agues and Fevers* (1682). Once instructions were in print, the use of cinchona spread throughout Europe in the later seventeenth and eighteenth centuries.

Steady demand for the bark—in part because of its value for military medicine—motivated efforts to obtain a secure supply and chemical experiments to identify the active ingredients. In 1820, French chemists Pierre-Joseph Pelletier and Joseph Caventou extracted and isolated quinine from bark and gave the alkaloid its name. Purified quinine increasingly became the desired malaria treatment, and the nations that controlled the plants were happy to sell bark. Access to live plants or seeds was another matter. Imperial Spain and then the governments of its former South American colonies (which had all achieved independence by 1825) prohibited these exports. At first, efforts to smuggle them out either failed outright or yielded plants of low quality. In 1854 a botanist sent to Peru by the Dutch government, J.K. Hasskarl, loaded dozens of plants onto the ship *Prins Frederik*, but only two seedlings survived the Pacific crossing to Dutch-controlled Java.[14] Eventually, another promising batch of seeds made its way to London in 1865 where a Dutch official purchased a portion. Java's climate and mountainous terrain suited cinchona, and the yield from these transplants contained an especially high quinine content.

Quinine caused appreciable side effects, especially nausea. The effort to coax citizens and soldiers to withstand quinine's discomforts and bitter taste would be a recurrent public health challenge (and the inspiration for gin and tonic, created when British soldiers added alcohol to "Indian tonic water"). Consistent access to the drug remained an important objective. During World War II, when Japan occupied Java, the lapse in supply motivated the Allies to produce synthetic substitutes. They turned to two chemical compounds developed in the 1920s and 1930s: atabrine and chloroquine. Atabrine proved unpopular because it caused skin to take a yellowish hue and was rumored to cause impotence. Chloroquine also had significant side effects, but after limited trials during World War II it came into general use in 1947.

In the meantime, however, quinine had shifted the prospects for European enterprises in warm climates throughout Africa and the Indian Ocean basin. As discussed in chapter 4, malaria, yellow fever, and other diseases snuffed out European efforts to penetrate the African interior before the 1840s. Even on the West African coast, nearly half of the British soldiers posted to Sierra Leone died every year.[15] A turning point was reached in 1854 when sixty-six men navigated the Niger River for four months without a single casualty from disease. The expedition's medical officer, William Balfour Baikie, proclaimed the value of quinine as a preventive as well as a cure.[16] Larger expeditions followed, including well-publicized journeys by Henry Morton Stanley across central Africa in the 1870s. The confidence European rulers soon felt in their dealings with Africa, on display at the Berlin Conference of 1884, would have been impossible without the successful use of quinine.

The beginning of cinchona cultivation in Southeast Asia roughly coincided with important changes to Britain's India colony. Since 1765, large parts of India had been controlled by the British East India Company. An uprising against Company rule in 1857–58 prompted the British government to assume direct control. Thereafter, colonial officials vastly expanded irrigation and water management projects to increase the amount of arable land, forestall the effects of famine, and provide profits for British financiers. Over decades, engineers and untold numbers of laborers accomplished astonishing feats. By the late 1920s, roughly 75,000 miles of canals provided water to 30 million acres of land.[17] The death toll from diseases was also staggering: between 1904 and 1909 an average of 4 million people reportedly died every year from "fevers," in all likelihood mostly from malaria or diseases that were worsened by a concurrent malarial infection.[18] Malaria vied with cholera as the greatest cause of mortality in the Indian subcontinent.

While malaria had been present in India long before the colonial period, aspects of the British development programs heightened its impact. Many irrigation canals were constructed without parallel drainage systems, resulting in fields that flooded during monsoon rains. Embankments created for roads and railways often had the same effect, and some newly irrigated regions had firm, claylike soil that resisted water absorption and caused formation of pools. The spread of standing water created breeding areas for *Anopheles* mosquitoes that conveyed malaria to new regions or increased its incidence in regions where it was already established. Immigrants who came to dig canals were especially susceptible to local variants of malarial infection. Some of these dynamics were noticed as early as the 1840s by British officials along the West Jumna (or Yamuna) Canal in northern India. By 1925, when malaria was distinguished from other causes of fever, sanitary official Charles Bentley noted that the rate of infection in Bengal paralleled the amount of railroad construction. In the most heavily developed areas of west Bengal, rates of infection among inhabitants exceeded 90 per cent and some other parts of the province were not far behind.[19]

However, relatively few other observers connected disease with British policies. As Mark Harrison has shown, throughout the nineteenth century colonial medical officials remained influenced by environmental approaches to disease that harkened back to Galenic miasma theories. They linked India's high rates of "fever" to its pronounced climate cycles and the abundance of rotting vegetable matter in its humid climate.[20] Over time, the focus of attention shifted to include Indian cultural and social arrangements. European observers, for example, often commented on the presence of ponds, known as "tanks," that provided a communal water supply in the center of villages. After 1817, recurrent cholera epidemics encouraged officials to investigate stagnant pools or ditches that might send poisonous effluvia into the air. In 1884, a team led by Robert Koch had famously located cholera bacilli in just such a pond (see chapter 5).

Later in the nineteenth century, shifting explanations of disease among experts did little to dislodge a European tendency to blame Indians themselves. Even in 1936, malaria expert J.E. Sinton faulted Indians for creating "man-made malaria" through neglect of sanitary precautions, and he estimated an annual incidence of 100 million cases. Sinton focused on ineffective sanitary practices rather than innate characteristics that made Indians susceptible to disease. Nonetheless, his observation was a variant of a pervasive Western belief that "civilized" peoples were in one way or another incompatible with "native" social and environmental land-scapes. As we have seen in earlier chapters, during the early twentieth century similar perceptions undergirded segregative practices in other regions controlled by Westerners, including the Panama Canal Zone, plantations in South America and West Africa, and in the emergent apartheid regime of South Africa.

By the 1910s, British India was one of the world's largest consumers of quinine. Efforts to promote its use among the Indian populace expanded substantially in the 1890s. Government officials took measures to ensure the quality of quinine products and attempted to establish supply chains that would reach to the village level.[21] Quinine's role in health promotion was redefined, as *Plasmodium* parasites were identified and malaria was distinguished from fevers with other causes. Robert Koch was one of the drug's most influential supporters. In 1901, after a quinine trial with plantation workers in New Guinea, Koch asserted that it destroyed malaria parasites and served to prevent transmission in a population. As quinine was recast from fever-reducing remedy to microbe killer, it remained unclear whether its prophylactic use—in other words, consumption of quinine by uninfected people—was still of value, as observers such as Baikie had claimed. British officials continued to encourage quinine prophylaxis but their efforts were only partially successful. As Harrison has noted, only a small urban minority in India truly embraced Western sanitary reforms, and even these supporters often were reluctant to finance sanitary measures with taxes.[22]

Alongside the shifts in quinine usage, by 1900 malaria was reframed in an even more fundamental way: the disease was increasingly defined by the mosquitoes that transmitted it. Beyond India, this would have important consequences for the public health strategies that took shape by the mid-twentieth century. Moreover, as engineers, entomologists, and chemists expanded the range of available tools to confront the disease, the transformation of physical and disease landscapes assumed an explicitly ideological character.

Malaria, the Vector-Borne Disease

As discussed in chapters 4 and 7, the investigation of tropical parasites and insect vectors was undertaken in the late nineteenth century by a small international cohort of scientists who applied techniques of the new microbiology. The partial unraveling of malaria's mysteries was a team effort that drew from comparative studies of nonhuman parasites as well as human-based research.[23]

In 1880, a French military physician in Algeria, Charles Louis Alphonse Laveran (1845–1922), decided to investigate samples of fresh human blood instead of dried smears that were stained. Laveran saw microbes in motion: tiny bodies with dancing, whiplike flagella. No one had ever seen protozoa inhabit human blood cells. Although other researchers were skeptical, Laveran's claim eventually was supported by research on bird and reptile parasites by a Russian researcher, Vassily Danilewski (1852–1939). By 1890, scientists accepted that malarial parasites invaded red blood cells and that several species of plasmodia caused types of disease with distinct symptoms.

But where did the parasites originate and how did they reach the human body? Comparative research with birds provided some answers. In 1896–97, two students at Johns Hopkins University in Maryland, William MacCallum (1874–1944) and Eugene Opie (1873–1971), found that sparrows and crows hosted gametocytes that, once they were ingested by a biting fly, reproduced sexually in the fly's stomach. While this offered a partial model for the transmission of malaria parasites, researchers continued to ponder how the parasites moved from birds to humans. Mosquitoes had long been considered a likely suspect. Some observers, such as Patrick Manson, thought that they might contaminate drinking water. In London, Manson dissected hundreds of insects, and he encouraged Ronald Ross, who was working for the Indian Medical Service, to perform similar research. Stationed in central India at Secunderabad, in August 1897 Ross observed the transmission of parasites from an infected man into mosquitoes that Ross had produced to feed on him. Thereafter, Ross moved to Calcutta where human malaria was infrequent, and he shifted his work to bird parasites and mosquitoes. More mosquito dissections revealed that rod-like parasite structures reached the insects' salivary glands from which they would be injected into a new bird host. Ross correctly guessed that human malaria worked the same way, but he would not be the first to prove it. In Italy, where human malaria was easy to find, between 1898 and 1900 researchers led by Giovanni Battista Grassi traced the entire parasite life cycle and, moreover, demonstrated that only female *Anopheles* mosquitoes transmitted malaria.

The proof that mosquitoes both ingested and transmitted malaria parasites offered a new avenue of attack against the ancient disease. In the preface of Ross's *Mosquito Brigades and How to Organise Them* (1902), he noted that people around the world took steps to avoid mosquito bites. Then he asked a simple question: "Rather than take so much trouble in protecting ourselves from the bites of these insects, would it not be better to get rid of them at once?"[24] Ross thought it was possible to eliminate *Anopheles* mosquitoes in limited areas, but such campaigns required military precision and a chain of command. Above all, Ross believed, mosquito warfare must be characterized by "energy, persistence, and an entire indifference to public or private opinion."[25] For seven years beginning in 1902, Indian officials tested his methods at Mian Mir, a military outpost in Punjab (present-day Pakistan). The chief measure deployed was to remove breeding sites in shallow irrigation channels and pools of standing water. After the trial was deemed a failure, Ross's further proposals mostly were ignored by India's colonial government, which instead promoted the use of quinine. However, his ideas were not ignored elsewhere. As noted in chapter 4, the essential ingredients described in *Mosquito Brigades*—a military mindset, single-minded focus on the vector insect, and a disregard of local civilians—had a lasting impact, and reinforced the authoritarian campaigns against mosquitoes elsewhere.

Indeed, the relative merits of vector control (i.e., killing mosquitoes), parasite control, and preventive therapy were debated around the world in the early twentieth century. Much depended on the local circumstances, especially the attributes and behavior of numerous *Anopheles* mosquito species in various environments. Not surprisingly, studies of this question—conducted either at private plantations (often by the Rockefeller Foundation) or by government and military officers—arrived at diverse conclusions. Visits by Robert Koch to the Dutch East Indies and New Guinea in 1900 reinforced his belief that parasite control was more practical than eliminating mosquitoes in a large territory. Accordingly, Koch commended the use of quinine to break chains of infection. In Italy, malaria eradication was a national priority after the peninsula was unified in 1870. Public health workers in the 1900s and 1910s combined land reform and agricultural development, rural education, and administration of quinine as both a preventive and a treatment. On the island of Taiwan, then under Japanese control, officials after 1906 implemented a combined strategy of blood testing and quinine alongside swamp drainage and cutting of bamboo thickets.[26] In the Panama Canal Zone during the 1900s, US Army officer William Gorgas favored military-style mosquito brigades as the American forces imposed measures against yellow fever and malaria. Colonial authorities found it difficult to enforce quinine consumption; often, they preferred to attack mosquitoes, particularly when armed forces could do the job. The link between malaria control and political transformation was especially explicit in Palestine, which became a protectorate under British administration in 1920 after the collapse of Ottoman rule in World War I. Drainage of the Huleh valley wetlands and anti-malarial measures became ideological rallying points for Zionists, who claimed to be "healing the land" as they attempted to carve a Jewish state out of the territory.[27]

Although India and some other regions such as southern Italy continued to use quinine, after 1920 large-scale campaigns increasingly targeted mosquitoes with arsenic-based chemical pesticides. The chemicals included Paris green, a compound of arsenic and copper that farmers had used in the United States for pest control since the late nineteenth century. In the 1930s, vector control was the instrument of choice in Brazil after malaria-carrying African mosquitoes (*Anopheles arabiensis*) hitched a ride across the Atlantic. Under the leadership of

Fred Soper, who had just orchestrated Brazil's yellow fever campaign for the Rockefeller Foundation, anti-mosquito squads once again fanned out to fumigate buildings, automobiles, and railway cars. Victory was declared after the teams vanquished the African mosquitoes from an area of 18,000 square miles, although other native *Anopheles* mosquitoes remained to transmit malaria plasmodia. In the 1930s and into World War II, mosquitoes were the visual embodiment of malaria's threat. The messages broadcast to soldiers traveling to tropical climes were sometimes light-hearted but always earnest: take your quinine, beware the treacherous female mosquito, and keep your shirt on.

DDT

In the early 1940s, vector control methods received their biggest boost from an odorless white powder with a long name: dichloro-diphenyl-trichloroethane. Its acronym, DDT, first became a symbol of scientific accomplishment and then, among environmentalists, a byword for dangerous pollution. DDT was first synthesized in 1874, but its history as an insecticide began in 1939 with Paul Müller (1899–1965), a Swiss chemist. He observed its remarkable properties as he searched for a way to protect crops from an invasive pest, the Colorado potato beetle. A few years later, Müller's employer, the chemical company J.R. Geigy, sent some DDT powder to New York. Tests soon revealed that DDT was far more powerful than any other insecticide. The lightest dusting would kill mosquitoes— plus flies, lice, and other insects—and the pesticide remained effective against larvae or mature insects for weeks or longer. Now a secret wartime weapon, DDT was produced in large quantities for use worldwide. It first proved its worth to the general public in the fall and winter of 1943, when German troops retreated from southern Italy and Allied forces took control of Naples. As a typhus outbreak swelled, supplies of DDT arrived. With assistance from the Rockefeller Foundation, dozens of delousing stations were set up to fumigate people and clothing on a massive scale. Between December 1943 and March 1944, more than 3 million people were dusted with DDT, and a catastrophe was averted.[28]

DDT was powerful, easy to manufacture, and cheap. After its initial success, the chemical swiftly served many disease control objectives. In May 1944, Soper took over malaria control in Egypt, after British officials failed to stop a devastating epidemic of *P. falciparum* malaria that cost more than 100,000 lives. A campaign with DDT rid the Nile River valley of the *A. gambiae* mosquito by the

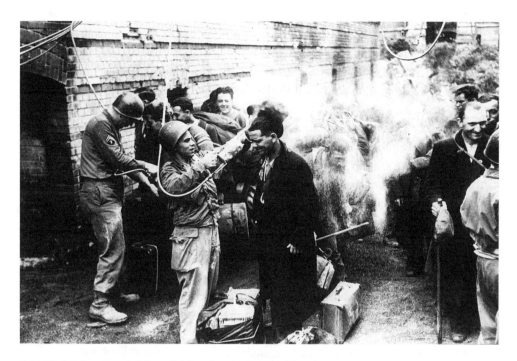

IMAGE 9.2 American soldiers disinfect freed prisoners. This photograph was taken in the spring of 1945. Through the end of World War II, Allied forces in southern Italy also treated domestic interiors with a solution of 10 per cent DDT and kerosene to combat malarial mosquitoes. To DDT's supporters, such measures linked disease prevention, American scientific prowess, and the renewal of peace and prosperity.

end of 1945.[29] During the invasion of France's Normandy beaches on 6 June 1944, legions of soldiers waded ashore wearing shirts impregnated with pesticide. Even Winston Churchill celebrated DDT's power and the prospect of its use by British troops fighting in Burma (now Myanmar). In the South Pacific, where casualties from malaria or dengue fever usually outnumbered wounds, the US Army outfitted bombers to spray island beaches before troops went ashore. Within the United States, the Office of Malaria Control in War Areas (MCWA) expressed concern in 1944 that returning soldiers would spread malaria and other diseases. Mosquito eradication was then funded under the MCWA, rechristened as the Center for Communicable Diseases (CDC), and embraced with enthusiasm by most Americans (CDC now stands for US Centers for Disease Control and Prevention). Not much malaria remained in the continental United States, but between 1947 and 1950 the CDC oversaw the spraying of 5 million homes. The campaign ended ahead of schedule when no more malaria could be found. DDT use continued in the United States for other pest control and agricultural purposes, reaching a peak in 1959 when 80 million pounds of DDT were applied alongside other chemicals. Even house pets were dusted with it to get rid of fleas.

Some of DDT's most visible successes came in Italy. After its surrender in early September 1943, retreating German troops destroyed water pumps and dikes that prevented salt water from reflooding the Pontine Marshes. As malaria encroached in the summer of 1944, planes used spray tanks fitted onto bomb racks to blanket the marshes with pesticide mist. Similar measures were undertaken further north around Venice and, most spectacularly, on the island of Sardinia from 1946 to 1951. The Sardinian campaign employed 14,000 peasants as scouts and sprayers in an effort to rid the island of its main malaria vector, the mosquito A. *labranchiae*. A few mosquitoes got away, but Sardinia's reported cases of malaria nonetheless fell from 75,447 cases in 1946 to nine in 1951. The entire country was considered malaria-free by 1962. After more than 2,000 years, a task was removed from the to-do list of the Italian peninsula.

While this success often was interpreted as a great victory for chemical pest control, historian Frank Snowden has argued that the Italian efforts built upon decades of community public health initiatives that had educated local populaces on the value of quinine distribution and the need to install metal screens to block mosquitoes. In the Littoria region around the Pontine Marshes, physicians and nurses assisted more than 100,000 people with malaria treatment and prevention even as the spraying got underway. Likewise, the Sardinia spraying campaign was simultaneously a public works project that provided thousands of jobs, access to needed food and clothing, and a focus for the "sanitary consciousness" that had been encouraged by years of health education. From this perspective, Italy's "conquest of malaria" reflected an integrated, community-based approach to disease control that unfolded over years, rather than the overpowering success of a pesticide sprayed from the air.[30]

This was not the main lesson that policy makers learned from DDT's success in the 1940s and 1950s. DDT's performance persuaded many people that chemical pesticides provided a cost-effective means to greatly reduce or even eliminate common scourges. In the United States and among western European nations, DDT was considered part of a suite of technological tools that could be used to foster development throughout the world and provide a counterweight in the global competition against Communist regimes in the Soviet Union and China. The addition of the anti-malarial drug chloroquine alongside quinine in the mid-1940s offered further support for large-scale eradication efforts. Between 1945 and 1965, malaria eradication programs made substantial advances and, in some cases, had lasting results.

Thereafter, as the prospects for the eradication of malaria receded, new voices were raised against DDT and the approach to human development that it represented.

Eradication Obstacles

Historians often describe pest eradication measures in the mid-twentieth century as an example of overconfidence in the power of science. But where malaria was concerned, many scientists discerned from the start that the program was a calculated risk. Researchers in Africa feared that eradication measures would cause populations to lose acquired immunity to *P. falciparum* malaria. These people would be helpless if malaria returned. By the late 1940s, researchers also recognized that insects soon developed resistance to chemical pesticides, although little was known about the variables that influenced this process.

Fred Soper and other proponents of eradication insisted on its feasibility, at least outside of tropical Africa. They pointed out that it was only necessary to kill enough mosquitoes to protect humans, not all the mosquitoes in a given region. The key technique was to spray DDT on indoor surfaces and outdoor roofs and walls where it would provide lasting protection without affecting natural environments. It was believed that if transmission of malaria could be interrupted for five years, no parasites would remain in human bodies for mosquitoes to ingest and spread. Where pesticide resistance was concerned, Soper's solution was to strike hard and fast to kill mosquitoes for the needed time frame. DDT had rid the United States of malaria, and it remained in widespread use. Its supporters failed to see why the rest of the world should be denied its benefits.

In 1955, the WHO launched an ambitious Malaria Eradication Programme (MEP). The plan was first to target regions where transmission was low to moderate and later to tame malaria in tropical Africa. As DDT was shipped around the world by the ton, hundreds of thousands of people were trained to go door to door bearing hand-held sprayers with pressurized tanks. In some regions of the world— the Balkans, Taiwan, parts of the Caribbean, northern Australia, and parts of northern Africa—malaria was eliminated and has never made a significant comeback. Progress was dramatic even in some areas with high rates of infection. The effort in India was a great short-term success: in the early 1950s, an estimated 75 million people contracted the disease and by the early 1960s this number had shrunk to about 50,000. Prosperous Western countries and some socialist nations with strong health care programs also achieved lasting elimination.

Elsewhere, the MEP was less successful. In much of South Asia and Latin America, the program failed to achieve large gains, and in most of Africa it never

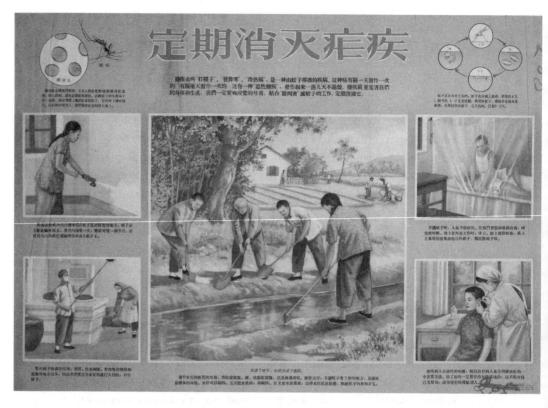

IMAGE 9.3 "To eradicate malaria within a certain time period." This public health poster was issued in 1956 by the Tianjin Health Propaganda and Education Institute in China. It depicts malaria control methods that were deployed throughout Asia. The centerpiece is effective irrigation with banks cleared of vegetation. Clockwise from top left, the flanking images depict pesticide spraying, mosquito bed nets, acupuncture therapy, and thorough cleaning. The two top images flanking the title depict mosquito transmission (left) and the plasmodium parasite life cycle (right).

got off the ground. One reason was the continued widespread use of DDT for crop protection. Particularly in southern Asia and Latin America, heavy crop spraying hastened the evolution of resistance in large mosquito populations. A host of local factors also influenced the spraying programs. For example, it was discovered that mud walls absorbed DDT and reduced its effectiveness.[31] The logistical obstacles ranged from government inaction and corruption to homeowners who refused to allow spraying inside. Funding for spraying programs often could not be sustained. As the landscape shifted, even India experienced a partial reversal: in the later 1960s and 1970s, reported cases of malaria climbed to a peak of 6.5 million in

1976, although the level dropped sharply when anti-malarial measures were resumed.

The MEP's biggest blind spot, perhaps, was its failure to account for the challenges that were created by migrant workers and other mobile populations. As workers traveled to new regions, their bodies were vulnerable to novel malaria parasites and they often received inadequate protection from available supplies of antibiotics. Drugs that failed to kill parasites fostered the evolution of drug-resistant mutations. In the late 1950s and early 1960s, this apparently took place among migrant mineworkers in Thailand who received insufficient doses of chloroquine. The workers spread drug-resistant malaria to surrounding areas and eventually throughout southern Asia.[32] In other cases, infected migrant workers restarted transmission in regions where elimination measures had ended. Some infected people had no visible symptoms, and without consistent blood screening many people who carried the parasites could not be identified. Although drug-resistant malaria parasites are of particular concern in this region, the problem reflects a growing crisis in the use of antibiotics for many diseases.

Politics and the New Environmental Movement

Shifts in Western political culture during the 1960s, particularly in the United States, had an outsized influence upon the funding that anti-malaria programs received. After World War II, the United States provided a large proportion of all funding for global health programs sponsored by the WHO and other agencies. In 1958, the US Congress allotted $100 million to the WHO for malaria eradication. By 1963, the sum had grown to $490 million, the rough equivalent of $4 billion in 2019.[33] However, the will did not exist for a long-term global campaign, and thereafter the United States halted its WHO funding and shifted resources to bilateral partnerships with individual nations. US aid drifted to projects that supported national objectives in Latin America or nondisease issues such as population control. By the late 1960s, these funding reductions adversely affected malaria eradication campaigns, notably in India and the neighboring island of Ceylon (now Sri Lanka). The waning US commitment confirmed the fears of eradication advocates. Fred Soper believed that resistance from bureaucrats endangered his plans as much as resistance in mosquitoes.[34]

By the mid-1960s, moreover, opposition to DDT had a new, powerful source of inspiration: as scientists continued to investigate the ecological impact of pesticides, Rachel Carson's *Silent Spring* (1962) crystallized opposition to toxic chemicals as a

Unnatural Selection: Antibiotics and Drug Resistance

Antibiotics—microbe-killing molecules derived from living organisms—are pervasive in the modern world, and their uses range far beyond infectious disease. They prevent infection during surgery, promote growth in animals, protect crops from pests, and disinfect all kinds of surfaces. However, other results are less benign: the spread of antibiotics throughout the globe has exerted selection pressure on bacteria and other microbes, thus accelerating the evolution of resistant strains. In many different contexts, antibiotic resistance poses an increasing threat to human health.

Since the widespread use of penicillin began in the 1940s, large quantities of antibiotic material—many millions of metric tons—have entered the soil, water, and air. In industrial farms, antibiotics are added to feed and enter the soil in manure and water runoff. Numerous industries either manufacture or use antimicrobial chemicals. Consumers in homes and hospitals excrete antibiotics in waste, and dispose of excess medications in landfills or sewage. Individual access to antibiotics and the frequency of use varies among countries, but experts believe that antibiotics are overprescribed worldwide, including in North America.[35] A recent study of seventy-six countries found that the defined daily doses of antibiotics increased 65 per cent between 2000 and 2015.[36]

How do microbes evolve resistance to antibiotics? In some cases, the potential for resistance apparently is present from the start. For example, in 1940 the first researchers to produce penicillin in large quantities found that some bacteria already had an enzyme that could destroy the antibiotic. Bacteria also evolve resistance when they mutate spontaneously. Once a trait is established and provides a survival benefit, the surviving bacteria pass it on to future generations. Most commonly, different strains of bacteria transmit genetic material to each other in a horizontal gene transfer (see figure 9.2). The transfer often takes place via a plasmid, a small ring of DNA that is separate from a chromosome. Since plasmids can replicate and spread on their own, they enable resistance genes to spread rapidly among bacteria. Microbes have evolved for billions of years, but antibiotics greatly accelerate the process by creating an environment that allows only resistant microbes to reproduce. In this respect, microbial evolution in the last century differs from the vast stretch of history that preceded it.

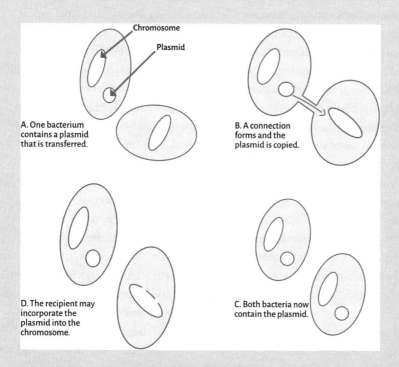

Chromosome

Plasmid

A. One bacterium contains a plasmid that is transferred.

B. A connection forms and the plasmid is copied.

D. The recipient may incorporate the plasmid into the chromosome.

C. Both bacteria now contain the plasmid.

FIGURE 9.2 Horizontal gene transfer

Antibiotic-resistant microbes complicate efforts to combat well-known diseases such as tuberculosis and malaria. However, other infections are more common in healthcare settings, where bacteria spread among people who have weak immune systems or whose bodies have lost defenses during medical treatments. Sometimes, the antibiotics themselves contribute to the emergence of disease. For example, a bacterium named *Clostridium difficile* colonizes the intestines of many patients after their natural bacteria have been weakened by antibiotics. In the United States alone, several hundred thousand infections occur each year and, in 2015, roughly 15,000 deaths were attributed directly to *C. difficile*.[37]

Many experts suggest that individuals and industries must reduce the consumption of antibiotics. The threat has also spurred interest in vaccines, which target the human immune system and do not encourage the evolution of drug resistance. However, for many dangerous infections the arms race of medicines and microbes will continue until other treatments are found.

means of engineering nature. A biologist and science writer, Carson had authored several popular books on ocean ecology. In *Silent Spring* she adopted a polemical tone, indicting chemical companies and lax government agencies for heedless contamination of the environment. The *New Yorker* first published the book in installments during the summer of 1962. The iconic opening pages of *Silent Spring* described a fictional town where harmony among humans and other life was disrupted by the blight of pesticides. Carson depicted insidious, creeping destruction: "There was a strange stillness. The birds, for example—where had they gone? Many people spoke of them, puzzled and disturbed. The feeding stations in the backyards were deserted. The few birds seen anywhere were moribund; they trembled violently and could not fly. It was a spring without voices."[38]

As *Silent Spring* arrived on newsstands, Americans also learned of terrifying deformities in infants that were caused by thalidomide, an anti-nausea medicine available in Europe. Against this backdrop, Carson cited scientific studies which showed that DDT caused weakened eggshells that destroyed robins, sparrows, and even bald eagles. Birds of prey, but also humans, were particularly vulnerable to toxins because DDT persisted in the environment and increased in concentration as the chemical moved up animal food chains. Carson also noted the ability of insects to swiftly develop resistance to chemicals and suggested that resistant mosquitoes already endangered malaria programs. Insect-borne diseases could not be ignored, Carson acknowledged, but she warned that indiscriminate use of pesticides would soon render them useless.

Chemical industry representatives protested—correctly—that no evidence demonstrated that normal DDT exposure caused cancer or other harm to humans. Corporate spokespeople attempted to disarm "Miss Carson" by suggesting that her arguments were rooted in emotional rhetoric rather than scientific fact. However, Carson's vivid account was not just about direct risks of exposure for people—she depicted DDT and other pesticides as insults to the web of life that had wide-ranging, dangerous repercussions. Her concerns were absorbed into broader, value-laden debates concerning the role of the United States in world affairs, the value of technological solutions to complex problems, and the unknown dangers of human impact on the environment. Fears about the impact of DDT were further amplified by the development of a new measurement technique, gas chromatography, which enabled scientists to detect trace amounts of chemicals. Evidence that DDT persisted in the environment did not, by itself, prove that it harmed humans or animals, but to environmentally conscious Americans a little knowledge was a frightening thing. *Silent Spring* helped galvanize a public outcry that culminated, in 1972, with the founding of the US Environmental Protection Agency (EPA). The agency soon canceled DDT's registration and implemented an almost total ban on its use in the United States.

Already by 1969, financial and practical challenges had forced the WHO to abandon malaria eradication as a goal and shift its focus to "control" of the disease. Millions of lives, or even tens of millions, had been saved or prolonged in the previous fourteen years. Nonetheless, the WHO's policy change was an admission of defeat for the MEP and, more broadly, for development schemes that imposed technical solutions without regard to local contexts. Many forces influenced the outcomes of the eradication program. However, the turn away from DDT in the United States undoubtedly made global access to the pesticide more difficult and for decades placed an effective anti-malarial measure out of reach for poorer nations. Eventually, public health advocates sought a middle ground for some regions where DDT could fill an urgent need. By the early 2000s, even some of DDT's most vigorous opponents, such as the Environmental Defense Fund, agreed that the pesticide could be used in indoor spraying programs without causing undue harm. In September 2006, the WHO recommended indoor residual spraying in areas with constant and high malaria transmission including throughout Africa.[39]

The assessment of DDT will undoubtedly evolve as assessment of the longer-term effects of pesticide use continues. There is still little evidence that DDT is a potent human carcinogen, and it remains effective as a pesticide in some contexts, but its worldwide diffusion has created challenges that its early proponents did not anticipate. DDT and other persistent organic pollutants (POPs) penetrate ecosystems far from where they are used after winds and water currents carry them to remote regions of the globe. POPs are of particular concern in circumpolar environments, where the toxins accumulate in large animals (whales, seals, and walruses) that traditionally have served important roles in the diet of northern Indigenous peoples.[40] DDT's costs and benefits are not reaped in equal measure around the world, and this creates a dilemma for global health strategists and advocates of environmental justice.

In the last twenty years, anti-malaria programs have profited from several innovations. Insecticide-treated bed nets have been distributed and sold by the hundreds of millions in parts of sub-Saharan Africa. The nets may not be environmentally neutral—one study claimed that mosquitoes developed insecticide resistance after they were introduced. However, they have markedly reduced infant mortality in malaria-prone regions.[41] In the late 1990s, drug companies began to distribute a derivative of artemisinin, a common herb known in English as wormwood. The drug is based on a traditional remedy used

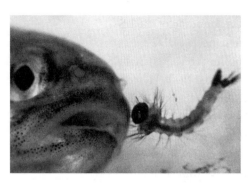

IMAGE 9.4 Mosquito fish feeding on a mosquito larva. This small *Gambusia* mosquito fish can consume its own weight in mosquito larvae each day. These fish have been introduced into waterways throughout the world to help control mosquito populations and reduce the threat of malaria and yellow fever.

in China for more than 2,000 years that was researched by pharmacologist Tu Youyou in the 1970s. Artemisinin derivatives are now a first-line therapy for malaria caused by *P. falciparum*; they are ideally administered in combination with other drugs to forestall the emergence of drug-resistant parasites. Vaccine research has also made recent strides. One candidate against *P. falciparum* malaria, the "RTS, S vaccine," has proceeded through clinical trials and, in 2018, was included in routine vaccination programs for several hundred thousand children in Ghana, Kenya, and Malawi. Several doses of the vaccine may reduce the incidence of *P. falciparum* malaria by 30–40 per cent, although total protection is not a foreseeable outcome. Finally, researchers have also explored the release of genetically modified (transgenic) mosquitoes that will resist malarial parasites. But after the uproar over pesticides, scientists are in no hurry to attempt another form of natural engineering.

Conclusion

There is no easy road to freedom from malaria. Although global eradication is sometimes proclaimed as a goal, public health experts are more apt to discuss pathways to control or elimination in certain regions. Malaria remains rooted in tropical Africa, and now also threatens parts of South America and Southeast Asia. Viewed over the long term, it may be said that the lasting achievement of the eradication programs was to banish malaria from temperate regions where it had encroached in the previous several centuries.

In important respects, however, the assaults upon malaria in recent times have created challenges that are novel in the long, intertwined history of humans, mosquitoes, and parasites. In the 1930s, J. E. Sinton considered "man-made" malaria to be the result of careless sanitary practices and inadequate water engineering. Certainly, such forces contributed to the incidence of malaria for many centuries, especially when colonizers attempted to fashion agricultural landscapes on ever-larger scales. Since the 1950s, however, humans have remade malaria in

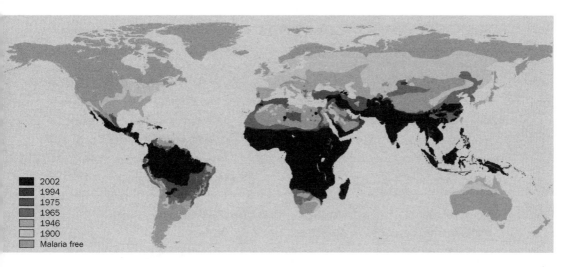

MAP 9.1 Global distribution of malaria risk, 1900–2002. In the second half of the twentieth century, the burden of malaria became increasingly concentrated in tropical regions.
Source: Simon I. Hay et al., "The Global Distribution and Population at Risk of Malaria: Past, Present, and Future," *The Lancet Infectious Diseases* 4, no. 6 (2004), https://doi.org/10.1016/S1473-3099(04)01043-6.

other ways. In the region surrounding the Mekong River (Southeast Asia), malaria parasites have developed resistance to artemisinin and other new drugs. Parasite resistance is encouraged when drugs are administered in improper doses or when just one drug is used alone. Moreover, many mosquitoes are now resistant to DDT and other pesticides. The ebb and flow of public health measures have also influenced the acquired immunities of millions of people. It can now be argued that human intervention has created many different malarias in contexts that have distinctive environmental and ecological features. Owing to rapid population growth in Africa, the number of people exposed to malaria is now greater than ever before. Is the current situation a result of scientific hubris that led to misguided programs or a failure of resolve that led global health programs to abandon effective tools? The answers will vary among observers and from place to place.

In 1955, the same year that the WHO commenced its malaria eradication campaign, ordinary families in the United States waged war against polio. By the millions, children bared their arms for a new vaccine developed by a team led by Jonas Salk. Only twenty years later the disease was almost eliminated from North America, but the activism of its survivors, who sought inclusion for the disabled, had barely begun.

WORKSHOP: MALARIA, DDT, AND THE ENVIRONMENTAL MOVEMENT

Scientific evidence offers interpretive challenges not only for historians but also for debates of current concern. Ideally, data can be verified by a community of scientists who agree on the validity of certain questions, methods of investigation, and experimental results. However, researchers are human—their topics of inquiry, tools, and means of presenting findings are all influenced by the societies that they inhabit. History offers many examples of scientific claims that reflect the interests of powerful social groups. For example, many ideas about racial characteristics that once were claimed to have an "objective" basis served to justify enslavement or coercion of Africans, Indians, and other colonized peoples.

For this reason, historical research that critically examines the formation of scientific knowledge can have great value. But the interrogation of science also creates a problem: the belief that scientific findings are not neutral—that evidence inevitably reflects an investigator's values or assumptions rather than unassailable truth—can undermine the ability of national or international communities to resolve conflicts or agree on common goals. In a globalized world, challenging questions often concern forces that operate on a vast scale, influence people around the world in different ways, or require specialized knowledge to understand. These factors can make it difficult to interpret scientific findings or even to decide what research questions should be asked in the first place.

The debate over DDT, which continues to this day, illustrates the problem perfectly. In the first half of the twentieth century, a new generation of chemical products were deployed for a wide range of domestic, industrial, and military purposes. The growing association of insects and parasites with destructive microbes increasingly seemed to call for scientific solutions. After World War II, hopes were especially high for the campaign against malaria, particularly since malaria was eliminated from the continental United States and Italy by the early 1960s. Health experts saw the prospect of dramatically reducing the global burden of malaria and perhaps even eradicating the disease altogether. Other public health achievements, notably the swift success of polio vaccination in the 1950s, contributed to a widespread faith in innovations such as DDT and the ability of science to find lasting solutions to basic problems.

Social currents began to change in the 1960s, reflected above all by a broad questioning of established institutions. In the United States, which exerted great influence in world affairs after World War II, the era was marked by a campaign for civil rights among African Americans and growing dissent toward military intervention in Vietnam. Environmental concerns—about radiation, carcinogens, and pesticides—symbolized a problem that was confronted as never before: the capacity of humankind to dramatically influence not only landscapes but also the fundamental fabric of the natural world.

DDT and other pesticides posed a knotty conundrum for scientists, officials, and the broader public. Many writers sought wide support, but debate revolved around concepts that were unfamiliar to laypeople and a wide range of evidence that was difficult, or even impossible, to independently verify. Ultimately, differing positions concerning DDT reflected not only contrasting approaches to the natural impact of chemicals (both known and potential), but also conflicting views of humanity's place in the natural world and the proper role of science in human affairs.

"Communications Create Understanding"—Robert White-Stevens (*Agricultural Chemicals*, October 1962)

A researcher in agricultural chemistry at the American Cyanamid company, White-Stevens vocally opposed Rachel Carson in print and on television. He and other industry advocates discerned a need for a concentrated media campaign to raise awareness of the benefits of chemicals in general and pesticides in particular. In this article written for professionals in his field, White-Stevens characterizes environmentalism as the product of urban elites who are unaware of the measures required to maintain an abundant and safe food supply. His writing reflects confidence in the value of human intervention in nature and belief in the importance of "assiduous attention to the truth and the facts" to combat what he considers distortions and misunderstanding. His remarks concerning the power of rapid communication—decades before digital communication became routine—appear prescient.

The single feature of our civilization to which can be attributed the largest credit for the incredible advances of man in the first half of the twentieth century is communications. Communication of information, both visual and verbal, has become virtually instantaneous all over the world; communication of goods and services has become completely worldwide, limited in time or place only by economics and politics. No longer is there separation between or within peoples except that forcefully imposed by man himself.

The tremendous advantages of such vast communication necessarily invokes concomitant disadvantages. There can no longer be secrets within or among nations or groups of people, and although efforts may be made to restrict and classify information, it is at best only a very temporary and transitory restraint ...

Another, and perhaps most significant, price we must pay for our modern system of communication lies in the tremendous responsibility it places upon us to use it wisely, truthfully, and with balance and restraint ... In a democracy such as ours, where legislation is often initiated and swayed and always executed in accordance with public opinion and acceptance, such assiduous attention to the truth and the facts, both in citation and interpretation, becomes doubly imperative.

Yet we have seen many cases in recent years where the welfare and livelihood of millions of people have been adversely affected by the deliberate misrepresentation of facts, and where our vast and penetrating communications system has been employed not to inform but to mislead. In former years, when our communications were less rapid and less ubiquitous, correction could the more readily catch up with error and maintain a favorable balance of understanding. Today, however, we often find that a false statement takes off like an ICBM [*an intercontinental ballistic missile*] and explodes in TV, radio, newspapers, magazines, and even in books, before a measured estimate of the facts in the matter can be assessed and presented objectively.

At the present time, our industry, among others, is sustaining just such an unjustifiable series of attacks. Small scraps of fact have been misrepresented and misquoted to the general public—usually the urban public that now constitutes the majority of our people—for the deliberate purpose of creating a false alarm and of influencing legislation....

We need now to tell the urban peoples in a thousand places and a thousand ways what scientific agriculture, including agricultural chemistry, has meant to their health, their welfare, and their standard of living. We should make it clear in schools, in service clubs, in church meetings, and in the hundreds of other groups to which our people attach themselves [*White-Stevens here lists achievements of scientific agriculture*]:

— that the entire cost of agricultural research by federal, state, and industry is less than the savings it brings in cost of food alone to the American people each year;
— that DDT alone has saved as many lives over the past fifteen years as all the wonder drugs combined;— that insecticides have been credited with extending the prospective life span in at least one Asiatic country [*he refers to a claim made for India*] from thirty-two to forty-seven years ...
— that agricultural science with all its disciplines working in close collaboration in the lab, in the college, in the field, in the factory, and out on the farm, has for the first time in man's long struggle against want procured the means to banish hunger from the earth in our time ...

[*White-Stevens then suggests that these benefits are not enough to capture the public's attention. Environmentalists such as Rachel Carson have seized the headlines with misleading rhetoric.*]

We need to tell our story with vividness and inspiration to catch the imagination of the urban masses.

Miss Rachel Carson has done it from the opposite side in her book *Silent Spring*, for she is a writer on biological subjects with an extraordinary, vivid touch and elegance of expression. She paints a nostalgic picture of Elysian life [*i.e., paradise*] in an imaginary American village of former years, where all was in harmonious balance with Nature and happiness and contentment reigned interminably, until sickness, death, and corruption was spread over the face of the landscape in the form of insecticides and other agricultural chemicals.

But the picture she paints is illusory, and she as a biologist must know that the rural Utopia she describes was rudely punctuated by a longevity among its residents of perhaps thirty-five years, by an infant mortality of upwards of twenty children dead by the age of five of every 100 born, by mothers dead in their twenties from childbed fever and tuberculosis, by frequent famines crushing the isolated peoples through long, dark, frozen winters following the failure of a basic crop the previous summer, by vermin and filth infesting their homes, their stored foods and their bodies, both inside and out ...

She ignores the fact that through the sciences she depreciates man can maintain himself today anywhere on earth. Within the past 100 years, man has emerged from a feeble creature, virtually at the mercy of Nature and his environment, to become the only being which can penetrate every corner of the planet, communicate instantly to anywhere on earth, produce all the food, fiber, and shelter he needs, wherever he may need it, change the topography of his lands, the sea and the universe and prepare his voyage through the very arch of heaven into space itself.

This is the stuff that science is made of, and man has learned to use it. He cannot now go back; he has crossed his Rubicon [*Julius Caesar's army famously crossed the Rubicon River before he assumed control of Rome*] and must advance into the future armed with reason and the tools of his sciences, and in so doing will doubtless have to contest the very laws and power of Nature herself. He has done this already by expanding his numbers far beyond her tolerance and by interrupting her laws of inheritance and survival. Now, he must go all the way, for he cannot but partially contest Nature. He has chosen to lead the way; he must take the responsibility upon himself.

"People and Pesticides"—Thomas H. Jukes (*American Scientist*, September 1963)

Jukes completed his PhD in biochemistry at the University of Toronto in 1933. In the 1960s, he worked at American Cyanamid alongside Robert White-Stevens before he became a professor of medical physics at the University of California at Berkeley. His work on nutrition helped pioneer the use of antibiotics in animal feed, and he later became a distinguished molecular biologist.

For a decade Jukes argued for the merits of DDT and other pesticides in numerous publications. He frequently debated claims made by Charles Wurster, a leading opponent of DDT whose writing is excerpted below. Jukes viewed DDT as an advance in technological prowess that could solve modern problems, above all the need to provide food for a rapidly expanding global population. His writings exhibited an underlying faith in American intervention in global affairs and a belief that natural resources should be managed for the benefit of humankind.

This article appeared in a popular science journal about a year after the controversy sparked by Rachel Carson's Silent Spring. *Although Jukes does not mention Carson or her book by name, allusions in his article unmistakably refer to fears that were provoked by her writings.*

The insecticide DDT (dichlorodiphenyltrichloroethane) has probably had a greater effect on disease and hunger than any other man-made chemical substance. The results produced by DDT are threefold: it has killed billions of insects and other arthropods that carry a number of diseases that have been the age-old scourges of mankind, it has controlled many of the insect pests that attack food crops, including codling worms, potato beetles, corn borers, thrips, aphids, and cutworms, and it has lowered the incidence of many bacterial diseases as a secondary result of its action against malaria and malnutrition.... The efficacy with which DDT and other chlorinated hydrocarbons have controlled these diseases is related to the vulnerability of their arthropod vectors to insecticides; the most susceptible are those that carry malaria, yellow fever, dengue, filariasis, and the louse-borne diseases. The sociological effects have been far-reaching, including reclamation of land for agriculture and urban expansion, decreases in absenteeism, higher earnings, and improved economic status....

[*Jukes later discusses the characteristics of DDT and cites reports of its ability to protect against malaria.*]

DDT is a stable substance and tends to leave persistent residues after spraying. This persistent quality has recently been criticized. Yet the residual effects are of essential importance in malarious regions, since the residues on the walls of sprayed buildings are sufficient to break the cycle of malaria by killing successive hatches of mosquitoes for several weeks. In Italy, 5,689 buildings in the Tiber delta region were sprayed with 5% DDT in kerosene, following which it was reported by Missiroli that Ostia [*an Italian city*] achieved a healthiness the like of which had not been seen there for 2,000 years. A campaign of residual spraying was then started throughout Italy in 1945 at a cost of 55 cents per inhabitant. In 1959, it was recorded by Simmons that not a single death had occurred from malaria in Italy since 1948, that large fertile areas had been converted from submarginal status to healthy, prosperous farmlands, and that the Pontine Marshes, for 2,000 years an uninhabitable morass of malaria, now were inhabited by 100,000 healthy people. In India it was reported by Pal in 1962 that since 1953 more than 147 million pounds [*of DDT*] have been used, with small amounts of benzene hexachloride and dieldrin [*two other pesticides*]. He estimated that during this period malaria in India had been reduced from 75 million cases to less than 5 million and that the average span of life in India is now forty-seven years as compared with thirty-two years before the eradication campaign ...

[*Jukes presents similar examples concerning the use of DDT to control typhus and bubonic plague. He then suggests that pesticides are no more harmful than natural residues or contaminants that modern scientific techniques can detect anywhere.*]

Small amounts of substances that are essentially foreign to the human body abound in our food, some originating from small quantities of bacteria, molds, and yeasts, some from the higher plants, some of universal origin from dust and soil, and some from the residues of agricultural chemicals. There is no evidence that any of the residues from pesticides are demonstrably harmful under the conditions that are normally encountered ... Most of us are relatively well inured to [*i.e., resigned to*] the fact that ... microbiological contaminants are everywhere, and the human alimentary tract serves as a home for potentially trillions of pathogenic bacteria. The advent of the scintillation counter [*an instrument, invented in 1944, that was used to detect and measure radiation*] has brought the realization that all biological material, including, of course, food, is inherently radioactive. One pound of DDT is a quantity sufficient to furnish 1 billion molecules per square foot of the United States. It is not suggested that the public should be told to ignore contaminants, but the facts regarding them should be more carefully and accurately explained than has been the case ...

[*The beginning of the following passage is an unsubtle reference to the rhetoric of* Silent Spring. *Jukes criticizes alarmism over pesticides, suggesting that other aspects of modern life are more destructive to wildlife. He addresses fears of the impact of DDT on bird populations by citing evidence that includes statistics collected by a conservation group, the National Audubon Society.*]

The image of a fragile and exquisite songbird dying in paralytic convulsions from the callous and unjustified application of a repulsive and deadly chemical sprayed broadcast over a defenseless landscape—this picture, regardless of the question of its possible authenticity, has a powerful effect on sensitive individuals. Many conservationists have expressed deep concern, since they view this image as part of a long train of events in which technology and weight of numbers have led man in North America to prevail with dire results in the struggle against Nature.

The spread of suburbs, industrial pollution, the drainage of marshlands, the building of superhighways, the increase in numbers of people, all have a disrupting effect on the population of wildlife compared with which pesticides are of minor significance. What are their effects on wild birds, for example? There is not room in this article to explore this at adequate length but a few points will be made. It is obviously possible to kill birds by direct exposure to a massive dose of pesticides. However, it has been reported that in the gypsy moth eradication project in Pennsylvania, "... not a single case of poisoning attributable to the DDT treatment at one pound per acre was reported. Officials of the National Audubon Society were satisfied that no damage was done to bird life, including nestling birds." [*The previous sentence refers to a US government program, conducted in 1957, that sprayed DDT over several million acres in Michigan, Pennsylvania, and New York.*]

Robins have been alleged to be victims of spraying programs due in part to their consumption of earthworms containing DDT. However, a recent report from the University of Wisconsin states that these birds were unaffected by thirty days of a diet of such earthworms which contained 26 ppm [*ppm = parts per million*] of DDT.... The transmission of avian diseases, including fowlpox and Newcastle disease [*viral infections of birds*], by mosquitoes, raises the question of possible protective effects on wildbirds resulting from the spraying of marshlands with insecticides. The red-winged blackbird, a denizen of marshes, jumped in the Audubon Christmas Bird Counts from 1.4 million in 1940 to 20 million in 1959.

[*Jukes concludes by suggesting that pesticide use will enable the necessary food supply for a rapidly growing global population. Leadership by the United States—in contrast to disastrous policies followed by an authoritarian regime in the Soviet Union—will be essential to this endeavor.*]

The inexorable upward extension of the world population curve continues at a rate of 5,600 per hour.... The best hope for coping with the need for food throughout the world lies in extending the superb agricultural technology of the United States into use in other countries. In the Soviet Union, the anti-scientific measures introduced by Lysenko [*Trofim Denisovich Lysenko, a Soviet scientist*] and fostered by Stalin, produced a big setback to agriculture. [*Soviet farming reforms in the 1920s and 1930s aggravated the impact of devastating famines in which millions of people died.*] Progress in American agriculture must not become similarly hamstrung by legislation resulting from inaccurate statements regarding the dangers of pesticides. The right to publish confers the obligation to tell the story without distortion, omission, misquotation, or innuendo. The issue is not one that merely involves 2 per cent of sales of the chemical industry; at stake is no less than the protection of the free world from hunger and disease.

"DDT Proved neither Essential nor Safe"—Charles F. Wurster (*BioScience*, February 1973)

Wurster completed his doctorate in chemistry in 1957 and became a professor at Stony Brook University in New York State. In 1967, he was a founding member of the Environmental Defense Fund that launched legal actions against the use of DDT. A generation younger than Jukes, Wurster specialized in the chemistry and biological impact of pesticides. This focus is apparent in the arguments that his writings advance to counter arguments in favor of DDT. Such evidence mounted in the 1960s as environmental and laboratory studies confirmed the pesticide's effects.

This article was written shortly after the Director of the US Environmental Protection Agency, William D. Ruckelshaus, ordered the cancellation of all registrations for DDT in the United States (in 1972). In large measure, the EPA's decision hinged on a relatively specific issue: the inability of DDT's manufacturers to prove that the pesticide would not harm organisms other than its targets. Underlying Wurster's criticism of DDT is a broader claim: nature must be protected from the worst effects of human intervention.

Last 14 June Administrator William D. Ruckelshaus of the Environmental Protection Agency (EPA), after scrutiny of the voluminous transcript of the seven-month hearing on DDT, concluded that DDT had outlived its usefulness and the costs and risks of continued use exceeded its benefit to society. Accordingly, he ordered almost all interstate sales of DDT halted by the end of 1972.

The DDT hearing and the ultimate decision did not arise from Rachel Carson's *Silent Spring* or from an "emotional" or "hysterical" public outcry, as the DDT industry has implied. Instead, litigation against DDT by the Environmental Defense Fund (EDF) and several other environmental organizations at the local, state and federal levels was supported by a large number of scientists, most of them research workers on insect control or on the effects of persistent pesticides on nontarget organisms and ecosystems ... The order [*by the EPA to halt sales of DDT*] applied only to DDT for specific reasons; at no time was this litigation directed at all pesticides. Its use abroad for malaria suppression also was never at issue.

[*Wurster then explains t*he rationale for the decision to ban DDT in all but extraordinary cases and why other pest control methods are preferable.]

Under federal law, the manufacturer has the burden of proving that his pesticide, when used as directed, will not harm nontarget organisms. DDT was banned because its proponents failed to demonstrate either its safety or its essentiality. To the contrary, scientists testifying for EPA and EDF confirmed the hazards and shortcomings of DDT in key areas.

Competent entomologists described integrated control [of pests and their predators] as an effective, economical and safe alternative to the outmoded and increasingly ineffective DDT approach. Integrated control blends biological techniques with selective use of nonpersistent insecticides, increasing crop yields and profits for farmers while decreasing pesticide usage.

DDT is incompatible with integrated control because it destroys the natural enemies of the pests, often leading to increased pest outbreaks. Farmers, consumers, and the environment all benefit from integrated control, but pesticide sales decline. The Ruckelshaus decision is especially encouraging because it will hasten conversion to these modern pest control practises. [*Wurster then outlines scientific findings concerning the environmental damage caused by DDT. He asserts that the claims of the pesticide's supporters do not disprove this evidence.*]

Numerous scientists at the hearing ... detailed the precipitous declines of various birds of prey and sea birds that have been caused largely by DDT. By affecting hormone and enzyme functions, DDT causes birds to lay thin-shelled eggs that break prematurely. The industry did not produce a qualified scientist who could refute this evidence. Their nearest attempt at "proving" DDT safe for birds came from observations of increased sightings at Hawk Mountain and on Christmas bird counts. Cross-examination revealed that the increases resulted from an increase in the number of observers rather than the number of birds.

The testimony of several scientists detail the hazards of DDT to fish and certain crustaceans. DDT lowers the reproductive success of fish by accumulating in the eggyolk and killing the fry shortly after they hatch from contaminated eggs.... The DDT proponents were unable to dispel the hazards of DDT to fish.

Authorities on chemical carcinogenesis, including two from the National Cancer Institute, testified that DDT is a cancer hazard for men because experiments in several laboratories have shown it to cause tumors in mice. Since agents cannot be tested for carcinogenic potential using human subjects, controlled experiments with mice using high dosages are the standard test method to warn of a potential human hazard.... Competent testimony that DDT is a cancer hazard for man was not successfully challenged by the industry....

The banning of DDT by Ruckelshaus was not a political decision. It was based on sound scientific information—probably the most comprehensive available for any pollutant. The DDT industry did not meet the burden of proof because it failed to establish either an essential need for DDT, or its safety for nontarget organisms including man.

INTERPRETING THE DOCUMENTS

1.   How does White-Stevens view the place of humans on earth and the role of technology in creating it? How do you think an environmentalist such as Charles Wurster would respond?

2.   Why does White-Stevens claim that "communications create understanding"? How would you evaluate that statement with regard to today's digital media environment?

3.   Both Jukes and Wurster appeal to scientific knowledge as a basis for understanding and decision making. How does each do so? What kinds of data does each find persuasive and relevant for the debate? Can the disagreement between them be resolved with scientific data?

MAKING CONNECTIONS

1.   What does the debate over DDT indicate about attitudes toward the natural world in the 1960s? How had perceptions changed since the views of Europeans in the fourteenth century? Since the turn of the nineteenth century?

2.   Compare the arguments made by White-Stevens and Jukes to the claims made for antimicrobial consumer products in the 1910s and 1920s. What arguments are made for the value of science (and scientists) in promoting human well-being?

For further reading: Elena Conis, "Debating the Health Effects of DDT: Thomas Jukes, Charles Wurster, and the Fate of an Environmental Pollutant," *Public Health Reports* 125, no. 2 (2010): 337–42.

Notes

1. Marianne Fedunkiw, "Malaria Films: Motion Pictures as a Public Health Tool," *American Journal of Public Health* 93, no. 7 (2003): 1056 n. 48.

2. Quoted in James L.A. Webb Jr, *Humanity's Burden: A Global History of Malaria* (Cambridge: Cambridge University Press, 2009), frontispiece.

3. WHO, *World Malaria Report 2018*, xii–xiii, https://www.who.int/malaria/publications/world -malaria-report-2018/report/en/.

4. CDC, "Anopheles Mosquitoes" (October 2015), https://www.cdc.gov/malaria/about/biology /mosquitoes/.

5. James L.A. Webb Jr, "Early Malarial Infections and the First Epidemiological Transition," in *Human Dispersal and Species Movement: From Prehistory to the Present*, ed. Nicole Boivin, Rémy Crassard, and Michael D. Petraglia (Cambridge: Cambridge University Press, 2017), 478–82.

6. Sunetra Gupta, "Mastering Malaria: What Helps and What Hurts," *Proceedings of the National Academy of Sciences* 112, no. 10 (2015): 2925–26.

7. Webb, *Humanity's Burden*, 20–27.

8. Webb, *Humanity's Burden*, 27–41.

9. Christopher Ehret, "Historical/Linguistic Evidence for Early African Food Production," in *From Hunters to Farmers*, ed. J.D. Clark and S.A. Brandt (Berkeley: University of California Press, 1984), 26–39.

10. Quoted in Sonia Shah, *The Fever: How Malaria Has Ruled Humankind for 500,000 Years* (New York: Farrar, Straus and Giroux, 2010), 64–65.

11. William Shakespeare, *Julius Caesar* Act I, Scene ii, quoted in Thomas H. Jukes, "People and Pesticides," *American Scientist* 51, no. 3 (1963): 356.

12. Mary Dobson, "'Marsh Fever'—The Geography of Malaria in England," *Journal of Historical Geography* 6, no. 4 (1980): 357.

13. Quoted in Mary J. Dobson, *Contours of Death and Disease in Early Modern England* (Cambridge: Cambridge University Press, 1997), 300–306, at 303.

14. Andrew Goss, *The Floracrats: State-Sponsored Science and the Failure of the Enlightenment in Indonesia* (Madison: University of Wisconsin Press, 2011), 37.

15. Philip Curtin, "Epidemiology and the Slave Trade," *Political Science Quarterly* 83, no. 2 (1968): 203, Table 1.

16. Fiammetta Rocco, *The Miraculous Fever-Tree: The Cure That Changed the World* (London: Harper Collins, 2004), 163–64.

17. Sheldon Watts, "British Development Policies and Malaria in India, 1897–c. 1929," *Past and Present* 165, no. 1 (1999): 150.

18. Watts, "British Development Policies," 161.

19. Ira Klein, "Malaria and Mortality in Bengal, 1840–1921," *Indian Economic and Social History Review* 9, no. 2 (1972): 132–60.

20. Mark Harrison, *Climates and Constitutions: Health, Race, Environment and British Imperialism in India, 1600–1850* (New York: Oxford University Press, 1999), 54–55.

21. Rohan Deb Roy, "Quinine, Mosquitoes and Empire: Reassembling Malaria in British India 1890–1910," *South Asian History and Culture* 4, no. 1 (2013): 67–69.

22. Mark Harrison, *Public Health in British India: Anglo-Indian Preventive Medicine, 1859–1914* (Cambridge: Cambridge University Press, 1994), 232.

23. Francis E.G. Cox, "History of the Discovery of Malaria Parasites and Their Vectors," *Parasites & Vectors* 3, no. 5 (2010): 1–9.

24. Ronald Ross, *Mosquito Brigades and How to Organise Them* (New York: Longmans, Green & Co., 1902), viii.

25. Ross, *Mosquito Brigades*, 13.

26. Robert Peckham, *Epidemics in Modern Asia* (Cambridge: Cambridge University Press, 2016), 170.

27. Sandra M. Sufian, *Healing the Land and the Nation* (Chicago: University of Chicago Press, 2007).

28. F.L. Soper et al., "Typhus Control in Italy, 1943–1945, and Its Control with Louse Powder," *American Journal of Hygiene* 45, no. 3 (1947): 319.

29. Soper et al., "Typhus Control in Italy," 27.

30. Frank M. Snowden, *The Conquest of Malaria: Italy, 1900–1962* (New Haven: Yale University Press, 2006), 198–207.

31. Randall M. Packard, *A History of Global Health: Interventions into the Lives of Other Peoples* (Baltimore: Johns Hopkins University Press, 2016), 159.

32. Randall M. Packard, *The Making of a Tropical Disease: A Short History of Malaria* (Baltimore: Johns Hopkins University Press, 2007), 167.

33. Alex Perry, *Lifeblood: How to Change the World, One Dead Mosquito at a Time* (London: Hurst & Co., 2011), 17.

34. Packard, *Global Health*, 143.

35. C. Lee Ventola, "The Antibiotic Resistance Crisis," *Pharmacy and Therapeutics* 40, no. 4 (2015): 277–83.

36. Eli Klein et al., "Global Increase and Geographic Convergence in Antibiotic Consumption between 2000 and 2015," *Proceedings of the National Academy of Sciences* 115 (2018): E3463–E3470, https://doi.org/10.1073/pnas.1717295115.

37. F.C. Lessa, L.G. Winston, and L.C. McDonald, "Burden of *Clostridium difficile* Infection in the United States," *New England Journal of Medicine* 372 (2015): 2369–70.

38. Rachel Carson, *Silent Spring* (New York: Houghton Mifflin Company, 1962), 2.

39. WHO, "WHO Gives Indoor Use of DDT a Clean Bill of Health for Controlling Malaria" (15 September 2006), http://www.who.int/mediacentre/news/releases/2006/pr50/en/.

40. David Leonard Downie and Terry Fenge, eds, *Northern Lights against POPS: Combatting Toxic Threats in the Arctic* (Montreal: McGill-Queen's University Press, 2003), 4–11.

41. Laura C. Norris et al., "Adaptive Introgression in an African Malaria Mosquito Coincident with the Increased Usage of Insecticide-Treated Bed Nets," *Proceedings of the National Academy of Sciences* 112, no. 3 (2015): 815–20.

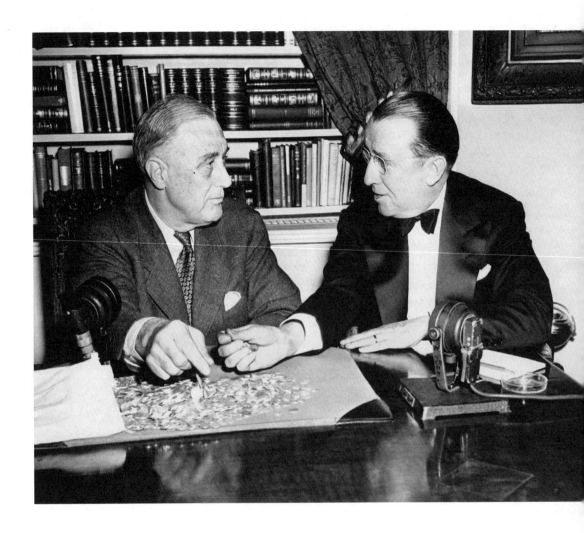

IMAGE 10.1 Franklin Delano Roosevelt and Basil O'Connor count coins at the White House (1944). Roosevelt served as United States president from January 1933 until his death in April 1945. He lent his personal prestige to polio fundraising campaigns led by the National Foundation for Infantile Paralysis (NFIP). Although he was paralyzed from the waist down by disease, Roosevelt concealed the full extent of his disability from the public. Basil O'Connor was Roosevelt's former law partner and confidante. He served as founding president of the NFIP.

ILLNESS, DISABILITY, AND
THE STRUGGLE FOR INCLUSION

10

n 1955, the philanthropic National Foundation for Infantile Paralysis (NFIP) chose Cyndi Jones, five years old, as a March of Dimes poster child for the region around her hometown of St Louis, Missouri. The little girl enjoyed the attention. The NFIP sent a photographer from New York to take her picture. She rode on parade floats and her picture appeared on billboards. The next fall, when Jones arrived in her first grade class, she saw a flyer that advertised a vaccination campaign. One photo depicted her smiling in a party dress as she leaned on her crutches. Above her, a headline read "VACCINATE YOUR FAMILY NOW AGAINST POLIO." The words "NOT THIS" were stamped next to Cyndi's arm; next to her, a boy and girl running hand in hand were labeled with an approving "THIS." As Jones later recalled, she wanted to hide under her desk. Instead, she went home and told her parents that the charity could no longer use pictures of her.[1]

The NFIP and the United States had reached a turning point in the long struggle against polio. For decades, the disease had haunted summer. It most often struck the young and was slightly more prevalent among boys, but beyond that its impact seemed disturbingly random. Sometimes polio killed by disabling the muscles that enabled breathing. Far more often, it caused paralysis in the limbs and torso. As scientists worked frantically, the incidence of infection rose to new heights in the early 1950s. Many communities closed public swimming pools, and a few towns even posted signs warning children to stay away. Then, in 1954, a massive trial tested a vaccine in children across the country. Church bells rang in celebration when positive results were announced in a press conference the following year. Polio vaccination became routine, and by the 1970s new cases of the disease almost disappeared in the United States and other Western countries.

However, hundreds of thousands of polio survivors such as Cyndi Jones were treated as a remnant for whom the vaccine had come too late. Many of these individuals—including Jones, who became an advocate for people with disabilities—refused to be defined by the disease and instead criticized attitudes and social structures that prevented their full membership in society. In the 1960s and 1970s, advocacy by polio survivors merged with a movement toward broader social inclusion for people with disabilities, African Americans, and women. Once considered objects of pity, polio survivors challenged prevailing social norms and encouraged other initiatives to acknowledge and embrace human diversity.

Since 2010, confirmed cases of polio worldwide have numbered only in the hundreds, but the push to eradicate the disease has encountered stubborn obstacles. The difficult drive to eradication illustrates how poverty, the fractured politics of conflict zones, and other barriers to effective communication continue to influence public health campaigns around the world.

Etiology and Early History

The term "polio" is an abbreviation of "poliomyelitis," which derives from the Greek words for "grey" (*polios*) and "marrow" (*myelon*) joined to a Latin suffix (*-itis*). Other names evoked the disease's most feared symptom: it was called "paralysis of the lower extremities" since the legs were often affected; "paralysis of the morning" because children sometimes went to bed and then awoke unable to rise; and, most commonly, "infantile paralysis." This latter term was a misnomer—children developed polio disease more often than adults but infants rarely experienced paralysis or other severe symptoms. However, the label connoted a lingering immaturity and deepened the stigma for polio survivors who faced lengthy recoveries or lifelong disability.

In the 1940s, researchers identified three distinct types of poliovirus. Type 2 poliovirus has now been eradicated, but the most common variant, Type 1, also causes the worst symptoms. The pathogen multiplies in mouth and nasal passages and the small intestine. It is expelled in feces, and usually enters a new host when it is ingested or (less commonly) inhaled. Fecal-oral contamination, which also fosters the spread of cholera, diphtheria, and typhoid, is more commonplace in cities that do not have consistent sewage treatment, water filtration, or chlorination. If the poliovirus is present in such settings, many people will contract it as infants when maternal antibodies limit the virus's replication and the severity of its effects. Individuals experience more severe symptoms if they contract polio after maternal antibody protection ends.

The effects of polio infection vary and many people experience few symptoms or none at all. During large outbreaks, roughly 4–8 per cent of infected individuals experience mild (or "abortive") poliomyelitis, which causes flu-like symptoms, stomach cramps, or a red, sore throat. In more severe cases of paralytic polio—less than 1 per cent of infections and sometimes as few as 1 in 1,000—the virus enters the spinal cord and damages the nerves that stimulate muscle contractions. Many people with paralytic polio recover because some nerve cells resist the virus or grow new connections to muscle fibers. However, if paralysis lasts for months the damage is usually irreversible.[2] In the bulbar form of poliomyelitis, which is fatal without intervention, the virus invades the brain stem and destroys the neurons that regulate the movement of the diaphragm and other muscles. For many polio survivors, it is now known that the disease often has after-effects. Decades after they contract the virus, more than a quarter of polio survivors experience post-polio syndrome (PPS), which manifests as chronic fatigue and progressive muscle weakness. The causes of the syndrome are not fully understood; its main effects are experienced in muscles that were weakened by the initial infection or by long-lasting spine and limb deformities.

Although polio may be induced in some mammals, including several monkey species, animals normally do not contract it and there is no nonhuman reservoir of infection in nature. Of course, this greatly increases the chance of success for eradication efforts. Smallpox, which was declared eradicated in 1979, also had no animal reservoir. Unlike smallpox, however, the great majority of people who contract polio experience no obvious symptoms. Poliovirus mostly inhabits the small intestine, and infected people excrete the virus in stool for weeks even when they are asymptomatic. This hinders case tracing and efforts to confirm that poliovirus is completely absent in a population that has not been fully vaccinated.

From Endemic to Epidemic Polio

A comparison between polio's (presumed) impact in the era before 1880 and in the twentieth century aptly illustrates why historians distinguish between *infection* with a pathogen and the physical or social manifestations of *disease*.

Until the turn of the last century, polio was probably endemic in much of the world—so ubiquitous, in fact, that the vast majority of city-dwellers contracted the virus in infancy. Many people "had polio"—that is, they hosted the poliovirus for a time—without realizing it. This state of affairs persisted until sanitary innovations altered the prevalence of polioviruses and the time of first exposure for some populations. At the end of the nineteenth century, a pathogen that was almost always benign when everyone was exposed as an infant became a dangerous threat when fewer women passed on maternal antibodies and children were exposed later in life. The common observation that polio is "a disease of poor sanitation" thus obscures the historical changes that caused polio epidemics to emerge when they did. Large outbreaks of paralytic polio resulted from *improvements* to sanitation that shielded individuals temporarily but failed to protect them from a later, more harmful exposure. For this reason, in the early twentieth century it was developed countries, and especially the United States, that faced the greatest incidence of polio.

References to characteristic symptoms of polio are infrequent before the nineteenth century. An ancient Egyptian stone engraving of a figure with a withered leg probably attests to its presence in the Nile River valley around 1400 BCE. Allusions in the Hippocratic writings and Galen to "acquired clubfoot" may also refer to polio, although similar physical conditions can either be congenital (i.e., present from birth) or caused by other diseases such as meningitis. From antiquity through the early modern era, polio's more severe manifestations did not stand out among the other causes of paralysis or disability such as leprosy, Pott's disease, or even poorly set bone fractures. In general, Europeans viewed the disabled with suspicion. It was often assumed that a person's physical deformity mirrored spiritual or moral corruption, and everyone, including medical practitioners, sought to avoid the disabled rather than investigate their afflictions.

Beginning in the late eighteenth century, European clinicians recorded polio-like symptoms and investigated minor outbreaks. From the 1880s forward, polio appeared more frequently in Scandinavia, England, and the United States. Many early episodes were in thinly populated rural areas such as Rutland County, Vermont (United States), which sustained 132 cases in 1894. The first major epidemic, in 1905, comprised more than 2,000 cases in Norway and Sweden. The dynamics of initial infections and transmission varied among communities and families. Research suggests that children in rural settings often were exposed to poliovirus relatively late, and were thus more vulnerable to severe symptoms. In some cases, crowded dwellings also increased the likelihood of severe infection.[3]

Investigation by Ivar Wickman (1872–1914), a Swedish pediatrician and epidemiologist, laid the groundwork for the later understanding of polio's epidemiology. Wickman used case tracing to demonstrate that polio was, in fact, a contagious disease, and he highlighted the role of schools in disseminating it through a community. He established that individuals with mild or asymptomatic cases of polio could spread the disease and that people who contracted polio were not potentially infectious to others right away. Wickman found that the **latency period** (the interval after persons are infected and before they are infectious to others) was three to four days for minor illness and eight to ten days for major illness.[4]

After 1905, as the number and size of polio outbreaks grew on both sides of the Atlantic, laboratory researchers began to investigate the disease. In 1908, a Viennese researcher named Karl Landsteiner (1868–1943) used a porcelain filter to isolate the poliovirus in serum, although the pathogen remained invisible under a microscope. At the Rockefeller Foundation in New York, Simon Flexner (1863–1946) experimented with monkeys to investigate polio's transmission and develop an antiserum or vaccine from an attenuated virus. In one important respect, Flexner's work was unlucky: he used the rhesus monkey, a species that does not host poliovirus in its digestive tract as humans do. Because Flexner relied on laboratory results, rather than evidence from human cases, he developed an incorrect theory that poliovirus entered through the nose and traveled straight to the spinal cord. Over time, Flexner's viral strain also became neurotropic—as it was passed from monkey to monkey, it adapted to nervous systems so that it could not replicate in the digestive tract at all. Doomed efforts to link this lab-created pathogen to real-world polio cases hampered investigators for decades.[5]

In the short run, therefore, scientists did little to allay public concerns about diseases that could strike vulnerable children. As discussed in chapter 6, by 1915 magazines and newspapers had popularized the notion that many diseases were caused by insidious, invisible germs. Researchers had also shown that malaria and yellow fever were spread by mosquitoes and that flies deposited germs on food. To observers in some communities, such findings justified a full-scale assault on offending insects. Already in 1906, Kansas public health officials adopted the motto "Swat that fly!"—baseball slang for hitting a fly ball—to refer to actual efforts to kill flies. Boy Scouts in Weir, Kansas, took the concept a step further by attaching squares of wire mesh to yardsticks, creating "fly bats" later known as "fly swatters." In 1913, the US city of Cleveland launched what one

writer described as an effort "to put the city on the map as a flyless city." Small
cards were printed for store patrons to anonymously inform shopkeepers of the
number of flies that were seen in their stores. City authorities even invited
participation from children. Schools distributed pamphlets as well as 200,000
swatters for obliging boys and girls to smite the flies that crossed their path.
Children were paid 10 cents for every hundred flies that they brought to "Anti-fly
headquarters" at the city hall.[6]

Defense against polio took on new urgency in the United States in 1916 when
a major epidemic caused roughly 27,000 cases and 6,000 deaths. New York City
alone sustained one-third of the nation's reported cases and mortality. As residents pondered what was to blame, health officials plucked thousands of stray cats
off the streets and euthanized them. Well-off inhabitants fled the city, and other
families were forbidden to shelter sick children at home unless they had a private
bathroom. Despite evidence that better-off households were affected as much as
lower-class ones, popular anxiety also focused on another familiar suspect:
immigrants and the filthy conditions in which they were assumed to live. In the
1910s, New Yorkers had heard the lurid story of "Typhoid Mary," an Irish cook
named Mary Mallon who spread typhoid fever to dozens of people. Tests confirmed that Mallon was an asymptomatic carrier of typhoid bacteria, but she
defied instructions to find another occupation and infected even more people.
Public health officers confined her to a cottage on North Brother Island in the
East River. As the number of polio cases mounted, hundreds of destitute children
were quarantined on the same island.[7]

More American children died from polio in 1916 than in any other year. As
discussed shortly, mortality dropped after artificial respirators were introduced
after 1928. However, observers who tracked the incidence of polio over years
noted an alarming rise in the total number of reported cases. Epidemics of
increasing severity interspersed with years of lower incidence. Nationwide,
46,215 polio cases were reported between 1920 and 1929, in 1930–39 the total
was 75,186, and in 1940–49 it was 173,680.[8] The growing number of young
children in the United States after 1948—the so-called "baby boom" after World
War II—contributed to the increase in cases.[9] Polio incidence peaked in the early
1950s; in just eight months between June 1952 and January 1953, more than
55,000 new cases were reported, a rate of over 35 people per 100,000. Although
American prosperity was approaching a zenith, polio offered a sign of communal
vulnerability and scientific impotence. The reported polio incidence in Canada
usually paralleled the numbers in the United States, but there were some

exceptions. In 1937, Canada sustained a much more severe outbreak than its southern neighbor, and nearly 1,000 people in Manitoba contracted polio in 1941. Christopher Rutty has suggested that the energetic response to polio, particularly in Ontario during the 1937 outbreak, propelled Canada toward state-sponsored healthcare that provided long-term treatment for polio and other chronic conditions as well.[10]

Polio sufferers who could not breathe or swallow posed an urgent challenge that required a mechanical solution. In the late 1920s and early 1930s, several independent groups of inventors designed tank ventilators that used negative air pressure to induce inhalation and exhalation. Sometimes, the devices could not be made fast enough—during the Ontario epidemic, technicians built them around the clock in the basement of Toronto's Hospital for Sick Children. A newspaper headline conjured an enduring image: "Massive Iron Lungs Grotesque, Glorious, Coax Life to Tots."

Such heroics did not end in the 1930s. When an epidemic struck Denmark in 1952, Blegdam Hospital in Copenhagen was inundated with bulbar polio patients. Negative pressure ventilators failed to prevent dozens of deaths. An anesthetist named Bjørn Ibsen (1915–2007) then applied a surgical technique: he inserted a tube into a patient's windpipe and used a bag with oxygen to provide positive pressure ventilation. "Bagging" saved lives but had to be done by hand, and so the hospital organized shifts of more than 2,000 students and nurses who attended the patients for months. Begun in desperation, Blegdam's polio care program evolved into a defined unit that integrated many types of expertise. These practices were emulated elsewhere as hospitals created units that were dedicated to the whole-body needs of critically ill patients. Intensive-care specialists today trace the origin of their discipline to the polio ward at Blegdam.[11]

Iron lung ventilators saved thousands of lives, but it is difficult to generalize about how polio survivors used them in the mid-twentieth century and, in rare cases, still use them today. A few paralyzed individuals lay prone in iron lungs for years, or even decades, but most users received breathing assistance for only a few weeks. Others used various machines for years but only for a few hours during each day or night. Finally, the needs of many polio survivors have evolved as they age, and in some cases muscle function requires more support later in life. As we consider polio's history, it is helpful to recognize the diversity of experiences *within* the community of survivors as well as the relationships between polio survivors, other people with disabilities, and members of the wider society.

SCIENCE FOCUS

A Breathing Space: The Iron Lung and Mechanical Ventilation

For decades, the iron lung has been a sobering, even frightening image—"the realization of the body's most dreadful fears," as the narrator in a recent novel described it.[12] However, the reality for iron lung users was often very different. Many of them described feelings of relaxation or release as the machine took over breathing functions that their body could not perform. The later developments in artificial ventilation technology continue to help millions of people.

After 1850, various inventors had designed machines that used negative air pressure to inflate lungs in a sealed chamber. Most devices were only tested on animals but, in 1864, Alfred Jones of Kentucky patented a box that enclosed a patient from the neck down and used a plunger to cause inhalation and exhalation. In 1928, Philip Drinker, Louis Agassiz Shaw, and Charles McKhann used similar techniques to design a tank ventilator (called a respirator at the time) for polio patients in Boston. Fears of polio ran so high that Drinker's team published an article in 1929 that explained how parents could build a machine with everyday items such as a vacuum cleaner tube and a wooden box. In 1931, John Emerson introduced a cheaper device with a sliding bed and side portals that enabled assistants to reach inside.

The simple design of Drinker and Emerson respirators imitated normal breathing. The device enclosed users in a sealed chamber with their heads protruding from one end. A crank moved a bellows attached to the other end to change the air pressure inside. When the bellows moved out and expanded the size of the chamber, negative air pressure expanded the users' lungs to cause inhalation. The opposite movement of the bellows reduced the size of the chamber and contracted the lungs for exhalation. Iron lungs saved lives, but also required constant vigilance. Nurses or other machines removed saliva when users could not swallow. The rubber gasket around the neck required monitoring to create a tight vacuum seal without chafing. Thunderstorms raised the possibility of power outages, and health care workers were often trained to provide breathing support manually.

Further innovations provided patients greater mobility and control. Beginning in the early 1950s, some patients used a rocking bed when they had milder symptoms or as they transitioned out of an iron lung. Beds relied upon gravity to perform the same function as the iron lung

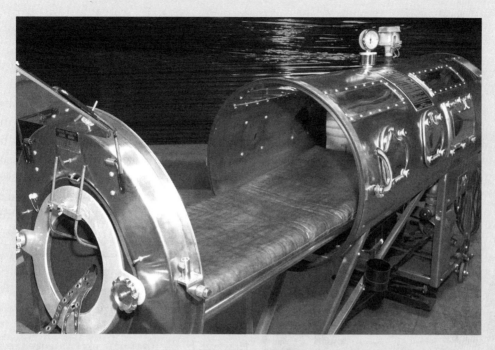

IMAGE 10.2 An Emerson respirator. The Emerson respirator was one of the devices known as an iron lung. Users were enclosed with their heads outside the circular opening. A bellows (at the far end) moved in and out to adjust air pressure and enable breathing. This respirator belonged to Barton Hebert of Covington, Louisiana, who used it from the late 1950s until his death in 2003.

bellows. They could be carried to different locations, and a few people even installed them in vans for long-distance travel. Individuals also traveled with a cuirass respirator (still in use today), which seals the user's torso in a chamber that resembles a turtle shell.

The high survival rates during the 1952 Copenhagen polio epidemic encouraged interest in positive pressure ventilation. Initially, the technique required an endotracheal tube inserted into the throat that gently pushed air into the lungs. This protected the airway from liquid secretions that would cause choking; later research suggested that positive pressure improved the exchange of oxygen and carbon dioxide in lung tissues. Air tubes had drawbacks—they were invasive and sometimes damaged the trachea—but in

the early 1980s nasal tubes were introduced that benefited many ventilation users.[13]

In 2003, during the global outbreak of SARS, hundreds of patients relied on mechanical ventilators. The crisis forced medical communities to consider preparedness for a larger pandemic. Concerns focused not only on the patients themselves but also on ventilators and building systems that might spread infection. In Toronto, where thousands of residents were quarantined during the outbreak, hospitals have responded by designing isolation pods, separate preparation rooms for staff, and air circulation systems that reduce the dispersion of infected aerosols. Such measures are important not only to counter SARS but also to prepare for future outbreaks of pandemic influenza or other respiratory diseases.

Therapy Debates and the Vaccine Quest

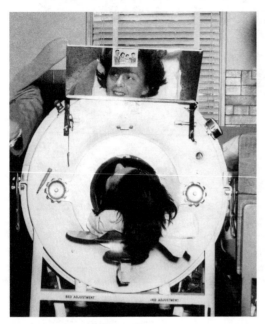

IMAGE 10.3 Iron lung user Virginia Lemke. Lemke was in an iron lung for six months. In the photograph she presents a stoic, even cheerful demeanor. Since such individuals were seldom photographed in distress, it is hard to know what the pictures reveal about their thoughts or feelings.

Most paralytic polio survivors did not have breathing challenges, but they faced other questions. How much mobility could their limbs regain? What was the best means of therapy? The answer to the first question varied. Some people recovered fully, but others relied on crutches or wheelchairs for the rest of their lives. In turn, practitioners passionately debated the second question. The more adventurous treatments included muscle stimulation with electric current and spinal taps to remove cerebrospinal fluid that was considered excessive or harmful. More often, doctors recommended massage and gentle exercise. Swimming pools or mineral springs were thought useful since the water's buoyancy made limbs easier to move. However, by the 1930s most experts agreed that limbs should be immobilized for weeks or months of recovery. Bedridden patients were strapped to a frame while splints and casts inclined their limbs to the desired position. As one doctor put it, a splint was like a stake that would straighten a growing rose bush.[14] In Ontario, a program was developed to manufacture and distribute standardized frames and splints free of charge. "Toronto splints" were used throughout North America and even stockpiled in New York in case of another epidemic.

Opposition to this style of therapy assumed an unlikely form: Elizabeth Kenny (1880–1952), an Australian nurse who reputedly found her gift for treating polio among patients in the remote outback. Untrained, outspoken, and determined, Kenny opened several clinics but then left Australia for the United States in 1940 after a government commission evaluated her work unfavorably. Kenny believed polio was a disorder of muscle spasms rather than nerves, and she prescribed heat and manipulation to relax and "reeducate" damaged muscles to their former movement. Experts found the theory absurd, but many patients and lay observers were inspired by Kenny's approach and outsized personality. Her autobiography, *And They Shall Walk* (1943), was a best-seller. Even a Hollywood movie, *Sister Kenny*, celebrated her challenge to medical orthodoxy. If nothing else, Kenny enlisted her patients as active participants in therapy, and she encouraged the swift recovery of movement whenever possible. As she once noted, "In the final analysis, it is the patient who must reopen the nerve path between the mind and the affected muscle."[15] Between 1940 and 1951, Kenny based her work in Minneapolis where she gave university lectures, established a foundation, and oversaw the creation of several more clinics. Although she was never esteemed by polio scientists, Kenny's work provided stimulus for the discipline of rehabilitation medicine.

The main focus of polio research was the quest for an effective vaccine. After World War II, this was seen as a test of scientific prowess as the United States competed with the Soviet Union in many arenas. However, to a remarkable extent, the endeavor was sponsored by private philanthropy rather than government agencies, and it drew much of its impetus from the image of one polio survivor, US President Franklin Delano Roosevelt (1882–1945).

Polio and the President

Roosevelt contracted polio in 1921 when he was thirty-nine years old.[16] He seemed an unlikely candidate for "infantile paralysis": tall, athletic, and wealthy, Roosevelt belonged to one of New York's best-known families. Polio paralyzed Roosevelt almost completely from the waist down and sidetracked his political ambitions, but the search for therapy trained his sights on new goals. In 1925, a friend touted the health benefits of a natural spring at the Meriwether Inn in rural Georgia. Roosevelt purchased the property. Rechristened Warm Springs, the run-down hotel soon evolved into a leading center for polio treatment and rehabilitation. It was also Roosevelt's personal retreat for the rest of his life. Although he carefully shielded the full extent of his disability from the public, at Warm Springs he mingled freely with the other "polios" and bobbed alongside them in the large, open-air swimming pool.

In 1928, New York State's governor, Al Smith, sought the US presidency and asked Roosevelt to pursue election as his replacement. Smith was defeated, but Roosevelt narrowly won, and then convincingly won re-election to the governorship in 1930. Two years later Roosevelt was elected president himself. He took office as the Great Depression caused widespread unemployment and hardship. Roosevelt no longer ran Warm Springs, but he remained deeply attached to the resort. When bankruptcy threatened, a public relations expert suggested a nationwide party in honor of the president as a fundraiser. Polio debuted as a national charity cause on Roosevelt's fifty-second birthday, 30 January 1934. In communities large and small, thousands of gala balls, square dances, card parties, and church suppers made just over 1 million dollars for Warm Springs. After several years of lucrative fundraising,

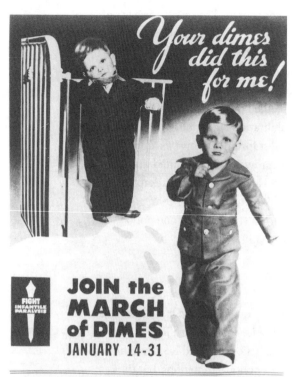

Your dimes did this for me!

JOIN the MARCH of DIMES
JANUARY 14-31

FIGHT INFANTILE PARALYSIS

THE NATIONAL FOUNDATION FOR INFANTILE PARALYSIS, INC.
FRANKLIN D. ROOSEVELT, FOUNDER

IMAGE 10.4 "Your dimes did this for me!" In 1946, Donald Anderson was the first official polio poster child for the NFIP. He is depicted at age three in a hospital crib with a neck brace, and at age six meeting life at full stride. The word "march" came to symbolize physical movement enabled by a metaphorical movement of charitable Americans. Note the reference at the bottom to Franklin D. Roosevelt as the organization's founder. See Richard J. Altenbaugh, *The Last Children's Plague: Poliomyelitis, Disability, and Twentieth-Century American Culture* (New York: Palgrave Macmillan, 2015).

in January 1938 the charity incorporated as the National Foundation for Infantile Paralysis (NFIP) and announced the treatment and cure of polio as its aims.

Although Roosevelt did not direct the NFIP's activities, he personally supported the charity in ways that later would be impossible for national elected officials. As its first fundraiser, the NFIP contrived a "march of dimes," inviting every American to send 10-cent coins to the president at the White House. The phrase played on the title of a popular current-events movie reel, the "March of Time," and it echoed the title of a familiar Depression-era song, "Brother Can You Spare a Dime." Thousands of envelopes flooded the White House; Roosevelt himself was photographed counting the coins. As a philanthropic strategy, the "march of dimes" was a master stroke. Previously, the wealthy had sponsored great causes—the Rockefeller Foundation and its ultra-rich founder are the prime example. During the Depression and World War II, greater fundraising potential lay, instead, in millions of small donations that were solicited in magazines, on radio, and eventually on television. There was no better symbol than Roosevelt, the man who "licked polio" and became a president who led the nation through dark times. Roosevelt died at Warm Springs on 12 April 1945, and the following year the US Treasury introduced a new dime that bore his likeness—a coin that was tailor-made for the next March of Dimes campaign.

Roosevelt's death prodded the NFIP to find other ways to keep polio in the public eye. In local drives, women went door-to-door collecting funds. NFIP staff solicited or wrote magazine articles. Polio-themed fashion shows showcased local or national celebrities. And in 1946, the foundation introduced regional and national poster campaigns that depicted disabled children accompanied by inspirational slogans.

The March of Dimes posters highlighted the resolve of children to recover and to overcome limitations imposed by their disabilities. After the eventual success of polio vaccines, the organization shifted its focus to emphasize the prevention of birth defects and infant mortality. In the 1940s and 1950s, however, the NFIP's fundraising prowess made it the largest financial sponsor of polio research in the world. Because of its prominence, it inevitably became enmeshed in controversies surrounding the development of a polio vaccine that had both scientific and political dimensions.

Scientific Rivalry and the American Vaccine Trial

The NFIP's financial support of polio science was crucial because the three decades of work that followed Simon Flexner's experiments had yielded few results. In the 1930s, numerous treatments and two different vaccines had failed, and no one really knew how polioviruses behaved in the body. Beginning in 1947, NFIP grants to universities and hospitals helped researchers study pieces of the puzzle. One team established that there were three types of poliovirus. This simple conclusion required tremendous labor and sacrifice—thousands of monkeys were injected with poliovirus in order to test and compare numerous samples. Other researchers demonstrated that polio entered humans through the mouth and further showed that the virus was present for a short time in the bloodstream before it attacked the spinal cord. This brightened prospects for a vaccine since the poliovirus could be targeted before it reached delicate nerve tissues. A third group demonstrated that poliovirus could grow in non-nervous tissue—a key correction to Flexner's work—and developed procedures for cultivating the virus in a test tube. For the first time, it seemed possible to safely grow large quantities of poliovirus for a mass vaccination program.

These innovations made vaccination the surest strategy for the defeat of polio. One important question remained: what type of virus preparation should the vaccine include? A rivalry unfolded among researchers with different approaches. Most experts believed that a live, attenuated form of the virus was required to mobilize the human body's immune defenses. However, Isabel Morgan (1911–1996) at Johns Hopkins University injected chimpanzees with a "killed virus" that was inactivated by formaldehyde.[17] Although Morgan left polio research in 1949, other researchers built on her insights. They included Jonas Salk, who had led the toilsome virus-typing project at the University of Pittsburgh. With help from the NFIP, Salk discreetly organized small tests of vaccines with inactivated virus at two nearby residential facilities, the D.T. Watson Home for Crippled Children and the Polk School for the Retarded and Feeble-Minded. As discussed in chapter 2, by the 1950s many scientists found the testing of vulnerable groups in institutions ethically questionable. However, standards of informed consent that would rule out such experiments were not yet imposed by law or enforced by other means. The experimental value of an enclosed population for vaccine trials was well established, and Salk was neither the first nor last researcher to use such methods. His tests indicated that the vaccine preparation with inactivated polio (IPV) was safe and effective against all three types of poliovirus.

Salk's association with the NFIP and the media attention he began to receive raised the hackles of older, more established scientists. Behind the scenes, experts that included Albert Sabin (1906–1993) argued for more time to develop a live-virus vaccine and suggested that scientists, rather than philanthropy bureaucrats at the NFIP, should be the ones to dictate the research agenda and pace of events. But a spike in polio cases during the summer of 1952 persuaded the NFIP that speed was essential to avert as much suffering as possible. The foundation cast its lot with the IPV and began organizing a large vaccine trial. The NFIP also recruited Thomas Francis, a pioneering researcher who had mentored Salk, to direct the trial. Francis accepted the job on the condition that an equal number of children would receive vaccine and placebo shots, thus creating a control group in order to measure the vaccine's effectiveness. In 1954, roughly 600,000 children stood in line for jabs in the arm (three separate shots were required). Francis's team analyzed the results for nearly a year. At a news conference on 12 April 1955—exactly ten years after Franklin Roosevelt's death at Warm Springs— Francis finally announced firmly positive results. As celebrations erupted around the country, the US Department of Health, Education and Welfare issued a license for the IPV within hours. Career scientists were chagrined by the excitement and unseemly rush, but history had been made.

This was a moment of triumph, but within weeks the halo that surrounded IPV began to dim. Cutter Laboratories, a small pharmaceutical company in Berkeley, California, produced and released thousands of vaccine doses containing virus that was not inactivated properly. Many children displayed symptoms of abortive polio, and the Cutter vaccines were blamed for five deaths and 51 cases of paralysis. Although some doses from other manufacturers apparently caused similar problems, Cutter found itself targeted by a lawsuit and at the center of a momentous legal battle. The laboratory claimed that it had followed appropriate procedures and pointed out that Salk had not furnished explicit instructions for how to produce the vaccines. Salk himself testified that the guidelines he provided were adequate. The lawsuit was tried by a jury and ended with an unusual ruling. The jury stated its view that Cutter's staff had not acted negligently when they produced the virus. However, instructions provided by the judge forced the jury to hold Cutter financially liable because the company had sold a product that caused harm to its users.

The "Cutter incident" had a lasting impact on the development of vaccines in the United States. Federal agencies quickly increased oversight and developed extensive guidelines for vaccine production. The CDC also greatly expanded its Epidemic Intelligence Service program, which still investigates outbreaks of diseases such as Ebola, West Nile fever, or AIDS. At the same time, as Paul Offit notes, "liability without negligence (fault) was born" as a result of the Cutter lawsuit. Companies could now be held accountable for harm even when they followed the best-available scientific practices and manufacturing standards. Offit suggests that the costs of liability insurance and high risk of litigation deterred companies from research and development of needed vaccines.[18]

Mass polio vaccination programs resumed in 1956 after experts reviewed the production procedures. However, fears of contaminated vaccines provided ammunition for Salk's critics, and several teams developed and tested live-virus vaccines later in the 1950s. Sabin, the most successful researcher, negotiated with officials from the Soviet Union to organize a large-scale trial in 1959. US-Soviet diplomatic tensions were set aside, and 10 million Soviet children received Sabin's oral polio vaccine (OPV) with drops or by eating prepared candy. Results of this trial were also positive, and in 1960 almost the entire Soviet population under twenty years of age received the vaccine (roughly 74 million people). OPV was "trivalent" because it included weakened material from all three poliovirus types; it was easier to prepare than IPV, did not require a trained practitioner to give shots, and was effective after only one dose. Public health experts perceived these advantages. OPV was licensed for use in 1962 and soon became the polio protection of choice in the United States and elsewhere.[19]

After 1962, more than 100 million Americans swallowed Sabin's vaccine. Indeed, the incidence of polio already had dropped sharply in North America, but OPV's convenience and effectiveness raised hopes that polio could be eliminated on the continent and eradicated worldwide. OPV did have one characteristic that would cause challenges. Since it used live virus, weakened forms of the pathogen would circulate in the environment after they were excreted by a vaccinated person. At first, this was not considered a serious drawback. Experts believed that most immune systems could defeat the weakened virus and persons who had not been vaccinated would develop antibodies that would protect them anyway.

However, viral material from OPV could, in rare cases, mutate over time into a dangerous pathogen. As discussed shortly, OPV would later contribute to the incidence of polio in regions where vaccination drives failed to reach large segments of a population and left opportunities for a mutated virus to cause disease.

By the 1970s, polio was becoming an afterthought in North America. The last outbreak of "wild" poliovirus, in 1978–79, struck individuals in Christian Mennonite and Amish communities who refused vaccinations out of religious principle. The outbreak originated in the Netherlands, and travelers brought polio to Canadian communities in Ontario and villages in the US state of Pennsylvania.[20] (As discussed in chapter 1, the rejection of medical interventions by these groups has some theological origins in the sixteenth-century Protestant Reformation.) After this incident, individual cases were rare, and by the mid-1980s polio had almost disappeared from western Europe as well. The remarkable success of the polio vaccines reaffirmed faith in laboratory science. Photographs of Salk, in particular, helped create an enduring image of the white-coated (male) scientist who works to benefit humankind.

However, the reported incidence of polio remained high in other parts of the world for decades after the 1950s. And Western nations also faced unfinished business: polio survivors, alongside other people with disabilities, faced physical and psychological obstacles to full social inclusion. We will consider both of these lingering challenges in turn.

The Global Challenge of Eradication

Reliable data concerning polio are not available from much of the world for the era prior to World War II. Initial reports from South America, sub-Saharan Africa, and Southeast Asia recorded relatively low rates of polio infection. However, studies of "lameness" that the WHO conducted between 1974 and 1982 suggested that rates of paralytic polio often were higher than experts had realized. Data gathered among children of grade-school age in the Ivory Coast, Niger, Somalia, and Burma (now Myanmar) yielded rates of poliomyelitis-related paralysis between 10 and 19 cases per 1,000 children. The actual incidence may have been substantially higher.[21] In 1977, the WHO launched the Expanded Programme on Immunization (EPI) to build on polio elimination measures that were already underway in most countries. The broader term **immunization** replaced the term "vaccination" that had been coined as a reference to the prophylactic use of cowpox material against smallpox.

In 1988, buoyed by the successful eradication of smallpox, the WHO committed more resources to polio eradication. Similar to smallpox, the poliovirus has no natural animal reservoir. However, other features of the disease create challenges that were absent during the smallpox campaign. Poliovirus usually does not spread through direct contact, and the majority of infections only cause symptoms that are subclinical (i.e., undetectable in a physical examination). Significant amounts of the virus may be excreted by unidentified individuals for weeks. Perhaps more importantly, polio has not caused sufficient mortality to elicit a high level of concern among wealthy nations. Between the late 1980s and the 2010s, war and social disruption interrupted eradication efforts and other public health measures. Nonetheless, WHO programs made tremendous progress in partnership with UNICEF and the business philanthropic organization Rotary International. The WHO reported a decline from an estimated 350,000 cases in 1988 to only 359 reported cases in 2014.[22] By the late 2010s, new polio cases were concentrated in the mountainous border country of Pakistan and Afghanistan, and in northern areas of Nigeria.

The stubborn obstacles to eradication in these two regions, both with majority Muslim populations, illustrate broader challenges that confront advocates of global public health. Traditional sources of Muslim teaching do not address immunization, but in Pakistan and Afghanistan, the procedure encountered some resistance on religious grounds. In the 2000s, Taliban leaders suggested that immunization efforts were part of a broader Western campaign to gather strategic intelligence or even to use injections to sterilize Muslims. One of these claims was not entirely groundless: in July 2011, it was revealed that the US Central Intelligence Agency used the pretext of an immunization campaign in order to confirm the location of terrorist Osama bin Laden. Some Pakistanis claimed that aerial drone attacks by US forces relied upon information gathered by immunization workers. As Robert Peckham notes, Western virologists compared epidemic surveillance to antiterrorism intelligence gathering and both enterprises relied upon similar global positioning technology.[23] These overlaps heightened suspicions among many ordinary Pakistanis, some of whom already perceived a conflict between their religious duty and Western medicine. Militants assassinated several health care workers and thwarted vaccination programs.

Religious objections to immunization have also played a role in Nigeria. Although many leaders in the country have supported immunization, some communities have relied on traditional practices including herbal medicines, prayer, and rituals that use passages from the Qur'an, the central sacred text of Islam. Other forces have also intervened: mistrust of government agents, who waged an ineffective campaign against measles in 2007, has contributed to a low degree of

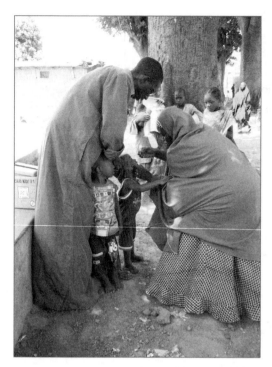

IMAGE 10.5 A health department worker administers oral polio vaccine. This photograph was taken in 2009 during a Sub-National Immunization Day in Zaria City, Nigeria. Elsewhere, campaigns have also relied upon trained community volunteers. Global eradication efforts against smallpox, rinderpest, and polio have all depended on the efforts of local collaborators as well as international agencies.

participation in immunization programs. In communities where some (but not all) children have received OPV, cases of vaccine-derived polio have troubled public health workers. Between 2005 and 2009, several hundred such cases were identified alongside several thousand cases caused by "wild" poliovirus.[24] As the strains continued to circulate in 2017, vaccine-derived polio cases were identified in the neighboring Democratic Republic of the Congo.[25] Most experts believe that the best course is to continue vaccination programs to reach a higher proportion of the population with safe vaccines. One part of this solution is to use "designer vaccines" that target particular types of polio but do not include other poliovirus material that might mutate. The WHO has also recommended the use of IPV, which uses killed virus that cannot spread to new hosts. The other, more difficult task is to reach populations in remote regions, including families who are reluctant to accept vaccines that are now associated with sickness. A general lack of primary health care resources and widespread skepticism of authorities have hampered immunization programs.

As the drive to vanquish smallpox demonstrated, the last stage of eradication is a hunt for dangerous pathogens that are on the move. The effort requires sustained community engagement at a grassroots level and funding for public education, surveillance, and vaccination. If polio eradication is not completed, a price will be paid by disadvantaged children who will encounter the virus with no immunities.

Polio, People with Disabilities, and a "Splendid Deception"

In North America, the social role of polio survivors shifted in the 1960s as large numbers of them grew into adulthood. Many found fulfilling lives; for others, however, discrimination eventually bred resistance and political activism. Authorities treated polio-related disability as a medical problem and focused on perceived impairments that prevented polio survivors from living "normal" lives. Polio survivors themselves argued that social structures, physical barriers, and attitudes were more disabling than the actual effects of the disease. They allied with other marginalized groups, including military veterans who sustained injuries in World War II, the Korean War, and Vietnam. In an era when civil rights advocacy took center stage, polio survivors formed a significant cohort and many led campaigns in support of inclusion.

As Amy Fairchild has suggested, some of the challenges that people with disabilities encounter may be traced to Franklin Roosevelt's influence in the 1940s and 1950s.[26] As the most famous polio survivor in America—and perhaps the world—Roosevelt presented the persona of a man who had conquered adversity and recovered good health. From the start, he controlled the public presentation of his illness. Even in the first days of his paralysis, journalists merely saw him smiling in repose rather than carried from place to place on a stretcher. As his political career progressed, stagecraft and cooperation by photographers allowed Roosevelt to sustain an illusion of mobility. He could move for short distances with his canes while swiveling his hips. He was often photographed standing behind a lectern, his leg braces concealed from view while his hands gripped the sides. Television would have made this illusion impossible, but there was no television. Roosevelt communicated with the public through occasional radio addresses, famously known as "fireside chats," that brought his direct, reassuring manner into millions of American living rooms. Roosevelt never denied that he was a polio survivor, and he adopted polio as a charitable cause, but he also perpetrated what one historian has called "a splendid deception," concealing his ongoing physical and mental struggles in ways that ordinary polio survivors could not imitate.[27] As a leader who was expected to emanate strength and vigor, Roosevelt did not attempt to reform widespread attitudes toward people with disabilities.

During his lengthy presidency (1933–45) and for years thereafter, Roosevelt's example inspired many individuals. However, as children grew older they no longer matched the plucky images that were projected by March of Dimes posters and other media. In memoirs, some polio survivors acknowledged feelings of anger and hopelessness when they failed to live up to Roosevelt's example. And for many, the celebration of Salk's vaccine on 12 April 1955 was a moment of deep disillusionment as they realized that little effort would be invested to find a polio cure. Author Wilfrid Sheed, who was attending college in England at the time, later described his reaction to the news:

I was surprised at the force of my irritation the day I first read about Dr. Jonas Salk and his famous vaccine. I could have sworn I knew better than that by this time—knew, for instance, that I wasn't going to get my legs back now, whatever anyone discovered; the switchboard in my spine had been dismantled years ago.... Yet here I was flinging the overseas edition of *Time* magazine against the wall of my Oxford sitting room so hard that the staples flew out. What had *taken* the man so long? ...

Well, this was *really* the end, baby. There'd be no more research now for sure, and no more gleams under the door, or hopes so small and crazy that I even hid them from myself.... We were *last* year's cover story now.[28]

Although Sheed experienced feelings of anger and isolation, as a disabled college student in the 1950s he was among the fortunate. Many paralytic polio survivors, born into prosperous middle-class lives, were forced to adjust their expectations for career achievement and family life. The obstacles were mundane, but nonetheless real: multistory buildings had no ramps or elevators, sidewalks had no curb cuts for wheelchairs, buses could not accommodate some passengers with disabilities, and only the wealthiest (such as Roosevelt) could afford modified cars that could be driven without foot pedals.

Even more pervasive was the widespread attitude that people with disabilities could not meet routine social obligations and, therefore, would accomplish less than "normal" individuals. This view was well represented among scholars and policy makers. For example, the leading sociologist Talcott Parsons (1902–1979) classified illness—what Parsons termed "the sick role"—as a form of deviance that prevented an individual from productively contributing to society.[29] This applied to polio as well: as Paul Longmore suggests, observers conflated the disabilities caused by polio with the disease itself. Polio survivors were considered "sick" people who were naturally dependent on others, rather than individuals who could be independent and productive when they received equal opportunity and respect.[30] Other people with disabilities faced similar stereotypes concerning the limited potential of "crippled" people.

Advocacy for the Disabled

In the early 1960s, several educational institutions became sites of activism for people with disabilities, including some with polio. The work of these individuals coincided with protests to secure equal rights for African Americans, which included marches and attempts to racially integrate public universities. Students at the University of Illinois formed an informal "wheelchair ghetto" that became a highly visible campus presence. Some clandestinely smashed sidewalk curbs to force the university to rebuild them with ramps. At the University of California, Berkeley, in 1964, a quadriplegic polio survivor named Edward Roberts (1939–1995) successfully sued for admission. Years of lobbying by Roberts and other students prompted the university to create a Disabled Students Program that enrolled nearly 400 students by 1977. Many activists drew on friendships they forged at rehabilitation centers such as Camp Jened in New York and Warm Springs.

Activists soon broadened their focus to include lawsuits and lobbying for national laws to guarantee access to public services. Some early cases ended in defeat because the United States Constitution did not provide people with disabilities the standing to sue against discrimination (unlike religious groups, for example, which enjoy some protections under the First Amendment of the Bill of Rights). In 1964, activists rallied under the motto "no taxation without transportation" and successfully petitioned Congress to enact the Urban Mass Transportation Act, which required accessible buses. A law enacted in 1968, the Architectural Barriers Act, required buildings that received federal funding to enable access for people with disabilities. This measure was drafted by Hugh Gallagher, a polio survivor who worked as an aide for Alaska senator E.L. Bartlett. In 1973, the Rehabilitation Act invoked the concept of "reasonable accommodation" for people with disabilities as a requirement for employers who received federal funding.

The Rehabilitation Act was intended to prohibit hiring discrimination by such employers as long as the applicants could perform the essential duties of an advertised job. However, mere passage of the law left a great deal undone. No rules for implementation were issued to clarify who was disabled, what constituted reasonable accommodation, or the means of enforcing the law. After years of delay, a draft of regulations languished in the Department of Health, Education and Welfare (HEW). On 5 April 1977, activists mounted demonstrations at eight HEW branch offices around the country. In San Francisco, Roberts and others staged a sit-in at an HEW office that lasted twenty-eight days. Members of the US Congress flew in from Washington to conduct a remarkable hearing in the occupied building, and the Rehabilitation Act rules were implemented shortly thereafter. Thirteen years later, Congress enacted the landmark Americans with Disabilities Act (ADA), which prohibited discrimination more broadly in hiring, public accommodations (such as hotels), transportation, and telecommunications.

In the last three decades, contrasting approaches to disability and civil rights have emerged in the United States and Canada.[31] Distinct traditions of jurisprudence in each country have influenced court rulings. Discussion has focused on the application of two key concepts: "reasonable accommodation" that must be

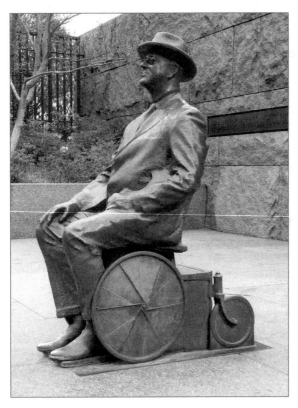

IMAGE 10.6 Statue at the Franklin Delano Roosevelt Memorial in Washington, DC. When the Roosevelt Memorial opened in 1997, it included a statue of a seated Roosevelt that concealed his wheelchair under a cloak, much as he had concealed it during his presidency. At the urging of historians and disability-rights advocates, funds were raised to place a second statue depicting Roosevelt in his wheelchair at the monument's entrance. The text behind him is a quote from Roosevelt's wife, Eleanor: "Franklin's illness ... gave him strength and courage he had not had before. He had to think out the fundamentals of living and learn the greatest of all lessons—infinite patience and never-ending persistence."

provided for a disabled individual and "undue hardship," an instance when providing accommodation would create an unfair burden to an employer or other party. In the United States, the Equal Employment Opportunity Commission has defined undue hardship as a "significant difficulty or expense" that would "fundamentally alter the nature or operation of a business." Employers assess on a case-by-case basis whether accommodations would cause undue hardship.[32] In legal challenges of these assessments, judges have attempted to balance the rights of people with disabilities against those of employers and other workers. In Canada, the legal landscape was transformed after the country adopted the Charter of Rights and Freedoms in 1982. The Charter provides "equal protection and equal benefit of the law" for individuals with mental or physical disability, and Supreme Court rulings have affirmed that workplace standards must incorporate conceptions of equality. Accommodation of disability, or of diverse abilities—in the case of male and female firefighters, for example—is the usual practice, and requests for exceptions must meet a high legal standard.

Polio survivors have deeply influenced these developments, which ultimately concern the nature of citizenship, equality, and participation in civil society. Through advocacy, polio survivors asserted control over the experience of disability and helped set in motion a transformation of many urban spaces and social institutions.

Conclusion

The history of polio remains relevant as the profiles of age and health status shift in populations around the world, and as technology shapes daily life and health care delivery. Just as the iron lung saved many lives, other medical advances extend life spans for people with chronic conditions (such as coronary heart disease or diabetes). Such conditions may cause impairment in one way or another, but computers, automated wheelchairs, and other assistive devices enable movement and social interaction in ways that were impossible fifty years ago. Indeed, terms such as "chronic," "impairment," or "disability" vary in usage according to context and no single approach fits every situation. Polio survivors have made a lasting contribution to this area of inquiry and practice: they were among the first to argue that their individual experience, knowledge, and goals, rather than standards imposed by others, should be the starting points for health-related measures and social changes.

Some polio survivors have spoken out in favor of childhood immunizations, reminding the public of the anxiety and suffering that vaccines have prevented. This topic began to receive greater attention in the 2000s as "vaccine hesitancy" increased in some British and North American communities.[33] While concerns about the safety of vaccination are as old as the procedure itself (see chapter 3), new concerns had emerged at the end of the twentieth century. In 1998, an article published in *The Lancet* medical journal alleged a link between a vaccine for measles, mumps, and rubella and the incidence of bowel disease and autism. However, the study was based on research with only twelve children, and other larger studies soon contradicted its findings. In 2010, *The Lancet* retracted the paper amid concerns that it was fraudulent and that the children had been subjected to unnecessary medical tests.[34] Experts believe that publicity about the study motivated many families to refuse vaccinations, thereby contributing to the risk of disease outbreaks in Britain and the United States. Other doubts arose concerning thimerosal, an ethylmercury compound added to some vaccines as an antibacterial agent. Several studies investigated a possible link between thimerosal exposure and autism and found no relationship.

These examples suggest that vaccine hesitancy can be caused by misinformation, especially when another, unexplained disorder such as autism raises anxiety. However, polio's history suggests that the proponents of vaccines must do more than debunk inaccurate claims with additional data. Polio vaccines have improved millions of lives, but, on rare occasions, harm has resulted from accidents (such as the Cutter incident) or, as in Nigeria, from vaccine-derived polio in a partially vaccinated community. Today, magazines or websites may magnify the perceived risks of other vaccines by presenting information selectively, inaccurately, or in a context that makes a threat appear imminent. The high standards that licensed vaccines must now meet may address some issues. Effective communication—careful listening to concerns about vaccines as well as the relay of information—may foster the success of public health programs even if some tensions remain unresolved.

Objections to immunization that are grounded in religious beliefs would seem to pose another intractable challenge. As the history of smallpox also illustrates, Christians, Hindus, Jews, and Muslims have all been represented among groups that reject vaccines. In many cases, however, such resistance to immunization has been amplified by cultural isolation, suspicion, or conflict rather than by particular religious tenets or standards of conduct. In the nineteenth century, it was the association of smallpox vaccination with imperial coercion, particularly by British forces in colonial India, that prompted communities to invoke religious or cultural objections. More recently, military conflict and mistrust of government have hampered immunization programs among Muslim communities in Nigeria and Pakistan. In contemporary North America, resistance to immunization in Amish or orthodox Jewish communities reflects a broader suspicion of intrusion from a dominant secular culture. Efforts must be made to understand the bases of principled resistance to immunization within specific historical, political, and social contexts.[35]

Polio caused widespread horror and hysteria in part because it struck middle-class families that occupied a central position in American society. By contrast, in the early 1980s, political elites responded slowly to AIDS as it emerged in gay communities in US cities and hospitals in West Africa. At first considered a threat to marginal or impoverished people, the AIDS pandemic has now assumed different profiles in many communities around the world. Forces that we have encountered in earlier chapters—colonization, urbanization, and technological change—have all influenced this uniquely modern disease.

WORKSHOP: POLIO AND SHIFTING PERCEPTIONS OF DISABILITY

Histories of disease, medicine, or public health frequently focus on the challenges that diseases cause and the responses to these challenges by professionals. The viewpoint of sick or disabled individuals often receives little attention. In the 1980s, some scholars, notably British historian Roy Porter, called attention to this limitation.[36] Medical practitioners acknowledged that they often failed to listen to their patients' accounts and deal adequately with their suffering.[37] Experts in these disciplines (and others) now recognize that sick or disabled individuals invest their experiences with meaning in ways that differ significantly from an external observer.

Prior to the twentieth century, most writers were laconic about illness, especially their own. Even in documents from the twentieth century, historians often encounter patients only through the writing of medical practitioners. Although such texts purport to represent patients in a neutral or scientific manner, they may also reflect important assumptions by the practitioner. Often, their observations (such as the first excerpt below) selectively describe and interpret the patients' attitudes and behavior in ways that reinforce a practitioner's point of view about the physical effects or social repercussions of a disease or disability.

Fortunately, polio survivors have written numerous published autobiographies and reflected on their experiences in other ways. This literature reveals the profound gap that once existed between medical approaches to polio and the diverse experiences of people with lifelong impairments. Polio survivor accounts cannot be reduced to "illness narratives." Their authors describe a struggle to live with circumstances that are framed by the structures of modern life as much as the effects of illness. In their efforts to conduct healthy lives on their terms, polio survivors and other people with disabilities have shifted widespread perceptions. Although challenges remain, impairment is no longer considered an insurmountable obstacle to a fulfilling life or to exceptional achievement.

Passage through Crisis: Polio Victims and Their Families—Fred Davis (1963)

This book is a short version of Davis's doctoral dissertation in sociology (University of Chicago) and is based on research he conducted with fourteen families in Baltimore beginning in 1954. The families were followed from shortly after their children contracted polio until fifteen months after their discharge from a recovery unit (roughly eighteen to twenty-four months total). News of the Salk vaccine did not significantly affect Davis's research.

Davis was influenced by Talcott Parsons's conception of a "sick role" that was a form of deviant behavior. In the chapter excerpted here, concerning the "Problem of Identity," Davis focused on nine families with children who experienced a range of disabilities. He identified serious psychological challenges that resulted from these "handicaps." In his view, stress and compensating strategies resulted from the families' inability to meet the expectations of normal behavior.

SOME REMARKS ON THE PROBLEM OF IDENTITY FOR THE HANDICAPPED

In considering the problem of identity confronting the handicapped person, one must view his situation alternately from the cultural and the individual standpoint. Unless he has been impaired from birth or early childhood, so that his primary identity is that of a handicapped person, it is more than likely that he will share, initially at least, many of the prejudiced and squeamish attitudes that are commonly shown toward the handicapped. He will tend, openly or secretly, to place a high value on many activities and pursuits that are closed to him because of his impairment. His attempts, if any, to be accepted by "normals" as "normal," are doomed to failure and frustration.... For the fact remains that, try as he may to hide or overlook it, he is at a distinct disadvantage with respect to several important values emphasized in our society: e.g., physical attractiveness; wholeness and symmetry of body parts; athletic prowess; and various physiognomic attributes felt to be prerequisite for a pleasant and engaging personality....

[*Davis suggests that polio families usually relied on one of two strategies to navigate the social world: "normalization," which is the attempt to participate while minimizing the importance of a disability, and "disassociation," which involved avoiding situations, as Davis puts it, "that might force them to recognize that others, and they themselves, regard the crippled child as 'different.'" Davis then presents case studies of two families, one that relied primarily on "normalization" strategies and one that relied primarily on "disassociation strategies."*]

The Pauluses—A Case of Pronounced Normalization

Six-year-old Laura Paulus was without doubt the most handicapped child in the group of nine. She wore full-length braces on both legs, a pelvic band, high orthopedic shoes, and, when traveling more than a short distance, had to use crutches as well.... Needless to say, from a purely physical standpoint Laura was extremely limited in what she could do....

In view of Laura's condition, it might be supposed that her situation was rife for dissociative tendencies; that, because of her grave inability to keep up with other children, she would soon be excluded, or would voluntarily withdraw, from the group of neighborhood children with whom she had played prior to her illness. But during the two years in which the Pauluses were seen, nothing of the kind happened, thanks chiefly to the efforts and personality of Mrs. Paulus, a young and energetic woman whom Laura admired immensely and whose guidance Laura seemed ever-ready to follow with equanimity and good cheer....

No sooner was Laura out of the hospital than Mrs. Paulus re-registered her in the school she had attended before her illness.... Mrs. Paulus also saw to it that Laura's play and social life were kept "as normal as possible."... Mrs. Paulus always encouraged Laura to go out and play with the neighborhood children, even though she knew it was difficult for Laura to keep up and that it was necessary for them to adapt games in order to accommodate her.... Later that year she enrolled Laura in the local Brownie troop [*i.e., Girl Scouts*], and although Laura could not, for example, go on hikes, on such occasions Mrs. Paulus would drive her to the camp site after the other children had arrived there on foot....

At least in her contacts with the project staff, Mrs. Paulus always exuded an air of optimism. Laura, she maintained, was "doing beautifully" and led "as normal and happy a life as any other child."... Mr. Paulus, although privately neither so optimistic nor so enthusiastic as his wife—once, for example, he spoke of his great disillusionment when he lifted one of Laura's legs and "it felt like a piece of rubber hanging there"—was careful not to express his misgivings before Laura or his wife....

Several incidents point up the "fatal flaw" of normalization as a deviance-correcting stratagem: the fact that others are frequently unable or unwilling to go along with it. Thus, for example, at an Elks-sponsored "kiddie show" at the local movie house, Laura was conspicuously given many more gifts than the other children. She was not permitted to take her seat until all the other children were seated, and after the film was over the children were made to remain in their seats until Laura departed. Again, when the Pauluses made a sight-seeing trip to Washington, DC, Laura insisted on negotiating the long flight of steps leading up to the Capitol without her parents' assistance. After watching her laborious ascent for several minutes, a bystander turned scoldingly on Mr. and Mrs. Paulus and said, "Are you going to make that poor child walk up all those steps by herself? ..."

The Harrises—A Case of Disassociation

Although eleven-year-old Marvin Harris was not so severely handicapped as several other children in the group (his right lower extremity was affected, and he wore a full-length brace and pelvic band), he and his family appeared to react more profoundly and with greater distress to Marvin's polio and subsequent impairment than did any other family in the study. This was evident from the very first interview, when Mrs. Harris wept and kept repeating, "I don't want my son to be a cripple." Mr. Harris wallowed in self-punitive memories of a polio-crippled acquaintance of his youth who, he said, was mean, embittered, and disliked by all who knew him....

On the doctor's recommendation, Mrs. Harris enrolled Marvin, very much against his wishes, in a school for handicapped children. Marvin not only resisted attending this school but, when it became apparent that he had no other choice, pleaded unsuccessfully with his father to drive him there every day so that he would not be seen in the company of the other handicapped children on the school bus....

The interviewer noted that Marvin did not so much deny his impairment as reject it.... During the summers, the Harrises made many trips to the beach. Marvin would refuse adamantly to go along if his parents made him wear the brace. Invariably, they gave in to the demand, and it was on one such occasion that Marvin broke his impaired leg, when a child running past caused him to lose his balance and fall.

In more calm and considered moments Mr. and Mrs. Harris would assert, as did Marvin, that he "really wasn't handicapped." Mrs. Harris stated, "He's nothing like those cerebral-palsy kids and children without arms and legs that go to school with him." Resorting to a kind of second-order normalization formula, Mrs. Harris would try to explain away Marvin's extremely negative and rebellious behavior by claiming "All boys his age are that way. My sister's boy gives her a lot of trouble too so I guess it's only normal."...

Although Marvin's condition had shown scarcely any improvement, when last seen Mr. and Mrs. Harris had found new hope in anticipating Marvin's imminent enrollment in a "regular" local high school. Marvin also was highly pleased with this development. His parents took the view that Marvin was at last receiving his due, since they—but more especially, he—were still inclined to maintain that he was "not really handicapped like the others." In apparent disregard of all that had happened during the year, Mrs. Harris remarked enthusiastically, "I think that when he goes to a regular high school, he'll feel that he's just like everybody else."

[*Davis's conclusion for the chapter summarizes his view of the dilemma faced by polio families and the limited success he perceives in their response to it.*]

The fundamental issue of identity confronting the families of the handicapped children was how to view, interpret, and respond to the many negative meanings imputed to a visible physical handicap in our society. Two broad stratagems of adjustment, normalization and disassociation, were found....

As regards their over-all interpretation of the quality and meaning of their situation, all the parents were wont to claim, despite much objective evidence to the contrary, that the experience had resulted in no significant change in their lives or in the attitudes and behavior of family members toward one another. This strong sense of continuity of identity in the midst of change doubtless betokens a high degree of social stability in these families. But from another vantage point, it perhaps also testifies to a failure of creative impulse—an excessive contentment with the familiar and known that inhibits the discovery of new meanings and purposes when important life circumstances change.

"The Second Phase: From Disability Rights to Disability Culture"—Paul Longmore (*Disability Rag*, 1995)

Longmore, who contracted polio as a child, was a leading disability rights activist and professor at San Francisco State University. This article, which was first published in a magazine devoted to disability activism, sketches a brief history of disability rights activism and suggests future directions for the movement.

Longmore and others attempted to shift the entire approach to the challenges faced by polio sufferers and others. This began with criticism of what Longmore calls "the medical model" that treats disability as a disease that forces people into dependency. Longmore points instead to the collective failure of medical professionals and others to tolerate difference and diversity. The "disability" problem did not lie with individuals who could not meet standards of behavior; on the contrary, it was a result of the standards themselves.

The movement of disabled Americans has entered its second phase. The first phase has been a quest for disability rights, for equal access and equal opportunity, for inclusion. The second phase is a quest for collective identity. Even as the unfinished work of the first phase continues, the task in the second phase is to explore or to create a disability culture....

While the medical model claims to be scientific, objective and humane, within its practice has lurked considerable ambivalence toward the people it professes to aid. In one respect, the medical model has been the institutionalized expression of societal anxieties about people who look different or function differently. It regards them as incompetent to manage their own lives, as needing professional, perhaps lifelong, supervision, perhaps even as dangerous to society.

The new disability perspective has presented a searching critique of the medical model.... Indeed, disability-rights advocates have argued that the implementation of the medical model in health care, social services, education, private charity and public policies has institutionalized prejudice and discrimination. Far from being beneficial, or even neutral, the medical model has been at the core of the problem.

In the place of the medical model, activists have substituted a sociopolitical or minority-group model of disability. "Disability," they have asserted, is primarily a socially constructed role. For the vast majority of people with disabilities, prejudice is a far greater problem than any impairment: discrimination is a bigger obstacle for them to "overcome" than any disability. The core of the problem, in the activists' view, has been historically deep-seated, socially pervasive and powerfully institutionalized oppression of disabled people.

To combat this oppression, the disability movement not only called for legal protection against discrimination, it fashioned a new idea in American civil-rights theory: the concept of equal access. Traditional rehabilitation policy defined accommodations such as architectural modifications, adaptive devices (wheelchairs, optical readers) and services (sign-language interpreters) as special benefits to those who are fundamentally dependent. Disability-rights ideology redefined them as merely different modes of functioning, and not inherently inferior....

The first phase sought to move disabled people from the margins of society to the mainstream by demanding that discrimination be outlawed and that access and accommodations be mandated. The first phase argued for social inclusion. The second phase has asserted the necessity for self-definition. While the first phase rejected the medical model of disability, the second has repudiated the nondisabled majority norms that partly gave rise to the medical model....

Those two phases are not separate and successive chronological periods. They are complementary aspects of the disability movement. The concept of equal access represents a politics of issues. It is the effort of Americans with disabilities to build an infrastructure of freedom and self-determination. The proclamation of disability and deaf pride and the elaboration of disability and deaf cultures express a politics of identity. It is an affirmation, a celebration of who we are, not despite disability or deafness, but precisely because of the disability and deaf experiences.

These two phases of the disability movement are reciprocal. Each is essential to the other. Together they declare who we are and where we intend to go.

"A Polio Patient's Story"—Marshall Barr (2008)

A native of Reading, England, Barr contracted polio as a child in 1949, but he did not have significant respiratory problems until years later. After several weeks of intensive care in 1971, Barr was able to return home where he slept in an iron lung at night. When Barr was interviewed in 2008, he had used various respirators for thirty-seven years.

Although Barr's account of the iron lung might be seen as an "illness narrative," he also describes how he integrated respirator technology into an independent life. Polio survivors adapted their routines over the years as technology changed and their bodies changed as well. The excerpt begins with Barr's description of life in an iron lung.

Then they said they were going to put me into an iron lung and I went 'Oh!!!' I did not know what an iron lung was, and had never seen one. But the relief of not having a respirator on my mouth and just laying flat on my back with the breathing taken over was quite relaxing. It was restful because there wasn't much for you to do in the iron lung.... The bit that you lay on actually pulls out like a tray. You would lay on it and get pushed inside. The mechanics are underneath the machine so you're laying on the pump. And of course you get the vibration underneath. Like: breathing, bump; breathing, bump. It was not quite like a smooth breath.

You can eat in the iron lung because your head is outside but the rest of your body is inside, although since you are flat on your back you really need to be careful when you swallow; you have to swallow in rhythm with the machine because it's pulling your diaphragm in and then pushing it out again. You just wait until it's breathing out and then you swallow....

The iron lung had port holes on the side which came in useful for physiotherapy. They had a rubber seal so you could open them on the down breath to put a hand in, to do physiotherapy or anything inside....

I have a brother and sister and I think if we had not had humor in the house I think it would have been a bit dire [*i.e., melancholy*]. My parents were probably worse off because my mother had to shut me in [*the iron lung*] every night. But it was fine and we just got into a routine. When she used to put the lid down, the only down side was, with your head outside and your arms inside, if you had an itch on your nose you couldn't scratch it. My mother's last job was usually to sort out any itches that I'd got....

[*Barr later describes the machines he has used and how the transition to different devices affected his routines.*]

I have never stopped using breathing machines. The iron lung, the 'old one' as I called it, I had from 1971 to 1986. The pump was getting worn out and by that time someone had invented a smaller type which I could operate myself. My mother obviously was getting older so I had that one instead. It was not as comfortable because it was much smaller, but it was convenient to be able to do it myself....

St. Thomas' [*a hospital that provided care and equipment*] were all geared up with iron lungs and such things. It was certainly beneficial from my point of view. They did make me this cuirass jacket. It was a shell-like thing that fits over your body and you just have a little pump that drives it. In the early days the world was wonderful. For short periods I could be without the iron lung. Anything was possible! And I did actually take it to Jersey [*a nearby island*]. I flew over to Jersey to stay with a friend....

Then in 1991 St. Thomas' got me another type of breathing machine which I still use now. It's called a 'Nippy' which is positive pressure. Just with a little thing over my nose and a black box about as big as a portable television, and it *is* portable. I mean, I have taken it away to stay with friends. Unfortunately now I need oxygen as well so it isn't so convenient but it's nice to be able to sleep in a bed....

I can't fault the medical profession. I know people get bad deals but I have never in my life had any bad deals. I have never asked for anything; whatever medical equipment I have been given has just been given because I need it. I am a bit cynical in some cases; people sometimes expect too much.

What is normal is doing what you can. You only have one life. OK, when I do go down [*i.e., encounter difficulty breathing*] I am ill. It is hard and it is difficult and sometimes you think it is sort of worth carrying on [*i.e., complaining*]. But I must say polio people have got that stubbornness; perhaps stubborn isn't the right word but they've got it. You have to get on with it you know.

INTERPRETING THE DOCUMENTS

1. Describe Fred Davis's viewpoint as a researcher. What assumptions does he make about polio sufferers and their potential for social involvement? Davis describes family members and their interactions—how do you think each of them would represent the obstacles created by polio-related disability?

2. In the 1940s and 1950s, do you think the experience of paralytic polio was different for males and females? Why or why not?

3. Davis suggests that polio families faced the challenge of "how to view, interpret, and respond to the many negative meanings imputed to a visible physical handicap in our society." How would Longmore characterize the challenge polio survivors and other individuals with disabilities faced? Or Barr?

4. How do changes in medical technology influence Barr's daily experience as a polio survivor? Would you describe him as disabled? Does he describe himself as disabled?

MAKING CONNECTIONS

1. Most of the people who contracted severe polio were children. How do you think this influenced the response and attempted treatments for the disease? How has the identity of "typical" sufferers played a role for other diseases such as tuberculosis or syphilis?

2. Consider how Longmore represents medical authority (and, by extension, scientific authority). How does his viewpoint compare with that of Rachel Carson or the scientists who debated the merits of pesticides? From what you can tell, did "scientific knowledge" have the same status in 1995 that it had in 1950? What changed?

For further reading: Amy Fairchild, "The Polio Narratives: Dialogues with FDR," *Bulletin of the History of Medicine* 75, no. 3 (2001): 488–534; Naomi Rogers, "Race and the Politics of Polio: Warm Springs, Tuskegee and the March of Dimes," *American Journal of Public Health* 97 (2007): 784–95.

Notes

1. Sherilyn Reus, "Change Agent," *Triton*, 3 May 2016, https://tritonmag.com/ada/.

2. Man Mohan Mehndiratta, "Poliomyelitis: Historical Facts, Epidemiology, and Current Challenges in Eradication," *Neurohospitalist* 4, no. 4 (2014): 1–4.

3. Heather T. Battles, "Differences in Polio Mortality by Socio-Economic Status in Two Southern Ontario Counties, 1900–1937," *Social Science History* 41, no. 2 (2017): 323–27.

4. M.R. Smallman-Raynor, A.D. Cliff et al., *A World Geography: Poliomyelitis. Emergence to Eradication* (Oxford: Oxford University Press, 2006), 95–102.

5. Naomi Rogers, *Dirt and Disease: Polio before FDR* (New Brunswick: Rutgers University Press, 1992), 23–24.

6. Jean Dawson, "Fighting the Fly in the Interests of Public Health: The Story of a Successful Crusade in Cleveland," *Scientific American* 111, no. 11 (1914): 209.

7. H.V. Wyatt, "Before the Vaccines: Medical Treatments of Acute Paralysis in the 1916 New York Epidemic of Poliomyelitis," *Open Microbiology Journal* 8 (September 2014): 145.

8. Sophie Ochmann and Max Roser, "Reported Paralytic Polio Cases and Deaths in the United States since 2010," https://ourworldindata.org. Data from United States Public Health Service, *Public Health Reports* (1910–51); and CDC, *MMWR* (1960–2010).

9. Michaela Martinez-Bakker, Aaron A. King, and Pejman Rohani, "Unraveling the Transmission Ecology of Polio," *PLOS Biology* 13, no. 6 (2015): 13.

10. Christopher J. Rutty, "The Middle-Class Plague: Epidemic Polio and the Canadian State, 1936–7," *Canadian Bulletin of Medical History* 13, no. 2 (1996): 305.

11. R.V. Trubuhovich, "In the Beginning: The 1952–53 Danish Epidemic of Poliomyelitis and Bjørn Ibsen," *Critical Care and Resuscitation* 5, no. 3 (2003): 227–30.

12. Philip Roth, *Nemesis* (New York: Vintage International, 2011), 8.

13. Arthur S. Slutsky, "History of Mechanical Ventilation: From Vesalius to Ventilator-Induced Injury," *American Journal of Respiratory and Critical Care Medicine* 191, no. 10 (2015): 1106–15.

14. Tony Gould, *A Summer Plague: Polio and Its Survivors* (New Haven: Yale University Press, 1997), 88.

15. David M. Oshinsky, *Polio: An American Story* (Oxford: Oxford University Press, 2005), 76.

16. Some scholars suggest that Roosevelt's age and symptoms were more consistent with Guillain-Barré syndrome, an auto immune disease. But Roosevelt considered himself a polio survivor and so do did everyone else. Armond Goldman et al., "What Was the Cause of

Franklin Delano Roosevelt's Paralytic Illness?" *Journal of Medical Biography* 11, no. 4 (2003): 232–40.

17. Oshinsky, *American Story*, 130–33.

18. Paul A. Offit, *The Cutter Incident: How America's First Polio Vaccine Led to the Growing Vaccine Crisis* (New Haven: Yale University Press, 2005), 154–77.

19. Oshinsky, *American Story*, 250–68.

20. Smallman-Raynor, Cliff, et al., *World Geography*, 463–66.

21. Smallman-Raynor, Cliff, et al., *World Geography*, 475–76.

22. Robert Peckham, *Epidemics in Modern Asia* (Cambridge: Cambridge University Press, 2016), 233.

23. Peckham, *Epidemics in Modern Asia*, 233–36.

24. Elisha P. Renne, *The Politics of Polio in Northern Nigeria* (Bloomington: Indiana University Press, 2010), 3.

25. WHO, "Circulating Vaccine-Derived Polio Virus Type-2—Democratic Republic of the Congo" (June 2017), http://www.who.int/csr/don/13-June-2017-polio-drc/en/.

26. Amy L. Fairchild, "The Polio Narratives: Dialogues with FDR," *Bulletin of the History of Medicine* 75, no. 3 (2001): 488–534.

27. Hugh Gregory Gallagher, *FDR's Splendid Deception: The Moving Story of Roosevelt's Massive Disability—And the Intense Efforts to Conceal It from the Public* (St Petersburg: Vandamere Press, 1999).

28. Wilfrid Sheed, *In Love with Daylight: A Memoir of Recovery* (New York: Simon & Schuster, 1995), 55–56.

29. Matthias Zick Varul, "Talcott Parsons, the Sick Role and Chronic Illness," *Body & Society* 16, no. 2 (2010): 72–94.

30. Paul Longmore, *Telethons: Spectacle, Disability, and the Business of Charity* (Oxford: Oxford University Press, 2016), 216.

31. Ravi Malhotra, "The Legal Genealogy of the Duty to Accommodate American and Canadian Workers with Disabilities: A Comparative Perspective," *Disabilities* 23, no. 1/2 (2007): 1–32.

32. United States Government, Equal Employment Opportunity Commission, "Enforcement Guidance: Reasonable Accommodation and Undue Hardship under the Americans with Disabilities Act" (October 2002), www.eeoc.gov/policy/docs/accommodation.html, under "General Principles."

33. Eve Dubé et al., "Vaccine Hesitancy," *Human Vaccines & Immunotherapeutics* 9, no. 8 (2013): 1763–73.

34. Jeffrey S. Gerber and Paul A. Offit, "Vaccines and Autism: A Tale of Shifting Hypotheses," *Clinical Infectious Diseases* 48, no. 2 (2009): 456–61; Fiona Godlee, Jane Smith, and Harvey

Marcovitch, "Wakefield's Article Linking MMR Vaccine and Autism Was Fraudulent," *British Medical Journal* 342 (2011), https://doi.org/10.1136/bmj.c7452.

35. Dubé et al., "Vaccine Hesitancy," 1773.

36. Roy Porter, "The Patient's View: Doing Medical History from Below," *Theory and Society* 14, no. 2 (1985): 175–98.

37. Arthur Kleinman, *The Illness Narratives: Suffering, Healing & the Human Condition* (New York: Basic Books, 1988).

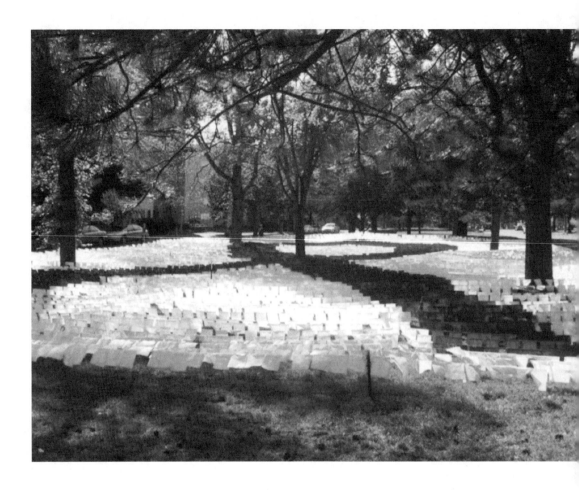

IMAGE 11.1 Community AIDS display in Victoria, Canada. The darker flags outline a ribbon. The red ribbon became an international symbol for AIDS awareness in 1992 after a campaign mounted by a group of concerned artists. Global mortality from AIDS has diminished since the 1990s because of increased public health measures and access to effective anti-retroviral drugs.

THE FACES OF HIV/AIDS

11

For decades, the CDC in Atlanta, Georgia, has published a weekly report of morbidity and mortality for the United States. In the 1980s, this bulletin's statistics and technical discussions were seldom of interest beyond a small circle of public health experts. The issue published on 5 June 1981 was no exception.[1] It included a report from Los Angeles about illnesses observed in five men during the previous eight months. All of them were "active homosexuals" who had contracted a rare form of pneumonia (*Pneumocystis carinii*), and two of them had died. All five, moreover, had a range of symptoms caused by human cytomegalovirus (HCMV). Harmless to most people, HCMV caused serious illness in individuals with weak immune systems such as infants or transplant patients. Now it seemed that gay men might be at risk, too. The picture was hazy, but an editorial accompanying the report suggested a link between cellular immune dysfunction, opportunistic infection with pneumonia, and "some aspect of a homosexual lifestyle or disease acquired through sexual contact."

That CDC article is the earliest known reference in medical literature to AIDS—acquired immunodeficiency syndrome.[*] It is the birth announcement, not of a virus or a disease, but of a pandemic that encompasses roughly 75 million infected individuals, 32 million related deaths, and the energies of countless family members, health care workers, scientific researchers, and government officials.[2] The human history of AIDS began at least decades before the earliest warnings of a new disease. But the outcry of the 1980s ended an era of optimism

---

[*] This is the wording most often used for the syndrome at present. The form "acquired immune deficiency syndrome" has also been in common usage since the 1980s and gave rise to the acronym AIDS.

in global public health. Initially considered a "gay plague" in North America, it is now clear that the impact of the pandemic transcends any social group.

As our history of other diseases has shown, epidemics often emerge when humans adopt new patterns within ecosystems or create agricultural and urban landscapes that cause exposure to various microbes. Bubonic plague spread along trade routes in the wake of climate change; yellow fever exploded among the newly created habitats of island plantations; and cholera struck early industrial cities that efficiently distributed contaminated water. In the case of AIDS, human technological and social changes not only created the potential for an epidemic, they vastly amplified the actual transmission of pathogenic material from one person to another. The emergence of AIDS is a remarkable parable of unintended consequences stemming not only from changes in sexual behavior and the sexual spread of disease but also, more fundamentally, from colonization, public health intervention, and globalization.

Etiology

Experts distinguish between infection with HIV (human immunodeficiency virus) and the clinical manifestations of AIDS that emerge in individuals who do not receive treatment. HIV refers to two distinct virus types, HIV-1 and HIV-2. Various forms of HIV-1 account for 95 per cent of HIV infections and are the chief cause of the global pandemic. HIV-2, which often results in a milder disease, has mostly been restricted to West Africa. Shortly after infection with HIV, many individuals experience a brief illness with fever, headache, and fatigue. A blood test can usually indicate **seropositivity** (the presence of antibodies for HIV) after several months. Without treatment, individuals who are infected with HIV-1 typically have few or no serious symptoms for about ten years. Thereafter, the damage to their immune systems manifests in a range of infections, particularly cancerous skin lesions known as Kaposi's sarcoma. Full-blown AIDS may also cause weight loss, chronic diarrhea, neurologic symptoms, and respiratory infections such as pneumonia or tuberculosis. Drug therapies have now greatly improved the prospects for many HIV-positive individuals, although drugs cannot cure the disease and no vaccine has been developed.

The complex transmission of HIV has created different profiles for the pandemic in populations around the world. The virus is usually transmitted by infected bodily fluids, especially blood, that pass through mucous membranes or broken skin.[3] Not every exposure transmits infection. Some of the factors that influence the likelihood of transmission are well understood, others are not, and several factors may work in combination to influence an individual's risk of infection. HIV is especially infectious for twelve weeks or so after it is contracted, and the risk of transmission in this interval is much higher than it will be during the next several years. In sexual intercourse, the higher exposure of mucous membranes in receptive partners places them at greater risk than insertive partners. The exposure of mucous membranes to HIV and other pathogens is also greater during anal sex than vaginal sex. The probability of transmission during any sexual contact rises dramatically when a participant has broken skin in the mouth, genitals, or anus, including ulcers caused by diseases such as syphilis or herpes. Male circumcision reduces the likelihood of transmission and has contributed to lower rates of HIV prevalence in many societies. Injection with a contaminated needle carries a high risk, and insufficient sterilization of syringes or other equipment also greatly magnifies the probability of transmission. Until blood screening procedures were widely adopted, the transfusion of contaminated blood products was especially dangerous and spread the virus in 90 per cent of exposures or more. HIV-positive mothers, unless treated, may infect newborns during pregnancy and childbirth or through breastmilk.

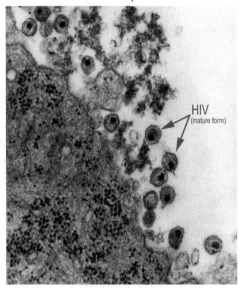

IMAGE 11.2 Human immunodeficiency virus. This highly magnified transmission electron micrograph indicates the presence of HIV in a human tissue sample. At the microscopic level, the disease is characterized by changes in the population of T-cell lymphocytes that play a key role in the immune system. Immune suppression leads to the clinical manifestations of AIDS. This image was captured in 1983, the same year that investigators first observed the HIV retrovirus.

HIV is a **retrovirus**, one of a family of pathogens that infect many types of mammals including sheep, horses, and simians (apes and monkeys). These pathogens are ancient in origin. Estimates based on recent samples suggest that retroviruses began spreading among small mammals more than 10 million years ago. Within the retrovirus family, HIV is classified in a genus of lentiviruses that cause a range of chronic, slow-developing diseases ("lentus" is a Latin term for "slow"). HIV's closest relatives are SIVs (simian immunodeficiency viruses), which are widespread among more than forty species of chimpanzees and monkeys, although infected animals do not always display symptomatic disease. SIV-1 is hosted by chimpanzees that are native to central Africa, while SIV-2 is hosted by sooty mangabey monkeys that are indigenous to West Africa.[4] Genetic analysis suggests that the types of SIV that led to HIV emerged between several hundred and 1,000 years ago and thereafter were transmitted to humans.

Retroviruses have distinctive characteristics that make them difficult for cells to repel. In most cells, strands of DNA make RNA that, in turn, makes proteins to perform various functions. Retroviruses reverse this process in the cells they enter. Viral RNA integrates with a host cell's DNA and uses it to replicate viral material. Over many generations, some cells undergo changes to inactivate such viruses and incorporate them into cellular genomes. And there the viruses stay: about 8 per cent of human DNA is now believed to contain endogenous retroviruses, or "fossil" viruses, left behind from encounters with pathogens long ago.[5]

Unfortunately, HIV is no fossil and it has developed other strategies to evade the human immune system. Like other retroviruses, HIV does not have a mechanism to correct genetic changes that occur during replication. Viewed from an evolutionary standpoint, such "transcription errors" are not really mistakes; they enable HIV to mutate about 1 million times faster than an organism that undergoes DNA replication. When more than one subtype of HIV is present in a host, the different viruses may combine to create a new form. More than eighty circulating recombinant forms of HIV have been identified, adding to the challenges of halting the spread of HIV.

The virus is also difficult to treat because of the type of cells it targets. In the human bloodstream, the virus attaches to a protein (CD4) that appears most frequently on the surface of T lymphocyte white blood cells, or T-cells. These cells normally help coordinate the body's immune functions, but HIV uses them to manufacture viral material that spreads to other cells and also to create reservoirs of dormant viral material. This latent HIV infection, which current drugs cannot destroy, is possible because T-cells normally are tasked with "remembering" previous pathogens and mobilizing a swift response if they reappear. The reactivation of these cells triggers a new phase of viral replication. HIV quickly evades any single drug that is used against it, but changing "cocktails" of several drugs can now hold replication at bay for many years.

Nothing was known of HIV until 1981. Thereafter, the emergence of AIDS became one of the great medical mysteries of the twentieth century. The first efforts to understand the disease became a race, both to alleviate suffering and to win prestige and profit from the discovery of a new pathogen.

Chasing an Unknown Disease

AIDS could not be identified as a distinct syndrome until laboratory tools became available that could identify its causal retrovirus. Because HIV's chief effect in the body is immune suppression, AIDS had no characteristic symptoms of its own. The first sufferers displayed the symptoms of opportunistic infections that HIV prevented their bodies from fending off. While laboratory research on the syndrome proceeded, public health officials attempted to track new cases. At the end of 1981, fewer than 1,000 possible cases were identified worldwide. By August 1989, the number of reported cases in the United States alone had reached 100,000, and the prevalence in Canada at the time was later estimated to be between 30,000 and 40,000 cases.[6] The initial findings led experts in North America to scrutinize gay men and other marginal social groups. The public discussion of AIDS that stemmed from this narrow focus obscured the full scope of the crisis for a critical period of several years.

Prior to the identification of HIV, researchers had begun to explore possible links between retroviruses and cancer. This investigation linked long-running lines of inquiry concerning the causes of disease. Since the mid-nineteenth century, scientists had suggested that some diseases were caused by abnormal behavior of human cells. In 1847, the influential pathologist Rudolf Virchow (1821–1902) described and named the blood disease "leukemia" (i.e., cancer of the blood cells) and, in 1865, Karl Thiersch (1822–1895) suggested that skin cancers were made of skin cells. After 1870, Louis Pasteur and Robert Koch steered most researchers to investigate microbes that entered the body. But a few remained interested in exploring the relationship between these invaders and the cells they targeted. In 1911, Peyton Rous (1879–1970) of the Rockefeller Institute transmitted tumor material between chickens and proved that a virus could induce cancer. His finding remained an isolated observation until the 1950s, when discoveries concerning the role of DNA and RNA allowed scientists to consider the relationship of viruses and cell genetics more fully.

Initially, molecular biologists believed that genetic information could flow in only one direction: DNA made RNA and RNA made proteins. Then, in 1970, it was shown that RNA from some viruses used an enzyme, labeled **reverse transcriptase**, to integrate with DNA. Knowledge of this enzyme raised the possibility that many forms of abnormal cell growth were caused by retroviruses. To cancer researchers, this was both a possible explanation and an exciting diagnostic opportunity. If the reverse transcriptase enzyme could be found in cells, it would signal the presence of pathogens that otherwise could not be detected. At the US National Cancer Institute, a team led by Robert Gallo (1937–) worked for years to refine a test for reverse transcriptase and identify a retrovirus that caused a type of leukemia. By the spring of 1981, the team had succeeded. Gallo named the first known human retrovirus "human T-cell leukemia virus" (HTLV).

The scientific research of the next several years was formative both for the expert understanding of AIDS and for public apprehension of the crisis. Although interest in retroviruses initially was spurred by cancer research, by the end of 1981 reports of worrisome infections shifted the research agenda. In addition to the pneumonia cases in Los Angeles, physicians in New York identified similar instances of pneumonia and a spike in cases of Kaposi's sarcoma. This skin cancer, usually considered fairly benign, had been associated primarily with darker-skinned older men. But the new cases appeared in young white men, almost all of them gay, and their cancers soon spread and turned deadly. As vague warnings about a "gay plague" circulated in the United States, European cities reported dozens of cases of the nameless syndrome, almost all among gay men with American sexual contacts. After initial suggestion that the syndrome might be named Gay-Related Immune Deficiency (GRID), the CDC formally introduced the more neutral term "acquired immune deficiency syndrome" (AIDS) in September 1982. By this time, some cases involving hetero-sexual transmission had been reported, but they received little attention and homosexuality remained an important diagnostic criterion for the disease.[7]

In 1982 and 1983, teams of microbiologists in the United States and at the Pasteur Institute in France hunted for evidence of retroviruses in cell cultures. Initially, the researchers worked under the assumption that the new pathogen belonged to the family of HTLV retroviruses identified by Gallo's team. However, early in 1983 the Pasteur Institute group, led by Luc Montagnier (1932–) and Françoise Barré Sinoussi (1947–), investigated lymph node tissue and isolated a retrovirus with characteristics that differed from HTLV. The French scientists named this isolate "lymphadenopathy associated virus" (LAV) and shared samples with Gallo's lab, although they were circumspect about its precise relationship to AIDS. A battle of acronyms began. Gallo defended the primacy of his research program, first by suggesting that LAV was unrelated to AIDS and then by announc-ing in spring 1984 that a retrovirus named HTLV-IIIB was the definitive cause of AIDS. Tests soon revealed that LAV and HTLV-IIIB were, in fact, the same; the French researchers had discovered the virus, while Gallo's team confirmed that it caused AIDS and developed a means of producing it in large quantities for antibody screening. A bitter argument over bragging rights and spoils ended with a profit-sharing arrangement for the diagnostic blood test and an agreement to share credit for the discovery. Scientists also agreed on a name for the virus that stuck: HIV, for human immunodeficiency virus.

Meanwhile, officials in the CDC interviewed physicians and patients nation-wide, considering every case of disease that might be relevant. Much attention focused on the large gay communities in New York, San Francisco, and Los Angeles. It was apparent that men in these centers were disproportionately affected, but how were their immune systems compromised? Did inhaled drugs or topical creams increase the risk of infection? Were some men genetically predisposed to immune suppression? Was it a new form of hepatitis B, which was relatively common among gay men? There were other leads as well. A New York study (published in May 1983) found immunodeficiency in "infants born to promiscuous and drug-addicted mothers."[8] French researchers focused on cases of disease among individuals from Africa and Haiti and concluded that heterosexual transmission was significant as well as same-sex transmission. By the fall of 1982, cases of the disease began to appear among hemophiliacs, leading to concerns about the nation's blood supply.

Many avenues of inquiry would later prove important, but as fears about AIDS rippled through North America, reports about one group of gay men greatly influenced the general perception of the crisis. In June 1982, the CDC published an article concerning cases of disease that were concentrated in Orange County, California (near Los Angeles). A subsequent "cluster study" of this group, published in March 1984, highlighted the role of one AIDS patient who was directly or indirectly connected to forty other cases.[9] The patient did not live in Orange County and received the confidential label "Patient O" to indicate an origin from "(O)utside of California." The designation "O" was misinterpreted as "0" (zero) when investigators numbered cases within the cluster according to the date of the patients' onset of symptoms.[10] Thus originated the notion of an AIDS "Patient Zero," a concept that took on new meanings and exerted an outsized influence once it moved beyond the research community at the CDC.

Some experts soon realized that the cluster study's depiction of the spread of AIDS and the central role of one patient was misleading. A guiding premise was mistaken: the study had assumed that the onset of symptoms took place on average about a year after initial infection. In 1985, a new blood test for HIV was applied to hundreds of archived samples. This analysis revealed that the interval between infection with HIV and the emergence of AIDS was actually several years or more. Therefore, the time frames that were cited between presumed dates of infection and the onset of symptoms were too short to plausibly account for the spread of HIV among the individuals in the study. The contact tracing that epidemiologists relied upon to track infections with short incubation periods was misleading for this novel disease. Where HIV transmission was concerned, no cluster existed.[11]

In the meantime, however, the cluster study had come to the attention of San Francisco journalist Randy Shilts (1951–1994). One of the few openly gay reporters in American media, Shilts sounded alarms about the indifference of both the gay community and US policy makers to the growing health crisis. In his best-selling book, *And the Band Played On* (1987), Shilts identified "Patient Zero" as Gaëtan Dugas (1953–1984), a Canadian flight attendant from Quebec who had many hundreds of sexual partners between the early 1970s and his death in 1984. Although the text of the book avoided an explicit accusation that Dugas had brought AIDS to America, Shilts left no doubt that he considered Dugas a representative of dangerous sexual excess in the gay community. In San Francisco, an epicenter of gay culture, many men frequented bathhouses that were a venue for casual, anonymous encounters. Shilts included a depiction of Dugas's conduct in a bathhouse that was more memorable to many readers than the book's passionate critique of public health authorities and politicians.[12]

When *And the Band Played On* was released in the fall of 1987, its publisher, St Martin's Press, circulated excerpts of the book that highlighted Dugas's role in spreading AIDS. Media reports concerning the book further insinuated that Dugas not only was at the center of an early cluster of AIDS patients in San Francisco but also that he played a key role in the introduction of AIDS to the United States. For example, on 15 November 1987 the popular news program *60 Minutes* broadcast a segment on AIDS that included an interview with Shilts. Anchorman Harry Reasoner's narration labeled Dugas as "Patient Zero—one of the first cases of AIDS; the first person identified as a major transmitter of the disease." For his part, Shilts claimed that the combination of Dugas's "unlimited sexual stamina" and mobility as a flight attendant contributed to the nationwide spread of AIDS. The fact that Dugas was Canadian further heightened suspicions in the United States. Newspaper headlines labeled him "the man who gave us AIDS" and he was depicted as an individual who knowingly, or even maliciously, spread disease without regard for the consequences. Shilts's reference to "Patient Zero" did not explain the source of AIDS; it did create a lasting meme that signaled the initial culprit in an outbreak of disease.[13]

Later studies would confirm the observation made in 1988 by San Francisco epidemiologist Andrew Moss that "the cluster study is a myth."[14] Genetic analysis of blood samples has now offered strong evidence that a viral subtype of HIV-1 arrived in the United States from the Caribbean in the early 1970s. Nonetheless, the legend of Patient Zero seemed to confirm the apparent connection between

AIDS and uncontrolled homosexuality that framed the early discussion of AIDS in North America. In US government circles, Shilts's account was read by key presidential advisors and referenced by lawyers who debated criminal penalties for HIV transmission.[15] The concentration of AIDS cases among gay men and intravenous drug users also discouraged attention to the crisis among social conservatives who influenced President Ronald Reagan's administration. Funding for AIDS research at the CDC suffered in comparison with the resources allocated to other projects, leading a US Congressman from California to fume that "if the disease had appeared among Americans of Norwegian descent or tennis players, rather than gay men, the response of the government and the medical community would be different."[16] Although the CDC warned in December 1982 of the possible transmission of disease through blood products, no review of the national blood supply was undertaken until the fall of 1984. Federal policies also failed to address the spread of AIDS and other diseases by unsafe drug injections. In 1988, US lawmakers banned the use of federal funding for needle exchange programs, a move that contrasted with the actions of European nations. At the time, the spread of a new form of solid cocaine ("crack") was a crisis of its own, and US politicians wished to avoid the criticism that they were enabling drug use by handing out needles.[17]

Gay community groups in large cities, such as the Gay Men's Health Crisis in New York (founded in January 1982) and AIDS Vancouver (founded in the spring of 1983), soon played a leading role by conducting awareness campaigns and handing out condoms. However, some gay men considered the vague linkage of AIDS and a "homosexual lifestyle" as an attempt to use medical science and public health surveillance to suppress their activities. Meanwhile, the potential for AIDS to spread among heterosexuals continued to receive little attention. When researchers in Africa attempted to publish evidence for heterosexual transmission in Zaire, a dozen scientific journals rejected the study before it finally appeared in the British journal *The Lancet* in the summer of 1984.[18]

AIDS was both poorly understood and highly politicized in the 1980s. Initially lost amid the controversies was a series of articles published in 1983–84 by researchers at the California Primate Research Institute in Davis, California. They documented several episodes of AIDS-like disease among captive monkeys at the facility, including one outbreak in 1969. Over the next several years, researchers collected samples of SIV that established relationships between SIV-2 and HIV-2 and later between SIV-1 and HIV-1. In 1993, the Smithsonian Museum in Washington, DC, conducted genetic tests on monkey tissue samples preserved in its archives. The museum found evidence of SIV earlier than previously known, possibly as far back as the 1890s. By 2000, as testing techniques improved and genetic samples from various times and places were analyzed, it became apparent that the pandemic's origins were at least several decades in the past. And evidence increasingly pointed to an African origin, although this claim remained hotly contested both inside and outside of Africa.

As HIV's beginnings were pushed further back in time, its historians faced a conundrum. To understand why, it is helpful to reconsider our understanding of HIV transmission in relation to the pandemic's origins. In the absence of open sores or broken skin, HIV will not spread by casual contact such as a hug or a handshake, and it does not survive for lengthy periods outside the body. Thus, under natural conditions (i.e., without needles or blood transfusions), HIV does not transmit as readily as diseases such as influenza, measles, or (formerly) smallpox. Even in the remotest parts of Africa, the chances of initial infection from a chimpanzee's bodily fluids were slim. On average, the human-to-human transmission of HIV required exchange of bodily fluids multiple times. Normal circumstances would therefore enable a few cases of HIV, or at most a few dozen, but not a spread of the disease around the globe. Why did the pandemic emerge when it did? What chain of events amplified the spread of HIV from a few individuals to tens of millions?

Seeking the Origins of HIV/AIDS

Many factors contributed to the origin and spread of HIV. Efforts by historians to explain its emergence have been equally multifaceted and interdisciplinary. In addition to first-hand accounts, government health reports, and clinical case histories, researchers have analyzed large collections of blood samples collected on other occasions, such as outbreaks of Ebola in Africa during the 1970s. The evidence base includes phylogenetic analysis of SIV samples among chimpanzees as well as cases of HIV. This has required work far from the laboratory or the library. To investigate the natural prevalence of SIV, in the early 2000s animal trackers roamed a large swath of forest in central Africa to search for chimpanzee feces. The viral DNA that was collected from more than 100 stool samples, when compared with material from human viruses, confirmed beyond doubt the geographic origins of HIV-1.

The known HIV-1 viruses fall into four groups, each of which originated with a separate cross-species transmission event. Phylogenetic analysis suggests that the ancestor virus of HIV-1 group M, the most widely spread group, was transmitted to a human host sometime between 1910 and 1930. However, it is not unlikely that the first human infection with an HIV-like virus took place several centuries ago. The simian virus that became HIV-1 in humans originated on the order of 1,000 years ago, and bush hunters who ate contaminated chimpanzee meat may have contracted it on more than one occasion. Since the population of central Africa was sparse, with relatively little mobility, over the centuries a few hunters and their intimate contacts probably lived and died anonymously with an AIDS-like disease. Likewise, slaves who were taken from West Africa did not have the opportunity to spread the disease widely and AIDS-like infections may have gone unnoticed.

What happened in the early twentieth century to start a pandemic? One scenario is that a bush hunter went to a colonial center—a city, or perhaps a railroad labor camp—and infected a sex worker with numerous clients who then spread the disease further. However, the overall probability that such an encounter played a decisive role by itself is relatively remote. Most rural men did not frequent cities, the ones who did would not always frequent sex workers, and numerous encounters were probably required to transmit the virus.

Jacques Pepin has recently suggested that needles were most likely involved in the early spread of HIV.[19] As explained in chapters 7 and 9, beginning in 1917 French doctors conducted intensive public campaigns to treat sleeping sickness, yaws, leprosy, and eventually malaria. This was carried out by mobile teams of practitioners who traveled among remote communities. Because many treatments required multiple intravenous injections of arsenical drugs, doctors and nurses walked from village to village on a circuit to administer weekly shots. Although efforts were made to maintain sanitary standards, little was known about viruses, and scant attention was paid to the possible transmission of unknown pathogens by parenteral means (i.e., through injection). Pepin suggests that some villages were rescued by the new medicines and the hard-working practitioners who brought them. Certainly, these campaigns reflected the desire to protect both African laborers and colonial officials. The sweeping French programs (and, to a lesser extent, those of doctors in the neighboring Belgian Congo) disrupted the landscape of diseases that had previously existed across central Africa.

SCIENCE FOCUS

Sticking Points: Injection Equipment and Modern Health Care

Needles are a uniquely modern technology. They have saved millions of lives but their use has also caused unintended harm and inspired controversy.

While the hypodermic needle (to break the skin) is a relatively recent innovation, its frequent partner, the syringe, has a longer history. Ancient sources document syringes used to inject or withdraw fluids for enemas and other procedures. From the seventeenth century forward, investigators conducted various experiments with animal bladders connected to quills or hollow wooden tubes. Europeans also used metal lancets to puncture the skin, usually for bloodletting but also for smallpox inoculations and then cowpox vaccinations.

In the mid-nineteenth century, interest in injection technology grew as chemists refined morphine, quinine, and other drugs into water-soluble powders. Morphine injections became preferred once it was demonstrated that the drug acted faster and with fewer obvious side effects when it entered the bloodstream via injection instead of being swallowed. As inventors independently tested various devices, in 1853 Frenchman Charles Pravaz (1791–1853) added a hollow metal needle to a silver syringe with a screw that controlled dosages. For the next century, glass and metal syringes worked in tandem with needles. Intravenous injection (into veins) became more common to enable swifter drug absorption and the administration of smaller doses.

After World War II, injection equipment adapted to support the vast immunization projects of the era. Disposable glass syringes, plastic syringes, and jet injector guns that used forced air all came into wide use during the 1950s. Only later did it become clear that such programs sometimes spread infections, particularly hepatitis C, when working conditions prevented health workers from adequately sterilizing injection equipment. Dirty needles were not the only problem: jet injector guns could be contaminated by fluids that splashed onto the nozzle or were sucked back into the gun when it was recocked. The largest known case of disease transmission by a public health program took place in Egypt from the 1950s to the 1980s. During a campaign to eliminate schistosomiasis—a parasitic infection caused by flatworms that live in freshwater snails—millions of Egyptians received injections that were contaminated with the virus that causes hepatitis C.

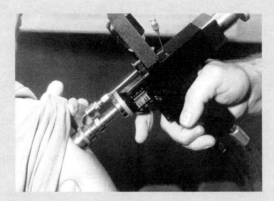

IMAGE 11.3a The "peace gun" (jet injection gun). These devices used forced air to deliver a stream of vaccine solution.

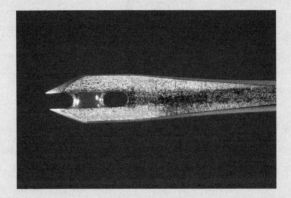

IMAGE 11.3b Bifurcated needle with vaccine solution. Alongside jet injection guns, bifurcated needles were instrumental in smallpox eradication campaigns.

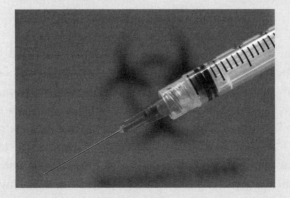

IMAGE 11.3c Metallic hypodermic needle and plastic syringe barrel. For immunizations, needles most commonly are used for intramuscular injection (into muscle tissue) or subcutaneous injection (between muscles and skin). Intravenous (IV) injection or therapy is used to introduce antibiotics, to replace fluids or blood products, or for chemotherapy.

At times, simpler methods have accomplished goals that more complex mechanical devices could not. During the smallpox eradication campaign, the jet injector guns required skilled maintenance and sometimes broke down. In many regions, they were replaced by the simple bifurcated needle, which held a drop of liquid vaccine in its clipped eye. Simpler to use, the needle also required less vaccine liquid than the gun to administer an effective dose. Immunization campaigns eradicated smallpox and greatly reduced the incidence of other diseases, particularly polio.

During the campaigns, health workers or trained volunteers managed needles, syringes, and drugs. In recent decades, medical laypeople have gained greater access to injection equipment in order to manage chronic conditions such as diabetes. This has reduced health care costs, and many individuals have benefited from the autonomy enabled by inexpensive and disposable "sharps." On the other hand, the availability of needles increases the potential for unintentional infection when equipment is not sterilized or transmission of infections when drug users share equipment. The danger is especially high for individuals who voluntarily or involuntarily are excluded from health care facilities that provide safe and sterile equipment and procedures.

While illegal drug use is not always involved in needle contamination, the politics of needle access reflects a broader controversy concerning the proper social response to substance use disorders. In 2016, the UN endorsed a statement recognizing that drug addiction is "a complex multifactorial health disorder characterized by chronic and relapsing nature," that nonetheless may be prevented and treated.[20] Health care advocates have considered whether public agencies should provide injection equipment to marginal groups to minimize the risk of disease transmission and drug overdose. In most of North America, proposed safe injection sites have faced legal hurdles and public resistance. Since 2015, however, rising mortality related to opioid use has encouraged some cities to reconsider the merits and drawbacks of such facilities. The increased availability of single-use injection equipment and other innovations may influence social policies at both local and national levels.

Small but powerful, needles undoubtedly will remain a topic of debates concerning medical necessity, public safety, and moral obligation.

The drugs, diseases, and injection techniques varied, but over several decades Western doctors administered tens of millions of shots throughout the region where HIV-1 would soon emerge. Infected individuals may then have reached the important center of Brazzaville, a city on the north bank of the Congo River (formerly in the French Congo and now the capital of the Republic of the Congo). This scenario rests on inferences from various sources rather than direct evidence. Some of the most suggestive findings come from recent assessments of elderly Africans who received medications by injection beginning in the 1920s. In 2010, studies of elderly residents of Cameroon and the Central African Republic demonstrated a connection between infection with hepatitis C and intravenous treatment decades earlier, either for malaria or sleeping sickness.[21] This is a clear indication that contaminated needles spread hepatitis C. Some scholars consider this strong circumstantial evidence that HIV spread the same way; it would have left no survivors to be found decades later. Skeptics of this view have pointed out that hepatitis C is much more infectious by parenteral transmission than HIV and that sexual intercourse has always been the main route of HIV infection in Africa.[22]

Historians are on somewhat firmer ground with their analysis of later events in Kinshasa, which lies directly across the Congo River from Brazzaville and is now the capital of the Democratic Republic of the Congo. Formerly known as Léopoldville (or simply Léo), the city gained prominence in 1923 when it became the capital of the Belgian Congo. Officials rigidly controlled immigration into the city and privileged the access of male workers over female ones. Men outnumbered women, at times by more than three to one. Although the gender imbalance eased over time, in the 1950s there were still three men for every two women in Léo. Sex work was highly profitable and widely accepted for both single and married women and probably contributed to the gradual spread of HIV. The Belgian colony also built a rail line that connected Léo to diamond mines further south and transported roughly 1 million people a year in the later 1940s.

In 1960, both the Belgian Congo and the French Congo gained independence and Léo's population exploded during a period of great social upheaval. Phylogenetic analysis suggests that around this time there was a marked increase in the rate of transmission and the genetic diversity of HIV-1 viruses in group M. This evidence is consistent with public health observations of the time that a new form of high-volume, high-risk sex work took hold, with some women servicing up to 1,000 clients per year.[23] Social unrest also increased the movement between Léo and Brazzaville; if the virus did not already have a solid foothold on both sides of the river, it certainly did by the early 1960s. Impoverishment and disintegration of the region's economy and political structure fostered the further spread of the virus.

Although HIV spreads less readily than many infectious diseases, once a few infected individuals reached one or more large communities, the possible routes of transmission grew rapidly. Syphilis lesions caused sex workers to transmit the virus more readily to clients, especially in the weeks just after an initial infection. Men or women treated intravenously for an STI could contaminate syringes that were used dozens of times or more without proper sterilization. Over time, mother-to-child transmission of HIV also spread the disease among the next generation. HIV-positive children did not contribute to the sexual transmission of the virus, but they may have received medical treatments that contaminated equipment and blood supplies. Contaminated blood was a particular danger in regions where malaria was endemic—which included Kinshasa—because young children often required urgent transfusions when malaria infection caused anemia. One study recorded that Kinshasa's Mama Yemo Hospital performed about 12,800 transfusions in 1985–86 and 560 children contracted HIV.[24]

These dynamics played out with additional contributing factors once HIV reached the western hemisphere, apparently first in Haiti during the mid-1960s.[25] Shortly after Congo became independent, the UN recruited technical advisors, including 4,500 French-speaking Haitians, to assist the country's leaders. At some point, a Haitian individual returned home and initiated HIV transmission in the country's sexual and health services networks. Haiti itself was relatively impoverished and its capital, Port-au-Prince, was a known destination for North American tourists in search of cheap sex. Because of the increasing availability of air travel for North Americans, it was a short trip to Port-au-Prince from Miami or New York. Air transport also facilitated another route for infection that may have been equally important: the growing trade in blood products for use by hemophiliacs. For eighteen months in 1971 and 1972, a company named Hemo Caribbean in Port-au-Prince exported thousands of liters of plasma each month to the United States. Haitian blood donors also numbered in the thousands, including many impoverished men who received a few dollars per week for their contributions. Again we are left with circumstantial evidence—Hemo Caribbean's records have vanished and there was no test for HIV contamination at the time—but the time frame of the company's activity corresponded to the first years of HIV in Haiti. Later transmission episodes involving blood products confirms that Haiti's blood supply could have contributed to the early dissemination of HIV in North America. Much evidence that might confirm this hypothesis was destroyed in order to protect health-care providers from lawsuits.[26]

In June 1981, it was not known that the latency period between HIV infection and the onset of AIDS could approach ten years. The cases of gay men that seized headlines in the United States were the visible tip of an iceberg. Below the surface were many thousands of infected individuals worldwide who had not yet displayed obvious symptoms or who lived without access to Western medicine and diagnostic services. In Africa, an epidemic was well underway before anyone realized that a new disease existed. This contributed to the apparently sudden beginning of the pandemic and, more than any other factor, may account for the later severity of the African HIV/AIDS pandemic.[27] Although transmission within a segment of the urban gay population played a role in North America, other forces—invasive medical treatments, the heterosexual sex trade, and upheaval in impoverished regions—were all more significant in the early spread of HIV.

HIV/AIDS around the World

In the mid-1980s and much of the 1990s, global measures to counter the pandemic were slowed by the stigma of sexually transmitted disease, electoral politics in the United States, and the bureaucracies of international organizations. Other nations were often no more willing than the United States to reckon with HIV/AIDS as a homegrown problem. As cases of the new disease mounted, the "social distancing" of marginal groups took various forms. For example, Johanna Hood has shown that Chinese media depictions in the early 1990s linked AIDS to *yuanshi*, a term that evoked a primeval origin for the disease among Africans whose societies were stereotypically associated with the jungle. Such depictions resembled notions of primitive peoples that many Westerners held in the early twentieth century. Public health posters and other media served to distance ethnic Han Chinese from AIDS, although young people, women, and especially sex workers were increasingly vulnerable to infection.[28]

Indeed, initial reports of AIDS in many Asian nations were subdued. India announced few cases, and the spread of HIV in the Philippines was attributed to American military servicemen rather than more widespread transmission. Only in Africa did the alarm bells ring loudly, as researchers in Kinshasa confirmed the heterosexual spread of HIV and suggested that the epidemic was wider in scope than had been recognized. Their warnings did not galvanize concerted action by wealthier nations or the WHO. Media reports of the SIV "monkey viruses" fostered the belief that Africa's disease was different from HIV in the wealthier northern hemisphere. Even among the WHO leadership, AIDS was not counted among the worst problems in Africa or elsewhere. On 13 July 1985, when a group of A-list rock bands staged an

African benefit concert for telecast around the world, it was famine relief, not AIDS, that claimed center stage.

This began to change in May 1986, when the WHO sponsored a Special (soon renamed Global) Program on AIDS that was directed by Jonathan Mann (1947–1998). Impassioned and charismatic, Mann did more than any other individual to raise the global profile of the AIDS crisis in the late 1980s. The Global Program focused on blood supply screening, clinical management of cases, public education, and prevention of discrimination. None of this happened too soon. When the Global Program concluded its first four years, an estimated 310,000 people had died from AIDS and roughly 8.9 million were living with HIV.[29] Rampant infection undermined the health of numerous communities. As immune-suppressed people experienced new cases or relapses of diseases such as tuberculosis or pneumonia, they also increased the danger of infection for others.

As we consider the progress of AIDS in the following quarter century, it is sobering to consider how an energetic response to early warning signs might have influenced the scope of the crisis. The following section will briefly describe several different trajectories that the pandemic has followed in various regions.

One Pandemic, Many Paths

Africa still carries the greatest burden of HIV/AIDS and merits particular attention. In 2004, sub-Saharan Africa had 2 per cent of the world's population but nearly 30 per cent of its HIV cases, as well as the world's highest rates of AIDS-related tuberculosis.[30] From its origins in central and West Africa, HIV spread east and south, following transportation routes used by laborers and long-distance truckers. In many regions, labor patterns that disseminated tuberculosis also fostered the spread of HIV; in turn, the immune deficiency caused by HIV elevated rates of tuberculosis. Another contributing factor was the high rates of a herpes simplex virus (HSV-2) that caused sores that facilitated transmission. By the 1990s, heterosexual transmission of HIV in Africa had outpaced other forms of transmission, and, as the epidemic progressed, a disproportionate number of women were infected. Botswana was especially hard hit: among its 1.7 million inhabitants, in 2000 HIV prevalence among adults was estimated by UNAIDS at 36 per cent.

The contrasting experiences of Uganda and South Africa illustrate the range of responses to the pandemic among Africa's diverse nations. Formerly controlled by Britain, Uganda in the early 1980s was emerging from a period of repression and social stagnation under the dictatorships of Idi Amin and Milton Obote. By 1986, when forces led by Yoweri Museveni (1944–) asserted control, the AIDS crisis had assumed a terrifying scale: later estimates suggested that, in one southern Ugandan district, more than 8 per cent of young people aged 15–24 contracted HIV *in a single year* (1987). In some truck-stop towns along the Trans-African highway, by 1990 one-half of the adult residents were infected with HIV.[31] Ugandan officials openly acknowledged the crisis and Museveni himself announced: "To not be open about AIDS is just ignorant. This is an epidemic. You can only stop it by talking about it—loudly, so that everybody is aware and scared."[32] Supported by the UN Global Program, Ugandan schools launched awareness initiatives, officials routinely discussed AIDS at public events, and funds were provided for blood screening, surveillance, and epidemiological research. Muslim and Christian organizations, which already offered care for many AIDS patients, were also enlisted to educate and promote responsible behavior. In 1989, Uganda's leading Muslim jurist, the Chief Qadi, proclaimed a *jihad* (sacred struggle) against AIDS, and progressive Muslim leaders urged an end to stigmatization and marginalization of the sick. By 2008, the prevalence of HIV was estimated to be around 6 per cent. This statistic may overstate Uganda's success, and certainly reflects a high death rate as well as a decline in new infections, but sustained government measures apparently influenced behavior among Uganda's younger citizens. Aspects of Uganda's national strategy were emulated by other African nations. The fact that Uganda's HIV prevalence increased slightly after the late 2000s indicated that continual efforts are necessary to avoid a resurgence in infections.

Colonialism and its aftermath played an especially prominent role in the response to HIV/AIDS in South Africa, which, in the 1980s, remained under an apartheid regime that legislated segregation among its citizens. Similar to the United States and western Europe, initial attention focused upon gay men, transfusion recipients, and hemophiliacs. However, heterosexual intercourse soon became by far the predominant means of HIV transmission. As in other southern African nations, the spread of AIDS was especially pronounced among women who were dependent upon males in a migrant labor system. Transactional sex between younger women and older men was widespread and contributed to the high rate of infection among pregnant women (estimated at 24.5 per cent in 2000). AIDS not only orphaned millions of children, it infected millions more from birth. By 2003, South Africa had an estimated 5 million individuals who had contracted HIV.[33]

South Africa's apartheid government paid relatively little attention to AIDS, and this did not change dramatically after the election of a democratic government led by Nelson Mandela (1918–2013) in 1994. The immense challenges facing the new regime discouraged it from addressing AIDS as a broader problem. Some leaders also resisted the scientific consensus concerning the causes and treatment of AIDS. For a time they advocated the use of a toxic industrial solvent, marketed under the name Virodene, as an alternative to anti-retroviral therapy. Mandela's successor Thabo Mbeki (1942–), who was elected in 1999, continued to cast doubt on the effectiveness of anti-retroviral therapy and, more broadly, on the legitimacy of an international medical community that he regarded with suspicion. In 2000, when the annual International AIDS Conference was held in Durban, South Africa, Mbeki infuriated many participants by focusing on poverty, rather than HIV transmission, as the primary cause of the pandemic. Although the Mbeki government eventually agreed to provide free anti-retroviral therapy in public health services, health minister Manto Tshabalala-Msimang (1940–2009) continued to promote untested remedies and nutritional advice. This contrarian position reached a low point at the Toronto International AIDS Conference in 2006, when South Africa's exhibition hall display featured beet root, garlic, and lemons as AIDS remedies instead of anti-retroviral treatments that had proven effective for millions of patients. Such advocacy, which was not representative of broader South African perspectives, revealed how the rejection of colonial injustice could take an extreme form of denialism against Western science and its presumed attitude toward African culture.

While transmission among heterosexual partners was the most significant driver of HIV transmission in Africa, elsewhere the pandemic assumed other profiles. Although new infections began to drop worldwide after 2004, dramatic increases were reported in eastern Europe and central Asia, where the collapse of the Soviet Union in 1991 had initiated a long period of social and economic upheaval. Here the predominant mode of HIV transmission was (and is) injected drug use, although the spread of HIV among men who have sex with men may be underreported.[34] The rate of infection has been especially high in Russia, where roughly one-fifth of known injection drug users tested positive for HIV in 2015. The Russian infections reported that year exceeded the combined total of all western European countries, and it was estimated that at least 1 million of Russia's 145 million inhabitants were HIV-positive. Russia's public health experts warned that the nation might move from a concentrated epidemic in an at-risk group to a generalized epidemic that would spread through the wider society.

The example of Romania, formerly a satellite state of the Soviet Union, illustrates how local circumstances have influenced the level of HIV infection in particular populations. In the 1980s, the regime led by Nicolae Ceausescu (1918–1989) encouraged population growth by forbidding abortion and contraception until women had given birth to five children. Since this policy was not paired with economic support for large families, numerous children were abandoned to the care of state institutions. Malnourished infants and children were routinely given small transfusions of whole blood. While this was considered a means to "boost immunity," unscreened blood and improperly sterilized equipment instead enabled the transmission of AIDS and other viruses. It is estimated that 10,000 children were infected between 1987 and 1991. Although these policies were discontinued after Ceausescu's dictatorship collapsed in 1989, a decade later Romania was still the site of 60 per cent of the pediatric AIDS cases registered in all of Europe.[35] Thereafter, however, the national government responded aggressively with assistance from the UN and private sponsors, and by 2003 it had become one of the few countries in the world to offer universal anti-retroviral therapy. A successful pediatric clinic in the city of Constanta also provided a model for a large-scale AIDS treatment program that was emulated by an even larger African clinic in Botswana, another epicenter of childhood AIDS cases.

In the large Indian subcontinent, the spread of AIDS is marked by distinct, yet overlapping patterns. In 2014, India had an estimated 2.1 million people living with AIDS, the largest number of any Asian country. In the southern states, where HIV prevalence was roughly five times as high as in the northern states, high rates of infection were identified among sex workers who initiated the spread of HIV among their clients and the clients' other sexual partners. Further north, intravenous drug use has played a prominent role in Myanmar, an important producer of opium and heroin. Among the smaller nations of Southeast Asia, Thailand has experienced the highest HIV prevalence, in part because its largest metropolis, Bangkok, is an established center of the sex trade. Although concentrated efforts to educate sex workers and the general populace encouraged a steep reduction in new infections, in 2012 it was estimated that 1.1 per cent of Thailand's inhabitants were infected with HIV. Unlike most other parts of the world, women who injected drugs had a higher estimated HIV prevalence (30.8 per cent) than men who injected drugs (24.2 per cent), probably because of the overlap between drug use and sex work.[36]

These brief examples underscore the diversity of experience in the AIDS pandemic and illustrate how political regimes and social conventions create distinct patterns within a general crisis. But what role has scientific research played in efforts to stop AIDS? So far, a vaccine has proven elusive, but HIV therapies with anti-retroviral medicines have greatly improved longevity and quality of life for PLHIV. The increase in the number of infected individuals, far from signaling a failure to stop the disease, indicates instead that a diagnosis of HIV infection is no longer considered a death sentence.

The Advent of AZT and HAART

On 13 August 1998, the *Bay Area Reporter*, a weekly newspaper in San Francisco, published a tall headline in bright red: "No obits." For the first time since 1981, there were no AIDS deaths for the paper to report that week. Many thousands of Bay Area residents were still infected with HIV but a turning point had been reached. In the 2000s and 2010s, highly active anti-retroviral therapy (initially known as HAART and then simply as ART) transformed AIDS into a chronic illness—at least for those with access to the drugs and the means to use them consistently.

The research that laid the groundwork for ART's success began immediately after the virus soon known as HIV was identified in the spring of 1984. Scientists investigated its genetic sequence and activity in order to block or interfere with its penetration of a cell, prevent the replication of genetic material, or interfere with the virus's "budding off" from one cell before attacking another. This research was accompanied by tests of drugs that had been developed previously for cancer treatment to see if they would also be effective against HIV. In summer 1985, it was found that one such drug, azidothymidine (AZT), suppressed the function of the reverse transcriptase enzyme that enabled the copying of viral RNA into cell DNA. Although AZT was a powerful drug, it had been shelved for many years because of its limited benefits and severe side effects, which included nausea and anemia. On average, AZT therapy could only prolong the life of AIDS patients for about a year, but, in the mid-1980s, AIDS was so lethal that any reprieve offered hope to many thousands of patients.

Controversy accompanied the approval of AZT by the FDA in March 1987 and continued for the next several years. One source of concern was the expedited approval process that was deployed in the clinical trials of AZT. Drug approval usually involves computer modeling, tests for safety and efficacy with a small group of patients, and a trial of its effects on a larger population. After a year of testing with a small group, government officials considered AZT's success sufficiently proven and the trial was halted. The pharmaceutical company Burroughs-Wellcome was allowed to market the drug (under the name Retrovir) without a large-scale trial. Although this decision was made to allow swift access to the drug for dying patients, Burroughs-Wellcome later faced criticism when side effects were noted among its many users. Another flashpoint was the drug's price and the control over its distribution. Initially, the retail purchase price for a year's supply of AZT was $8,000 or more. Since no other effective treatment could be had, activists argued that drug providers were extorting profits from vulnerable patients. The AIDS advocacy group AIDS Coalition to Unleash Power (ACT UP) staged protests at the headquarters of the FDA and Burroughs-Wellcome that brought attention to the plight of AIDS patients. Other critics pointed out that the research and drug development had been conducted by government agencies funded by taxpayers (alongside additional tax breaks to Burroughs-Wellcome).[37] The company successfully defended its patent, but vocal protests encouraged it to lower the cost, although the annual price tag was still thousands of dollars. With later AIDS drugs as well, concerned groups sought to reconcile the competing priorities of public safety, swift approval, and equitable access.

As the use of AZT increased, researchers also developed several protease inhibitors that blocked the formation of proteins that HIV requires to mature and move from one cell to another. Beginning in 1996, protease inhibitors were used in combination with AZT or similar agents to dramatically reduce the viral load in AIDS patients. The results of the combined therapy were remarkable: weak and emaciated individuals swiftly revived, and for the first time some AIDS patients could contemplate the prospect of many years with their disease under control. Lower levels of the virus also reduced

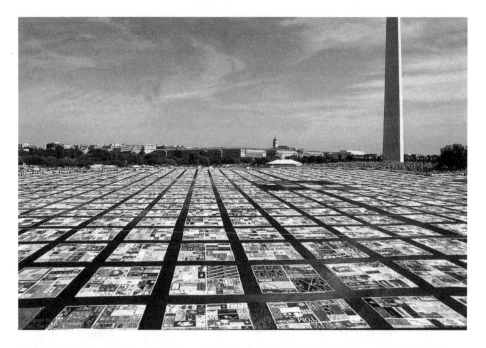

IMAGE 11.4 Panels of the AIDS Memorial Quilt on display at the US National Mall, Washington, DC. Begun by San Francisco AIDS activist Cleve Jones, the AIDS Memorial Quilt was first displayed in Washington on 11 October 1987 (shown here in 2011). The full quilt now comprises more than 49,000 panels that each measure 3 feet by 6 feet. It is the largest work of community art in the world.

the likelihood of further transmission. Worldwide, less than 3 million people had access to anti-retrovirals in 2005, but ten years later this figure had grown to 17 million. The increases in access were especially marked in southern and eastern Africa, where more than 10 million people received ARV therapy by 2015.[38]

Conclusion

The WHO has announced a goal to greatly reduce the global impact of AIDS by 2030. However, this is only one possible outcome. Worldwide, the annual decline in new infections has slowed, and an estimated 1.7 million individuals contracted HIV in 2018.[39]

What will it take to rid the world of HIV? Further reduction in HIV transmission will require sustained international commitment and efforts that are adapted to local values and norms. This challenge has political and cultural dimensions as well as public health ones. Some countries have laws that allow the criminalization of HIV infection, and millions of people face the loss of health care or other opportunities if they disclose their HIV status. Needle distribution and exchange programs, although linked to reductions in disease transmission, remain a topic of heated debate. The lack of clean needles poses a serious obstacle to HIV prevention in eastern Europe and central Asia. In this region, and particularly in Russia, reported cases of infection rose by more than 25 per cent between 2010 and 2018.[40] In central and southern Africa, gender inequality, economic insecurity, and lack of access to condoms contribute to the high prevalence of AIDS among women and adolescent girls. Since the financial and human costs of treating full-blown AIDS far exceed the expense of ARV treatment, there is positive incentive to meet this challenge. Vaccine research has also proceeded, although a shot that approaches 100 per cent effectiveness, such as the smallpox vaccine, is a remote prospect. A large-scale trial that began in South Africa in the fall of 2017 should yield results in 2020.

The campaign against AIDS in North America requires outreach to disadvantaged groups who historically have experienced social exclusion, economic inequality, and lack of access to public health services. African Americans consistently face higher rates of HIV infection than other residents of the United States, especially in the southeastern region that has a history of slavery and racial discrimination. By some estimates, the HIV prevalence among African American gay men is comparable to the level in southern Africa. In Canada, although data are not available from every province and territory, Indigenous residents in 2014 were estimated to be roughly 2.7 times more likely to contract HIV than non-Indigenous Canadians.[41] In North America overall (as well as central and western Europe), gay men and other men who have sex with men remain the population with the highest rates of infection. While many of these individuals are socially and economically secure, the blame that was initially assigned to gay men for AIDS has reinforced distrust of health authorities and their prescriptions.

For gay men, and the overlapping groups of individuals who inject drugs, perform sex work, and live without stable housing, early detection and rapid treatment requires inclusion in public health services. It has been shown that new HIV infections decline significantly when these services are provided in a supportive environment free of stigma and discrimination. While North American jurisdictions have often criminalized drug use, the city of Vancouver opened the first legally sanctioned supervised injection site on the continent in September 2003. Thereafter, the facility enjoyed substantial local support but also faced spirited opposition from politicians and antidrug advocates who questioned the morality of enabling drug use.

Although moral discourses about drugs and sex influenced the discussion of AIDS from the start, the history of the syndrome's origins carries broader lessons concerning humanity's capacity to inflict disease on itself. The spread of HIV was enabled by human actions on several levels. In large central African populations, widespread medical interventions at the village level, gendered immigration policies in colonial centers, and the disruptions of decolonization all encouraged the transmission of infections. While many facts about the early diffusion of HIV will always remain obscure, injected drugs (both therapeutic and illicit), transfusions, and other procedures involving blood exchange contributed significantly to its spread, alongside high-volume prostitution in urban centers. In North America, HIV transmission was also facilitated by expanding air travel and the loosening of sexual restraints and patterns of sexual behavior in gay and heterosexual networks. But the emergence of AIDS cannot be attributed solely, or even primarily, to the actions of a particular social group. Many forces have contributed to its spread.

The human experience of HIV/AIDS has progressed through several stages: the undetected spread, for many years, of disease caused by an invisible pathogen; its emergence, in the 1980s, as a global epidemic and focus of social anxiety; and as a pervasive scourge, sometimes managed as a chronic disease, that assumes various profiles in communities around the world. As the pandemic progresses, its diverse trajectories reveal the impact of government policies, preventive strategies, and treatments. In an era in which international collaboration is tenuous, and gross disparities exist between countries, can the pandemic be brought to an end without a new level of international collaboration?

WORKSHOP: AIDS, MEDICINE, AND COLONIALISM
IN MODERN SOUTH AFRICA

"With medicine," wrote the Afro-Caribbean philosopher and political theorist Frantz Fanon, "we come to see one of the most tragic features of the colonial situation."[42] This observation from 1965, drawn from Fanon's observation of Algeria's decolonization from France, applies to the experience of sub-Saharan Africa in the early era of AIDS.

In the year 2000, for the first time, the annual international conference on AIDS was to be held in Africa. While advocates hoped that the summit would highlight Africa's AIDS crisis—the estimate of HIV-positive individuals in sub-Saharan Africa was roughly 24 million—the run-up to the conference was marked by controversy.[43] As evidence mounted concerning the need for anti-retroviral drugs, some prominent figures in the country of South Africa, including its president Thabo Mbeki, had refused even to acknowledge that AIDS was caused by a virus. Mbeki assumed the presidency of South Africa in June 1999 as the successor to Nelson Mandela. His appointee as minister of health, Manto Tshabalala-Msimang, also proclaimed the value of a healthy diet and herbal remedies and was widely criticized by the international scientific community. Critics blamed the slow adoption of anti-retroviral therapy for unnecessary deaths, particularly since treatment can reduce the transmission of AIDS from a mother to an unborn child.

Mbeki has been roundly criticized for his refusal to accept a scientific consensus that HIV causes AIDS and for supporting treatments that were ineffective or even harmful. However, we must recognize the historical roots of AIDS denialism in South Africa. For many Africans, the legacy of Western public health interventions was mixed. Smallpox vaccinations, anti-malarial campaigns, and other measures saved many lives but were also associated with Western imperialism and the ceding of medical authority to outsiders. The inadequate initial response to HIV/AIDS in South Africa should be considered in light of its apartheid past and the broader colonial forces that this book has explored in earlier chapters.

> **"The Durban Declaration"** (*Nature*, 6 July 2000)
>
> *This proclamation was published to coincide with the opening of the XIII International AIDS Conference and specifically to respond to Mbeki and other authorities who had not acknowledged the causal role of HIV in the spread of AIDS. More than 5,000 researchers and health care professionals, including eleven Nobel Prize winners, were among the signatories. After outlining the scientific arguments for the causal role of a virus, the document announces that "HIV causes AIDS" and urges that "emphasis must be placed on preventing sexual transmission."*

AIDS spreads by infection, like many other diseases, such as tuberculosis and malaria, that cause illness and death particularly in underprivileged and impoverished communities. HIV-1, which is responsible for the AIDS pandemic, is a retrovirus closely related to a simian immuno-deficiency virus (SIV) that infects chimpanzees. HIV-2, which is prevalent in West Africa and has spread to Europe and India, is almost indistinguishable from an SIV that infects sooty mangabey monkeys. Although HIV-1 and HIV-2 first arose as zoonoses—infections transmitted from animals to humans—both now spread among humans through sexual contact; from mother to infant; and via contaminated blood. The evidence that AIDS is caused by HIV-1 or HIV-2 is clear-cut, exhaustive and unambiguous, meeting the highest standards of science. The data fulfill exactly the same criteria as for other viral diseases, such as polio, measles and smallpox:

- Patients with acquired immune deficiency syndrome, regardless of where they live, are infected with HIV. If not treated, most people with HIV infection show signs of AIDS within 5–10 years. HIV infection is identified in blood by detecting antibodies, gene sequences or viral isolation. These tests are as reliable as any used for detecting other virus infections.
- People who receive HIV-contaminated blood or blood products develop AIDS, whereas those who receive untainted or screened blood do not.
- Most children who develop AIDS are born to HIV-infected mothers. The higher the viral load in the mother, the greater the risk of the child becoming infected.
- In the laboratory, HIV infects the exact type of white blood cell (CD4 lymphocytes) that becomes depleted in people with AIDS.
- Drugs that block HIV replication in the test tube also reduce virus load in people and delay progression to AIDS. Where available, treatment has reduced AIDS mortality by more than 80 percent.
- Monkeys inoculated with cloned SIV DNA become infected and develop AIDS.

Further compelling data are available. HIV causes AIDS. It is unfortunate that a few vocal people continue to deny the evidence. This position will cost countless lives. There are many ways of communicating the vital information on HIV/AIDS, and what works best in one country may not be appropriate in another. But to tackle the disease, everyone must first understand that HIV is the enemy. Research, not myths, will lead to the development of more effective and cheaper treatments, and, it is hoped, a vaccine. But for now, emphasis must be placed on preventing sexual transmission. There is no end in sight to the AIDS pandemic. But, by working together, we have the power to reverse its tide. Science will one day triumph over AIDS, just as it did over smallpox. Curbing the spread of HIV will be the first step. Until then, reason, solidarity, political will and courage must be our partners.

**Thabo Mbeki's speech at the opening of the 13th International AIDS Conference
(Durban, 9 July 2000)**

*South Africa's president was an avowed skeptic of Western medicine, including anti-retroviral
therapy for HIV. Events prior to his Durban speech influenced the way that conference
delegates interpreted his remarks.*

*In April 2000, Mbeki sent an open letter to United States President Bill Clinton and other
addressees. He asserted that the relatively modest spread of AIDS among gay men and lesbians in
North America did not correspond to Africa's circumstances. He termed his nation's crisis "a
uniquely African catastrophe," and argued that it would be counterproductive to impose Western
solutions on an African problem. Mbeki pointedly linked his critics to the forces of apartheid, noting:*

*Not long ago, in our own country, people were killed, tortured, imprisoned and prohibited from
being quoted in private and in public because the established authority believed that their
views were dangerous and discredited. We are now being asked to do precisely the same thing
that the racist apartheid tyranny we opposed did, because, it is said, there exists a scientific
view that is supported by the majority, against which dissent is prohibited.*

*In contrast, many South Africans urged access to AZT and other drugs, particularly for
pregnant women. On the afternoon before the conference opened, Nelson Mandela's former wife
Winnie Madikizela-Mandela led a rally with thousands of supporters at the Durban city hall to
protest Mbeki's position and urge pharmaceutical companies to reduce prices for the drugs.
Hours later, Mbeki gave his opening address to the assembled conference attendees. His remarks
did not identify AIDS as a virus-caused syndrome. He emphasized the overall problem of poverty
rather than specific measures that most experts deemed necessary to slow the spread of HIV.*

Once more I welcome you all, delegates at the 13th International AIDS Conference, to Durban, to
South Africa and to Africa, convinced that you would not have come here, unless you were to us,
messengers of hope, deployed against the spectre of the death of millions from disease....

Let me tell you a story that the World Health Organization told the world in 1995. I will tell
this story in the words used by the World Health Organization. This is the story [*here Mbeki
gives an extended quote*]:

The world's biggest killer and the greatest cause of ill-health and suffering across the globe is
listed almost at the end of the International Classification of Diseases. It is given the code
Z59.5—extreme poverty.

Poverty is the main reason why babies are not vaccinated, why clean water and sanitation
are not provided, why curative drugs and other treatments are unavailable and why mothers die

in childbirth. It is the underlying cause of reduced life expectancy, handicap, disability and starvation. Poverty is a major contributor to mental illness, stress, suicide, family disintegration and substance abuse. Every year in the developing world 12.2 million children under 5 years die, most of them from causes which could be prevented for just a few US cents per child. They die largely because of world indifference, but most of all they die because they are poor....

This is part of the story that the World Health Organization told in its World Health Report in 1995. Five years later, the essential elements of this story have not changed. In some cases, the situation will have become worse....

As an African, speaking at a Conference such as this, convened to discuss a grave human problem such as the acquired human deficiency syndrome, I believe that we should speak to one another honestly and frankly, with sufficient tolerance to respect everybody's point of view, with sufficient tolerance to allow all voices to be heard. [*Mbeki pointedly omits reference to immune deficiency. This was consistent with his rejection of global health experts and his claim that poverty, not a pathogen, was the underlying cause of AIDS in Africa.*] Had we, as a people, turned our backs on these basic civilised precepts, we would never have achieved the much-acclaimed South African miracle of which all humanity is justly proud. [*Mbeki refers here to the peaceful end of legal apartheid in South Africa.*]

Some in our common world consider the questions I and the rest of our government have raised around the HIV/AIDS issue, the subject of the Conference you are attending, as akin to grave criminal and genocidal misconduct. What I hear being said repeatedly, stridently, angrily, is—do not ask any questions!

The particular twists of South African history and the will of the great majority of our people, freely expressed, have placed me in the situation in which I carry the title of President of the Republic of South Africa.

As I sat in this position, I listened attentively to the story that was told by the World Health Organization. What I heard as that story was told, was that extreme poverty is the world's biggest killer and the greatest cause of ill health and suffering across the globe. As I listened longer, I heard stories being told about malaria, tuberculosis, hepatitis B, HIV/AIDS and other diseases. I heard also about micro-nutrient malnutrition, iodine and vitamin A deficiency. I heard of syphilis, gonorrhea, genital herpes and other sexually transmitted diseases as well as teenage pregnancies. I also heard of cholera, respiratory infections, anemia, bilharzia, river blindness, guinea worms and other illnesses with complicated Latin names.

As I listened even longer to this tale of human woe, I heard the name recur with frightening frequency—Africa, Africa, Africa! And so, in the end, I came to the conclusion that as Africans we are confronted by a health crisis of enormous proportions. One of the consequences of this crisis is the deeply disturbing phenomenon of the collapse of immune systems among millions of our people, such that their bodies have no natural defense against attack by many viruses and bacteria. Clearly, if we, as African countries, had the level of development to enable us to gather accurate statistics about our own countries, our morbidity and mortality figures would tell a story that would truly be too frightening to contemplate.

As I listened and heard the whole story told about our own country, it seemed to me that we could not blame everything on a single virus. It seemed to me also that every living African, whether in good or ill health, is prey to many enemies of health that would interact one upon the other in many ways, within one human body. And thus I came to conclude that we have a desperate and pressing need to wage a war on all fronts to guarantee and realize the human right of all our people to good health....

I am pleased to inform you that some eminent scientists decided to respond to our humble request to use their expertise to provide us with answers to certain questions. Some of these have specialized on the issue of HIV/AIDS for many years and differed bitterly among themselves about various matters. Yet, they graciously agreed to join together to help us find answers to some outstanding questions. I thank them most sincerely for their positive response, inspired by a common resolve more effectively to confront the AIDS epidemic....

As I visit the areas of this city and country that most of you will not see because of your heavy program and your time limitations, areas that are representative of the conditions of life of the overwhelming majority of the people of our common world, the story told by the World Health Organization always forces itself back into my consciousness. The world's biggest killer and the greatest cause of ill health and suffering across the globe, including South Africa, is extreme poverty. Is there more that all of us should do together, assuming that in a world driven by a value system based on financial profit and individual material reward, the notion of human solidarity remains a valid precept governing human behavior!

On behalf of our government and people, I wish the 13th International AIDS Conference success, confident that you have come to these African shores as messengers of hope and hopeful that when you conclude your important work, we, as Africans, will be able to say that you who came to this city, which occupies a fond place in our hearts, came here because you care. Thank you for your attention.

Nkosi Johnson's speech at the opening of the 13th International AIDS Conference (Durban, 9 July 2000)

At age eleven, Nkosi Johnson (formerly Xolani Nkosi) addressed thousands of delegates at the opening of the conference. Born to an HIV-positive mother, Johnson had been a focus of controversy when his school, in violation of South Africa's constitution, discriminated against him on medical grounds by refusing to admit him. His adopted mother, AIDS worker Gail

Johnson, successfully sued for the school to reverse the decision and prompted schools throughout South Africa to revise their admissions policies. Gail and Nkosi Johnson founded Nkosi's Haven, an HIV/AIDS care centre devoted to mothers and children. After Nkosi's death in 2001, Nelson Mandela hailed him as "an icon for the struggle for life."

Johnson's reference to AZT medications was widely considered a rebuke to Thabo Mbeki. The South African leader rose and left the assembly while the boy was speaking.

Hi, my name is Nkosi Johnson. I live in Melville, Johannesburg, South Africa. I am eleven years old and I have full-blown AIDS. I was born HIV-positive.

When I was two years old, I was living in a care center for HIV/AIDS-infected people. My mommy was obviously also infected and could not afford to keep me because she was very scared that the community she lived in would find out that we were both infected and chase us away. I know she loved me very much and would visit me when she could. And then the care center had to close down because they didn't have any funds. So my foster mother, Gail Johnson, who was a director of the care center and had taken me home for weekends, said at a board meeting she would take me home. She took me home with her and I have been living with her for eight years now. She has taught me all about being infected and how I must be careful with my blood. If I fall and cut myself and bleed, then I must make sure that I cover my own wound and go to an adult to help me clean it and put a plaster on it. I know that my blood is only dangerous to other people if they also have an open wound and my blood goes into it. That is the only time that people need to be careful when touching me.

In 1997 mommy Gail went to the school, Melpark Primary, and she had to fill in a form for my admission and it said does your child suffer from anything so she said yes: AIDS. My mommy Gail and I have always been open about me having AIDS. And then my mommy Gail was waiting to hear if I was admitted to school. Then she phoned the school, who said we will call you and then they had a meeting about me. Of the parents and the teachers at the meeting 50 percent said yes and 50 percent said no. And then on the day of my big brother's wedding, the media found out that there was a problem about me going to school. No one seemed to know what to do with me because I am infected....

And in the same year, just before I started school, my mommy Daphne died. She went on holiday to Newcastle—she died in her sleep. And mommy Gail got a phone call and I answered and my aunty said please can I speak to Gail? Mommy Gail told me almost immediately my mommy had died and I burst into tears. My mommy Gail took me to my mommy's funeral. I saw my mommy in the coffin and I saw her eyes were closed and then I saw them lowering it into the ground and then they covered her up. My granny was very sad that her daughter had died.

Then I saw my father for the first time and I never knew I had a father. He was very upset but I thought to myself, why did he leave my mother and me? And then the other people asked mommy Gail about my sister and who would look after her and then mommy Gail said ask the father. Ever since the funeral, I have been missing my mommy lots and I wish she was with me, but I know she is in heaven. And she is on my shoulder watching over me and in my heart.

I hate having AIDS because I get very sick and I get very sad when I think of all the other children and babies that are sick with AIDS. I just wish that the government can start giving AZT [*anti-retroviral therapy*] to pregnant HIV mothers to help stop the virus being passed on to their babies....

When I grow up, I want to lecture to more and more people about AIDS—and if mommy Gail will let me, around the whole country. I want people to understand about AIDS—to be careful and respect AIDS—you can't get AIDS if you touch, hug, kiss, hold hands with someone who is infected. Care for us and accept us—we are all human beings. We are normal. We have hands. We have feet. We can walk, we can talk, we have needs just like everyone else—don't be afraid of us—we are all the same!

INTERPRETING THE DOCUMENTS

1. Thabo Mbeki asserted that AIDS had created a "uniquely African catastrophe." Why would he make this claim? What arguments could be made in support of this view, or against it?

2. Mbeki rejects the analysis offered by most scientists concerning the cause of AIDS. How does the implicit debate over scientific knowledge compare to the discussion of evidence in the debate over DDT?

3. Nkosi Johnson was described by Britain's newspaper *The Guardian* as "the boy who publicly scolded a president and woke up a nation." Why would Johnson's speech have had this effect?

MAKING CONNECTIONS

1. Between its apparent emergence in the 1980s and the early 2000s, AIDS was frequently compared to the Black Death or to bubonic plague in general. How do you consider this comparison today (both in terms of the impact of AIDS and what we know about the behavior of the two diseases)? Are there analogies to other diseases in history that seem more useful?

2. How was AIDS depicted in the North American media in the 1980s? How do various media influence your own perception of AIDS and other diseases today?

3. Should we still refer to an "HIV/AIDS" pandemic? How have HIV infection and AIDS assumed different profiles in various societies around the world?

For further reading: Didier Fassin and Helen Schneider, "The Politics of AIDS in South Africa: Beyond the Controversies," *British Medical Journal* 326 (2003): 495–97; Peter Piot, Sarah Russell, and Heidi Larson, "Good Politics, Bad Politics: The Experience of AIDS," *American Journal of Public Health* 97, no. 11 (2007): 1934–36.

Notes

1. CDC, "*Pneumocystis* Pneumonia—Los Angeles," *MMWR* 30, no. 21 (June 1981): 1–3.

2. UNAIDS, *Fact Sheet—Global AIDS Update 2019*, 1. The figures are estimates that fall within a statistical range. Extensive global and regional data are compiled in UNAIDS, *Data 2019*, https://www.unaids.org/sites/default/files/media_asset/2019-UNAIDS-data _en.pdf.

3. CDC, "HIV Transmission" (31 October 2018), https://www.cdc.gov/hiv/basics/transmission .html.

4. Steven C. Stearns and Jacob C. Koella, *Evolution in Health and Disease* (Oxford: Oxford University Press, 2007), 174–77; Paul M. Sharp and Beatrice H. Hahn, "Origins of HIV and the AIDS Pandemic," *Cold Spring Harbor Perspectives in Medicine* 1, no. 1 (2011), https://doi. org/10.1101/cshperspect.a006841.

5. Kalliopi Doudou and Paul Whiteley, "We Are All Part Virus—The Role of Human Endogenous Retroviruses," *Pharmaceutical Journal* 292, no. 7799 (2014): 244.

6. Dennis H. Osmond, "Epidemiology of AIDS in the United States," HIV InSite (March 2003), http://hivinsite.ucsf.edu/InSite?page=kb-01-03; D. Boulos et al., "Estimates of HIV Prevalence and Incidence in Canada, 2005," *Canada Communicable Disease Report* 32, no. 15 (2006): Figure 1.

7. Mirko D. Grmek, *History of AIDS: Emergence and Origin of a Modern Pandemic*, trans. Russell C. Maulitz and Jacalyn Duffin (Princeton: Princeton University Press, 1993), 23, 38; CDC, "Epidemiologic Notes and Reports: Immunodeficiency among Female Sexual Partners of Males with Acquired Immune Deficiency Syndrome (AIDS)—New York," *Mortality and Morbidity Weekly Report* 31, no. 52 (1983): 697–98.

8. Arye Rubinstein et al., "Acquired Immunodeficiency with Reversed T4/T6 Ratios in Infants Born to Promiscuous and Drug-Addicted Mothers," *Journal of the American Medical Association* 249, no. 17 (1983): 2350–56.

9. D.M. Auerbach et al., "Cluster of Cases of the Acquired Immunodeficiency Syndrome: Patients Linked by Sexual Contact," *American Journal of Medicine* 76 (March 1984): 467–92.

10. Michael Worobey et al., "1970s and 'Patient Zero' HIV-1 Genomes Illuminate Early HIV/AIDS History in North America," *Nature* 539, no. 7627 (2016): 98.

11. Richard A. McKay, *Patient Zero and the Making of the AIDS Epidemic* (Chicago: University of Chicago Press, 2017), 77–81.

12. Randy Shilts, *And the Band Played On: Politics, People and the AIDS Epidemic* (New York: St Martin's Press, 1987), 198.

13. David S. Barnes, "Targeting Patient Zero," in *Tuberculosis Then and Now*, ed. Flurin Condrau and Michael Worboys (Montreal: McGill-Queen's University Press, 2010), 51.

14. Andrew R. Moss, "AIDS without End," *New York Review of Books* 35, no. 19 (1988): 60.

15. Richard A. McKay, "'Patient Zero': The Absence of a Patient's View of the Early North American AIDS Epidemic," *Bulletin of the History of Medicine* 88, no. 1 (2014): 185–89.

16. The congressman, Henry Waxman, served as a representative from California between 1975 and 2015. Quoted in Laurie Garrett, *The Coming Plague: Newly Emerging Diseases in a World Out of Balance* (New York: Farrar, Straus and Giroux, 1994), 303.

17. Michael Hobbes, "Why Did AIDS Ravage the US More Than Any Other Developed Country?" *New Republic* (12 May 2014), https://newrepublic.com/article/117691/aids-hit-united-states-harder-other-developed-countries-why.

18. Peter Piot et al., "Acquired Immunodeficiency Syndrome in a Heterosexual Population in Zaire," *The Lancet* 324 (1984): 65–69.

19. Jacques Pepin, *The Origins of AIDS* (Cambridge: Cambridge University Press, 2011). Theories of HIV emergence are also discussed in: Tamara Giles-Vernick et al., "Social History, Biology, and the Emergence of AIDS in Colonial Africa," *Journal of African History* 54 (2013): 13–18.

20. Nora D. Volkow et al., "Drug Use Disorders: Impact of a Public Health Rather Than a Criminal Justice Approach," *World Psychiatry* 16, no. 2 (2017): 213.

21. Pepin, *Origins of AIDS*, 139–42.

22. Polly R. Walker et al., "Sexual Transmission of HIV in Africa," *Nature* 422, no. 6933 (2003): 679.

23. Jacques Pepin, "The Expansion of HIV-1 in Colonial Léopoldville, 1950s: Driven by STDs or STD Control?" *Sexually Transmitted Infections* 88, no. 4 (2012): 307–12; Nuno R. Faria et al., "The Early Spread and Epidemic Ignition of HIV-1 in Human Populations," *Science* 346, no. 6205 (2014): 59–60.

24. R. Charbonneau, *IDRC Reports* 19, no. 2 (1991): 22–23.

25. M. Thomas P. Gilbert et al., "The Emergence of HIV/AIDS in the Americas and Beyond," *Proceedings of the National Academy of Sciences* 104, no. 47 (2007): 18566–70.

26. Garrett, *Coming Plague*, 363.

27. John Iliffe, *The African AIDS Epidemic: A History* (Athens, OH: Ohio University Press, 2006), 1.

28. Johanna Hood, "Distancing Disease in the Un-black Han Chinese Politic: Othering Difference in China's HIV/AIDS Media," *Modern China* 39, no. 3 (2013): 280–318.

29. UNAIDS, "UNAIDS Data 2017" (August 2017), http://www.unaids.org/en/resources /documents/2017/HIV_estimates_with_uncertainty_bounds_1990–2016.

30. Iliffe, *African AIDS Epidemic*, 33.

31. Iliffe, *African AIDS Epidemic*, 67–95, at 71–72.

32. Iliffe, *African AIDS Epidemic*, 67.

33. Didier Fassin and Helen Schneider, "The Politics of AIDS in South Africa: Beyond the Controversies," *British Medical Journal* 326 (March 2003): 495.

34. Jade Fettig et al., "Global Epidemiology of HIV," *Infectious Disease Clinics of North America* 28, no. 3 (2014): 8–9.

35. Karen Dente and Jamie Hess, "Pediatric AIDS in Romania—A Country Faces Its Epidemic and Serves as a Model of Success," *Medscape General Medicine* 8, no. 2 (2006): 11.

36. Fettig et al., "Global Epidemiology," 5–6.

37. Victoria A. Harden, *AIDS at 30: A History* (Washington, DC: Potomac Books, 2012), 133–38.

38. UNAIDS Global Update (31 May 2016), http://www.who.int/hiv/mediacentre/news/global -aids-update-2016-news/en/.

39. This estimate lies in a range of 1.4 million to 2.3 million new infections with HIV. *UNAIDS, Global AIDS Update 2019*, 1.

40. UNAIDS, *Data 2019*, p. 8, Figure 2.6. The available data suggest that new infections in the Russian Federation account for the region's increase.

41. "Canada's 2016 Global AIDS Response Progress Report," 6, http://www.unaids.org/sites /default/files/country/documents/CAN_narrative_report_2016.pdf.

42. Frantz Fanon, *A Dying Colonialism* (New York: Grove Press, 1965), 121.

43. UNAIDS, *Report on the Global HIV/AIDS Epidemic* (June 2000), 124, http://data.unaids.org /pub/report/2000/2000_gr_en.pdf.

CONCLUSION

I n 1992, a committee of leading disease experts in the United States issued a
seminal report entitled *Emerging Infections*, which addressed health threats
that were soon categorized as "emerging and reemerging diseases." In tandem
with the growing global awareness of AIDS, the report sounded an alarm for
scientists and the public. It predicted the emergence of many new diseases in
the future. Notably, the report forecast that the majority of emerging diseases
would stem from zoonotic infections occasioned by activities that disrupt boundaries between humans and other animals or reshape physical relationships among
them. The report also suggested that efforts to perceive, detect, understand, and
respond to new threats should be grounded in the history of disease.[1]

Apart from AIDS, which is the most widespread "emerging" disease, scourges
of older vintage that include malaria, tuberculosis, and cholera continue to cause
the most morbidity and mortality. The term "reemerging" implies that these
diseases once had a much reduced impact, or even disappeared, but have now
returned. This reflects Western perceptions—in most regions, such diseases were
never tamed completely. To a large extent, their global resurgence reflects the
increased human impact upon physical landscapes and microbial environments.
For example, drug-resistant strains of malaria and insecticide-resistant mosquitoes are legacies of unsuccessful eradication attempts. Likewise, tuberculosis's
most worrisome manifestations are cases that are extensively drug-resistant
(XDR-TB), caused by bacterial strains that have evolved resistance to both first- and
second-line drugs. Infection with such pathogens is especially dangerous when

they are coincident with HIV, which spreads through contaminated injection equipment as well as sexual intercourse. Air travel recently brought cholera from Nepal to Haiti, where it had never been before, and there is the potential for warming oceans—widely acknowledged as a result of human-induced climate change—to jolt the evolution of cholera vibrios in their host plankton. So pervasive are the social determinants of disease that tuberculosis, malaria, and AIDS all assume distinct profiles according to social conditions in communities around the world. Similar to influenza in 1918, these diseases are global burdens that pose challenges that vary with local circumstances. As the authors of *Emerging Infections* realized, such health threats turn us to history in order to understand both the unity and the diversity of our current complaints.

Where emergent diseases are concerned, several crises of recent years have also confirmed the warning in the *Emerging Infections* report and posed new challenges for control. In early spring 2003, an outbreak of pneumonia-like illness—soon named SARS (severe acute respiratory syndrome)—originated in China's Guangdong province. Later research established that Chinese horseshoe bats naturally host a SARS-like virus and that the human infection came through an intermediate host, a cat-like civet, that was sold in an open-air food market. The spread of SARS eventually caused a reported 8,100 cases and 774 deaths in thirty-seven countries. In Toronto, Canada, which sustained the largest outbreak outside of Asia, authorities quarantined roughly 30,000 people. Although this measure was almost entirely voluntary, critics argued that it unnecessarily diverted resources away from more urgent tasks and raised public anxiety concerning Asian immigrants. When the University of California, Berkeley, banned Asian immigrants from its summer school, critics compared the decision to the anti-Chinese sentiment that accompanied San Francisco's response to bubonic plague in 1900.

The debate over health resources, safety, and human rights was even more urgent a decade later when EVD caused more than 11,000 deaths in a West African region at the edges of Guinea, Liberia, and Sierra Leone (2013–15). First identified in 1976, Ebola viruses normally are hosted by fruit bats and cause disease in other mammals, including chimpanzees, gorillas, and possibly monkeys. Ebola is highly contagious; it spreads through contact with infected bodily fluids, and it is believed that outbreaks begin most often after exposure to contaminated bushmeat. Once a person is infected, the virus usually causes death with profuse bloody hemorrhaging that can continue transmission. During the 2013–15 epidemic, the disease killed more than half of the infected individuals.

The nations involved did not have adequate infrastructure for a strong public health response and resorted to control measures that harkened back to earlier centuries. In August 2014, they created a *cordon sanitaire* of armed guards around a region of roughly 4,000 square miles. Liberian troops also isolated a large neighborhood in the capital city, Monrovia. Despite the need to protect neighboring regions, experts warned that the strict quarantine might cause dangerous food and water shortages and actually hamper disease control. The African nations also relied heavily on foreign aid workers and medical personnel. Ebola's reputation was so fearsome that many of these workers found themselves in quarantine for weeks after returning home. A subsequent outbreak in the Democratic Republic of the Congo that began in the summer of 2018 had caused roughly 1,000 deaths by May 2019. Although by this time a promising vaccine and experimental treatments were available, armed conflict between the government and local militias stymied medical attempts to address the crisis.

While these episodes revived questions concerning the effectiveness and legitimacy of quarantines, in 2015 researchers linked alarming birth defects to infection with the mosquito-borne Zika virus. The virus is named for the Zika forest in Uganda where scientists first isolated it from a monkey in 1947. The Zika virus is usually hosted by *Aedes*-genus mosquitoes such as *Aedes aegypti*, which is the main vector for yellow fever and dengue fever. The virus may also be transmitted sexually. Until the 2010s, scientists considered Zika infection relatively harmless, and most infected people still experience mild symptoms or none at all. Within the last few years, however, a strain of the virus has mutated so that it can damage developing brain cells after a pregnant mother passes the virus to her unborn child.[2] The resulting abnormalities include microcephaly, a condition in which a baby's head is abnormally small and the brain is not properly developed. By February 2017, roughly 2,300 Brazilian children with microcephaly were identified. Smaller numbers of cases were reported elsewhere, including the mainland United States and Puerto Rico. Similar to SARS and Ebola, the Zika threat motivated an energetic response. In February 2016, more than 200,000 Brazilian troops were mobilized to conduct a public information campaign to encourage residents in affected regions to eliminate standing water that created mosquito breeding grounds. The epidemic reignited an international debate over the use of DDT for mosquito control, which Brazil had discontinued in public health campaigns in 1999.

These three episodes from West Africa, China, and Brazil illustrate the zoonotic character of most emerging infections. But they further highlight the factor that most observers believe is the key dilemma of global health: the growing disparity among nations in resources, infrastructure, and access to health care that is a characteristic feature of the modern world.

Many observers have highlighted poverty as an important factor that contributes to the spread of infectious disease. This claim applied to the industrial cities of the nineteenth century; it applies today to low-income countries that cannot provide consistent access to clean drinking water and sanitation. Such conditions often reflect a legacy of colonial exploitation. We might broaden the claim concerning poverty to suggest that social exclusion—of which poverty is one form—is a more fundamental factor that increases the danger of infectious diseases and other undesirable health outcomes. For example, the stigma encountered by gay men in the 1980s undoubtedly contributed to the inattention that surrounded HIV/AIDS, and African Americans and Indigenous Americans still encounter barriers to health care that are only partly related to economic poverty. Elsewhere in the world, the risks of disease increase for refugees from war or those displaced by environmental disaster. Reducing economic inequality will foster global health, but it is also necessary to address determinants of disease that stem from other forms of deprivation, discrimination, and exclusion. Notably, governments in former British colonies such as Canada, Australia, and New Zealand must collaborate with Indigenous communities to create equitable models for health care delivery.

In fact, a commitment to inclusion enabled the greatest public health successes of the twentieth and early twenty-first centuries: the eradication programs for smallpox and rinderpest. WHO Director-General Halfdan Mahler called smallpox eradication a "triumph of management"—arguably, the biggest triumph was the ability of public health workers to reach individuals around the globe and persuade them to participate. Likewise, rinderpest eradication workers solicited the support of rural tribal herdsmen by effectively connecting immunization of their cattle to their own well-being. A similar commitment has informed polio immunization efforts, but these have foundered when war or religious conflict prevent full involvement. Such programs require tremendous persistence and respect on all sides. In order to succeed, health advocates cannot treat everyone the same, or assume that every community should adopt identical values and objectives.

"Inclusion" has a definite meaning when it applies to a product or treatment, such as a vaccine, that is made available to everyone. As a broader statement of purpose, however, the word can seem bland and empty. After the WHO proposed its own version of inclusion in 1978—the slogan of "Health for All by the Year 2000"—it was later criticized for focusing on a vague mirage. But lofty goals can be a starting point for change if they point the way to concrete steps—and improvement in the health of people around the world is a change that will benefit us all.

When we consider the burden of diseases, it can be helpful to contrast the human standpoint with the imagined perspective of a microbe. Human achievements in statecraft, technology, and medicine have enabled sweeping transformations of the planet. Advances such as diphtheria antitoxin, penicillin, and vaccines have improved quality of life. They relieve suffering and enable survival for many who otherwise would perish. These changes are experienced as progress, especially in wealthy nations that have reaped the greatest benefits and shifted various costs of development onto less powerful nations. But for microbes, there is no progress. Each human innovation simply brings disruptions and, quite often, new opportunities to survive and propagate. Modern transport systems, which are the sinews of a global economy, ensure that a virulent pathogen anywhere has the potential to travel everywhere. Industrial poultry farms that raise a chicken for every pot also offer vast potential for genetic exchange among viral and bacterial strains. Antibiotics and chemicals destroy many microbes, but the ones that survive are more resilient. Humans write history, but microbes have history, too. A full reckoning of past events and future solutions must take account of how one history depends on the other.

Notes

1. Committee on Microbial Threats to Health, Institute of Medicine, *Emerging Infections: Microbial Threats to Health in the United States* (Washington, DC: National Academy Press, 1992). The report outlined the need to (1) perceive the potential for epidemics, (2) detect specific threats through surveillance, (3) understand the threats through research concerning pathogens, and (4) respond vigorously. See also Frank Snowden, "Emerging and Reemerging Diseases: A Historical Perspective," *Immunological Reviews* 225, no. 1 (2008): 9–26.

2. William Wan, "Zika Was a Mild Bug; A New Discovery Shows How It Turned Monstrous," *Washington Post*, 28 September 2017.

BIBLIOGRAPHY OF
WORKSHOP TEXTS

CHAPTER 1

"Ordinances against the Spread of Plague," Duane Osheim, trans. Italian text in
Alberto Chiappelli, ed., "Gli ordinamenti sanitari del comune di Pistoia contro la
pestilenzia del 1348," *Archivio Storico Italiano* 4, no. 20 (1887): 8–22.

"An Account of the Plague in Florence," Duane Osheim, trans., Latin text in Marchione
di Coppo Stefani, *Cronaca Fiorentina*, Niccolo Rodolico, ed., *Rerum Italicarum
Scriptores 30* (1913), Rubric 643.

"Report of the Paris Medical Faculty," in *The Black Death*, ed. and trans. Rosemary
Horrox (Manchester: Manchester University Press, 1994), 158–62.

"Medical Treatise of John of Burgundy," in Horrox, *The Black Death*, 34–35. Passages
in this workshop have been lightly edited for clarity and to standardize spelling.

CHAPTER 2

William Clowes, *Lues Venerea* [*Venereal Disease*] (London, 1579), Air–Aiiiv.

Steven Gosson, *Pleasant Quippes for the Upstarte Newfangled Gentlewoman* (London,
1595), A3r–B3v.

William Shakespeare, *Timon of Athens*, Act IV, sc. iii (London, 1734), 48–51. Some
spellings have been changed for clarity.

CHAPTER 3

Reuben Gold Thwaites, ed., *The Jesuit Relations* (Cleveland: Burrows Bros,
1896–1901), vol. XIII, 112–13; vol. XV, 177–79; vol. XVI, 16–17; vol. XIX, 87–92.

CHAPTER 4

Benjamin Johnson, ed., *An Account of the Rise, Progress, and Termination of the
Malignant Fever Lately Prevalent in Philadelphia* (Philadelphia, 1794), 3–10.

Jean Devèze, *An Enquiry into, and Observations upon the Causes and Effects of the Epidemic Disease, Which Raged in Philadelphia from the Month of August till Towards the Middle of December, 1793* (Philadelphia, 1794), 18–40.

Absalom Jones and Richard Allen, *A Narrative of the Proceedings of the Black People, during the Late Awful Calamity in Philadelphia, in the Year 1793: and a Refutation of Some Censures, Thrown upon Them in Some Late Publications* (Philadelphia, 1794), 8–15.

CHAPTER 5

William Farr, "Influence of Elevation on the Fatality of Cholera," *Journal of the Statistical Society of London* 15, no. 2 (1852): 155–83.

John Snow, *On the Mode of Communication of Cholera* (London, 1855), 38–55; 97–98.

William Farr, "Report on the Cholera Epidemic of 1866 in England, Supplement to the 29th Annual Report of the Registrar General" (London, 1867–68), xxxi–xxxv.

CHAPTER 6

Robert Koch, "On the Etiology of Tuberculosis (1882)," Thomas Brock, trans., *Reviews of Infectious Disease* 4, no. 6 (1982): 1270–74.

"Formamint—The Germ-Killing Throat Tablet," *Scientific American* 112, no. 5 (1915): 109.

"5 Spots Where Germs May Lurk," *The Ladies' Home Journal* (February 1922): 72.

"Don't Ignore the Menace of the Deadly Fly," *The Ladies' Home Journal* 36 (July 1919): 73.

CHAPTER 7

Both sources are excerpted from:

Cape of Good Hope Dept of Agriculture, *Report of the Colonial Veterinary Surgeon and the Assistant Veterinary Surgeons for the Year 1896* (Cape Town: W.A. Richards & Sons, 1897).

Jotello Festiri Soga, "Mr. Soga's Report (6 February 1897)," 135–38.

Anon. [Duncan Hutcheon or John Borthwick], "Resolutions Passed at Rinderpest Conference," 24–28.

CHAPTER 8

Two selections are archived at PBS Online, *American Experience*, http://www.pbs.org /wgbh/americanexperience/features/primary-resources/influenza-letter/.

"3000 Have Influenza at Devens," *Boston Post*, 17 September 1918, 9.

Roy Grist, "Letter from Camp Devens, Mass," 29 September 1918.

"Showing the Courage of Soldiers," *New York Times*, 5 November 1918, 12.

G.R., "Letter to the Editor," *American Journal of Nursing* 19, no. 3 (1918): 203–204.

CHAPTER 9

Robert H. White-Stevens, "Communications Create Understanding," *Agricultural Chemicals* 17 (October 1962): 34–38.

Thomas H. Jukes, "People and Pesticides," *American Scientist* 51, no. 3 (1963): 55–61.

Charles F. Wurster, "DDT Proved Neither Essential Nor Safe," *Bioscience* 23, no. 2 (1973): 105–106.

CHAPTER 10

Fred Davis, *Passage through Crisis* (Indianapolis: Bobbs-Merrill Press, 1963), 138, 149–52.

Paul Longmore, "The Second Phase: From Disability Rights to Disability Culture," *The Disability Rag* 16 (September–October 1995): 3–11.

Marshall Barr, "The Iron Lung—A Polio Patient's Story," *Journal of the Royal Society of Medicine* 103, no. 6 (2010): 256–59.

CHAPTER 11

"The Durban Declaration," *Nature* 406 (6 July 2000): 15–16.

Thabo Mbeki, "Speech at the Opening of the 13th International AIDS Conference (Durban, 9 July 2000)," *AIDS Bulletin* 9, no. 3 (2000): 4–7.

Nkosi Johnson, "Speech at the Opening of the 13th International AIDS Conference (Durban, 9 July 2000)," *AIDS Bulletin* 9, no. 3 (2000): 8.

GLOSSARY

(**bold** in the definitions denotes another term in the glossary)

adaptive or **acquired immunity** An immune response that the body develops in response to a **pathogen**. In humans, **T and B lymphocytes** play key roles in this complex process. The primary goal of vaccines is to prompt an adaptive immune response.

antibiotics Medicines derived from living organisms that fight **bacteria**. Different classes of antibiotics work in various ways. Some rupture bacterial cell walls (penicillin); some inhibit the synthesis of proteins or acids (tetracycline); and others stop the replication of DNA or RNA (ciproflaxin and rifampin).

antibodies Proteins manufactured by **B lymphocytes** that respond to foreign material. Antibodies bind to foreign proteins (**antigens**) and prevent **pathogens** from attacking cells.

antigenic drift Genetic changes to the makeup of a **virus** that affect its surface proteins. Over time, mutations accumulate and make the virus more difficult for **antibodies** to recognize.

antigenic shift Abrupt change in a **virus**, either because it jumps to a new host (e.g., from pig to human) or because it exchanges genetic material with another virus. Antigenic shift makes the new virus very difficult for an immune system to recognize and resist.

antigens Proteins that a body recognizes as foreign.

antiseptic Procedures implemented at the end of the nineteenth century to limit the invasion of microbes, especially during and after surgical procedures. Carbolic acid and other chemicals were often applied or sprayed to protect against **infection**.

arbovirus A virus that is hosted and transmitted by an **arthropod**. Arboviruses include yellow fever virus and Zika virus.

arthropod A phylum of animals with segmented bodies and jointed limbs that includes insects, spiders, and crabs. Some arthropods—such as mosquitoes, flies, and lice—host microbes and are **vectors** of disease.

aseptic Procedures implemented to remove all pathogenic material from an area such as a surgical operating room. Aseptic environments often rely upon heat sterilization of implements or sealed chambers.

atoxyl An arsenic compound that was used to treat **trypanosomiasis** in animals. Although it was found to be too toxic for human use, interest in the drug motivated Paul Ehrlich's research that ultimately resulted in the anti-syphilis drug arsphenamine.

B lymphocyte A type of white blood cell responsible for manufacturing antibodies. Some B "memory" cells speed up **antibody** production when they recognize a **pathogen**.

bacillus Latin for "little wand," the term was once used in a generic sense to describe some of the earliest observed **pathogens**, including *Y. pestis* (plague) and *B. anthracis* (anthrax). It now refers to a genus of rod-shaped **bacteria** that also includes *E. coli* and *C. diphtheriae* (diphtheria).

bacteria Single-celled organisms that do not have a membrane-bound nucleus.

bejel A bacterial disease that causes mouth sores, skin disfigurement, and sometimes bone damage. Its causal **treponeme** bacteria strongly resembles the agent of venereal syphilis, but bejel usually spreads by casual contact.

bifurcated needle A needle designed to administer a drop of vaccine between two prongs. It was used for subcutaneous smallpox **vaccinations** during the eradication campaigns.

Catholic A form of Christianity whose adherents traditionally have acknowledged the authority of the pope, encouraged the actions of celibate monks and nuns, and proclaimed the power of saints. The Catholic church traces its origins to antiquity but, in the sixteenth century, it also defined itself in opposition to emerging **Protestant** traditions.

chancroid A sexually transmitted bacterial infection that causes painful genital ulcers.

Columbian exchange The wide-ranging exchange of flora and fauna (including microbes) between Europe, the Americas, and Africa that followed the arrival of Europeans in the western hemisphere in the 1490s.

consumption Term for a "wasting disease," especially one involving the lungs. It was often interchangeable with the Greek term **phthisis**. Cases of consumption probably included pulmonary tuberculosis and perhaps other diseases with similar symptoms.

contact tracing The identification, examination, and follow-up of individuals who may have had contact with a person infected with a given disease. Contact tracing may help establish the characteristics of a novel **infection**, such as its **latency period** and its typical clinical symptoms.

contagion A Latin term used in various ways since the Middle Ages to refer to the spread of disease among persons or objects. In the early modern period it often was used to contrast with the notion that diseases spread by atmospheric **miasmas** rather than direct contact. Today, "contagious" is often used interchangeably with "communicable," especially to refer to diseases such as influenza that pass easily from one person to another.

cordons sanitaires Barriers to overland travel or trade that are intended to separate or isolate regions that are affected by an outbreak of contagious disease.

Creutzfeldt-Jacob disease A degenerative nerve disorder caused by abnormally formed proteins. It is classified with BSE (mad cow disease) in a group of "spongiform encephalopathy disorders." They are so named because sponge-like lesions in brain tissue are a characteristic symptom.

cytokines Protein secretions from cells in the immune system that help coordinate the activities of other cells.

dengue (or **dengue fever**) A flu-like viral **infection** that is spread primarily by *Aedes aegypti* mosquitoes. Although not always lethal, severe dengue remains a leading cause of serious illness and death in some countries of Asia and Latin America.

diphtheria Bacterial infection that affects mucous membranes in the nose and throat. Among other symptoms, it destroys tissue in the mouth and creates a coating or "pseudomembrane" that can block the throat and impede breathing.

dysentery A state of intestinal inflammation and diarrheal disease that may be caused by various **enteric bacteria**.

El Niño The periodic formation of a band of warm water in the Pacific Ocean off the coast of South America. It is the warm phase of a recurring climate pattern, the El Niño Southern Oscillation.

elimination Where the prevalence of disease is concerned, the term denotes complete (but not necessarily permanent) removal of a disease from a given region or continent.

endemic The term refers to human diseases that persist in a given region, often at a low level of **incidence**.

enteric bacteria Bacteria that inhabit the stomach and the intestines. They include *V. cholera* and other **pathogens** that cause diarrheal illnesses.

enzootic Similar to **endemic**, the term refers to animal diseases that persist in a given region, often at a low level of **incidence**.

epidemic Used historically to refer to substantial episodes of disease that develop rapidly in a city or region. Technical definitions define epidemics in terms of the number of cases of a disease above an accepted baseline in a given time interval.

epidemiology The study of the distribution of diseases (their **incidence**, **prevalence**, transmission, and other variables) and the conditions that influence health and disease within defined populations.

epizootic An outbreak of disease among nonhuman animals.

eradication The complete removal of a disease from nature. Human intervention has accomplished this feat with smallpox and rinderpest.

etiology The cause(s) of a disease or manner in which a disease originates.

filariasis A disease caused by microscopic roundworms. Sufferers experience profound liquid retention (lymphedema) in limbs or groin that is disfiguring and can be disabling.

general paresis A neurological condition observed among some sufferers of late-stage syphilis in which brain damage causes erratic behavior, loss of control over limbs, or mental incompetence.

gonorrhea Sexually transmitted **infection** caused by the **bacteria** *Neisseria gonorrhea*. Untreated, the disease may damage reproductive organs and cause infertility in women or men.

guaiac A hard, resinous wood indigenous to parts of South America and the Caribbean. It was used in therapeutic potions and salves for the cure of the pox in early modern Europe.

Guinea worm disease (dracunculiasis) An **infection** caused by parasitic worms that may be several inches long. The worms migrate through the body before emerging (usually from the feet) and causing painful sores.

herd immunity A threshold that a community reaches when the level of immunity among its members is sufficiently high to prevent a disease from causing a large outbreak. The level required for effective herd immunity varies among diseases.

humanism A European intellectual movement that attempted to renew society and culture by emulating classical learning and literature. Beginning among the learned elite of fourteenth-century Italy, scholars retrieved ancient Latin and Greek works and commented on their value, often in contrast to medieval "scholastic" approaches to knowledge. Humanist scholarship and values informed numerous debates concerning politics, religion, medicine, and other fields.

humors (doctrine) Ancient medical framework that considered four fluids (blood, phlegm, yellow bile, and black bile) to be the basis of physiology and pathology. Good health emerged from a proper balance of the humors. Regimens and medicines were conceived to maintain or restore this balance.

immune competence The suite of physical characteristics that contributes to a person's ability to resist disease.

immunization Often used synonymously with **vaccination**. It is the broadest term used to refer to the use of vaccines or antitoxins in the body in order to produce resistance or full immunity to a **pathogen**.

incidence The occurrence of new cases of a disease in a given time frame and geographic area. See also **prevalence**.

incubation period The interval between the arrival of a **pathogen** in the body and the emergence of symptoms. It can be related to **latency period**, but the two are not necessarily the same.

infection Similar to **contagion**, the term referred historically to the spread either of disease or of the factors that caused disease. The term is now usually deployed more narrowly to indicate disease that is spread through the action of microbes.

innate immunity Mechanisms for resisting disease that do not reflect a body's previous exposure to a **pathogen** or medical interventions that influence immunity (such as a vaccine). Innate immune responses include inflammation, destruction of foreign cells, and the destruction of body cells that have been compromised. There are intricate links between innate immune responses and **adaptive** immune responses.

inoculation The introduction of diseased material beneath the skin to induce a mild case of the disease. It was correctly believed (although a precise explanation was lacking) that the procedure would stimulate resistance in the body when it was exposed to the diseased material again. With respect to smallpox, the term was often used interchangeably with **variolation**.

lancet A pronged instrument (usually with five points) used through the nineteenth century for surgical procedures or for **inoculation**.

latency period The interval between the arrival of a **pathogen** in the body and the time that one person is infectious to another. This can be related to the **incubation period**, as symptoms (such as coughing) may also transmit **infection**.

leprosy From late antiquity through the Middle Ages, this referred to a stigmatizing condition marked by deformed extremities and cartilage, disfiguring skin conditions, and a hoarse voice. Uncertainty persists concerning its actual prevalence in the distant past. Modern cases, which are named Hansen's disease, are identified by the presence of the **bacteria** *Mycobacterium leprae*.

lock hospitals Facilities that were dedicated to the treatment and control of individuals who had the pox. The term "lock" apparently has its origins in late medieval London and evokes the overlap in space and function between earlier facilities created for lepers and pox houses.

lymph A fluid that circulates through lymph vessels and performs various functions related to blood circulation and immune function. It transports **bacteria** to lymph nodes and moves fats, proteins, and interstitial fluid around the body.

lyophilization Techniques of freeze-drying blood plasma or vaccine materials. Its use enabled the transport of vaccines to remote areas without cold storage. This contributed to the eradication of smallpox and rinderpest.

macrophages Cells that are specialized to detect and consume foreign microbes, their products, and dead cells.

measles A highly infectious viral disease that was ubiquitous among children prior to the introduction of **antibiotics**. Symptoms, which may include high fever and rash, ensue after an incubation period of about ten days. Measles also causes immune suppression and may contribute to increased **morbidity** and **mortality** from **opportunistic infections**.

Medieval Climate Anomaly An era (ca 950–1250) of relatively warm and dry weather worldwide. Historians of climate suggest that it coincided with high crop yields and population expansion.

miasma A cloud of unhealthy or noxious air or gas that was considered a cause of disease. Historically, the spread of plague, malaria, and other diseases was often attributed to miasmas.

microbiome The array or community of microbes (**bacteria, viruses,** fungi, etc.) that live in an ecosystem or an organism. Human microbiomes contain trillions of microbes that inhabit almost every body part.

molecular clock hypothesis The assumptions that DNA and proteins evolve over time at a relatively constant rate and that such molecular evolution will occur at a similar rate in closely related organisms. By inference, the genetic differences between two species of organisms (such as **viruses**) will be related to the time that has elapsed since they last shared a common ancestor.

morbidity Measure or rate of a particular disease or ill health.

morbillivirus A genus of viruses that includes measles and also included rinderpest. Morbilliviruses spread by a respiratory route, are highly contagious, cause immune suppression, and may cause large outbreaks among previously unexposed populations.

mortality Measure or rate of death.

neuraminidase inhibitors Used to combat influenza. Drugs that block the action of the neuraminidase enzyme prevent the **virus** from replicating.

opportunistic infection An infection that develops after a person's degree of immunity or resistance has been lowered by a previous stress that causes immune suppression. Pneumonia and tuberculosis are opportunistic infections that commonly affect people who live with HIV.

pandemic A human disease event that involves a wide geographic area such as a continent or even the entire world. The influenza pandemic of 1918–19 is the outstanding example of a global pandemic.

panzootic An animal disease event that involves a wide geographic area such as a continent or even the entire world. The African rinderpest panzootic of the late nineteenth century is an outstanding example.

paracultivation Food procurement practices that involve the replanting of wild plants in or near their original habitat, as opposed to clearing land and creating fields dedicated to crops.

pasteurization The treating, usually with heat, of packaged or bottled foods to destroy **bacteria** and inactivate enzymes that lead to spoilage.

pathogen A Greek word that literally means "producer of suffering." Today, the term usually refers to disease-causing microbes such as **bacteria**, **viruses**, or **protozoa**.

penicillin A mold that has **antibiotic** properties. In the 1940s, pencillin became the first living microbe to be used to destroy harmful **bacteria**.

phthisis An ancient Greek term for lung disease, used until the nineteenth century. Over the centuries, the term referred to cases of pulmonary tuberculosis and a range of other diseases with similar symptoms.

phylogenetic analysis A procedure for discerning evolutionary relationships among organisms or populations. In the study of microbes, variations in DNA are used to construct trees with branching orders that characterize lineages. This provides a framework for understanding changes over time in a microbe's traits or geographic movement.

plantation complex An economic and political order that was based on slave plantations, such as the network of island outposts in the Caribbean during the early modern period. Controlled in Europe, with slaves from Africa and trading interests in India, the impact of this plantation complex spanned the globe.

polymerase chain reaction A procedure in molecular biology to make millions of copies of a given segment of DNA. An enzyme and a primer are added to a DNA strand and subjected to heating and cooling to prompt a chain reaction of DNA manufacture.

polytomy This term is used in **phylogenetic analysis** to indicate a divergence of one evolutionary branch into three or more lineages. As with the **bacteria** Y. pestis, it may refer to the emergence of several strains or species of an organism from a common ancestor.

prevalence A measure of the individuals affected by a disease at a particular time.

Protestant Several branches of Christianity that originated from dissent within the European church in the sixteenth century. Protestants rejected the authority of the pope, advocated reading the Bible in vernacular languages, and rejected withdrawal from the secular world by monks and nuns.

protozoa Single-celled animals that have a membrane-bound nucleus (in contrast to **bacteria**, which do not have one).

quarantine Isolation measures to separate people or goods thought to be contaminated (or at risk of contamination) with harmful poisons or diseases. Used consistently in Europe since the fourteenth century, quarantine measures long predated modern understandings of **infection**.

quinine A chemical compound containing nitrogen that occurs naturally in the cinchona plant. Quinine neutralizes malarial parasites at various stages of their development.

quorum sensing The ability of **bacteria** to adjust their behavior in response to signals from other bacteria. Quorum sensing bacteria release chemical signals that enable them to assess the size of their community and to adjust their gene expression once a threshold is reached.

retrospective diagnosis The attempt to identify diseases of the past in terms of modern diagnostic categories.

retrovirus A virus composed of RNA that uses a **reverse transcriptase** enzyme to recruit a cell's DNA to manufacture more genetic material. The enzyme lacks a "proofreading" ability for transcription of genetic material, which is one reason that retroviruses mutate swiftly. Because retroviruses include DNA in their replication cycle, they are not classified as **RNA viruses**. HIV is a retrovirus.

reverse transcriptase An enzyme that enables an **RNA virus** to manufacture complementary DNA that can then integrate into the host organism's own genome.

RNA viruses Viruses that have ribonucleic acid (RNA) as their genetic material. RNA viruses generally mutate rapidly because their polymerases do not have the same "proofreading" ability that DNA polymerases do. This characteristic makes it more difficult to devise effective vaccines for diseases caused by RNA viruses. Ebola, SARS, influenza, **measles**, and the common cold are all caused by RNA viruses.

sanatorium Institution devoted to the care of people who suffered from **consumption** or tuberculosis.

sanitarian In nineteenth-century Britain, a supporter of measures taken to reduce dirt and filth, and therefore to foster lower rates of disease. Outstanding sanitarians included Edwin Chadwick (1800–1890) and Florence Nightingale (1820–1910).

seasoning A term formerly used to describe acclimation to climate and environment by immigrants to a region. Slaves and colonists were considered "seasoned," and thus more resistant to local maladies, after they withstood one or more episodes of (often tropical) disease.

sebaceous glands Skin glands in mammals that contain sebum, an oil that provides moisture and protection for skin and hair.

seropositivity Refers to blood samples that react positively to tests for **antibodies**. The presence of specific antibodies indicates that the body has been exposed to a particular infectious agent such as a **virus**. For people who have contracted HIV, a test that indicates seropositivity is an early sign of the need for medical intervention.

single nucleotide polymorphism (SNP) A variation that occurs at a precise position in a genome when an allele is changed, deleted, or added. Evolutionary biologists use SNPs to trace the history of organisms, especially microbes with small genomes that can be fully reconstructed and analyzed.

Sitala Ancient Indian goddess of healing for poxes, sores, and other maladies.

social construction An approach to history (of science and medicine in particular) that stresses the influence of social context upon perceptions of disease or other aspects of nature.

streptomycin A soil microbe with antibiotic properties. Isolated in the 1950s, streptomycin was the first of a class of "–icin" **antibiotics** that remain in wide use.

sulfa drugs (sulfonamides) These antibacterial agents were created from synthetic chemical compounds. In wide use during the late 1930s and 1940s, sulfa drugs were often replaced by **penicillin** and other **antibiotics**, but they remain in use for some therapies.

T lymphocytes White blood cells that perform various functions for the immune system.

trachoma A bacterial **infection** that affects the inner eyelid. Although treatable with **antibiotics**, the infection can lead to blindness if untreated.

treponemes Spiral-shaped **bacteria** that cause venereal syphilis and several other human diseases.

trypanosomes A genus of single-celled **protozoa**. In Africa, trypanosomes are hosted by tsetse flies and cause diseases among both humans and mammals.

trypanosomiasis The diseases of animals and humans that are caused by **trypanosomes**. The severe form of Human African Trypanosomiasis (HAT), commonly known as sleeping sickness, occurs when the **protozoa** invade brain tissue to cause sleep disorder, seizures, and death.

typhoid (or typhoid fever) Caused by the **bacteria** *Salmonella typhi*, typhoid is contracted from food and drinking water contaminated by feces. It is possible to host and spread the bacteria without displaying obvious symptoms.

typhus A group of diseases caused by related **bacteria**. Epidemic typhus is caused by *Rickettsia prowazekii* and spread by discharges from body lice that host the bacteria. The disease can be lethal, and its symptoms include high fever and chills, headache, aching muscles, and a rash that begins on the back or the chest.

vaccination Historically, the term first described Edward Jenner's substitution of cowpox material for smallpox material in **inoculation** procedures. Often interchangeable with **immunization**, it now refers more broadly to the introduction of similar vaccines into the body.

variolation Often used interchangeably with **inoculation**. It describes the formerly widespread practice of introducing smallpox *Variola* into the body to induce an immune response. The procedure was superseded by **vaccination** with cowpox material.

vector An organism, such as an insect, that transmits a **pathogen** to another organism. The vector organism may host a stage of development in the pathogen's life cycle and participate in a cycle of transmission. For example, malarial **protozoa** mature and reproduce in mosquitoes, the offspring develop further in humans and reproduce again, and immature forms return to mosquitoes.

viremia Denotes a stage of illness in which **viruses** enter the bloodstream.

virgin soil epidemic Refers to the impact of a disease when it encounters a new population. The concept rests on the assumption that populations without prior exposure to a **pathogen** will face far higher **morbidity** and **mortality** than experienced populations.

virulence In the context of disease, the term refers to a **pathogen's** capacity to damage the health of an individual.

virus A microorganism that typically consists of nucleic acid in a protein sheath. Viruses are smaller than **bacteria** and cannot grow or reproduce apart from a living cell.

yaws A disease caused by **treponemes**. Often a disease of children in tropical regions, the disease initially causes skin ulcers and later bone damage.

zoonoses Infections that originate in animals and jump to humans.

SUGGESTED
READING

The following texts provide suitable starting points for further investigation of many topics. Some of the listed works are cited in the chapters, and others are additional resources.

Introduction

Two encyclopedias offer broad essay collections with abundant citations: Mark Jackson, ed., *The Routledge History of Disease* (New York: Routledge, 2016); and Kenneth Kiple, *Cambridge World History of Human Disease* (Cambridge: Cambridge University Press, 1993). Also useful: James L.A. Webb Jr, "Globalization of Disease, 1300–1900," in *The Cambridge World History*, eds Jerry H. Bentley, Sanjay Subrahmanyam, and Merry E. Wiesner-Hanks (Cambridge: Cambridge University Press, 2015), 54–75. Two articles discuss issues pertaining to history in a global framework: Mark Harrison, "A Global Perspective: Reframing the History of Health, Medicine, and Disease," *Bulletin of the History of Medicine* 89, no. 4 (2015): 639–89; and the more skeptical view of Sarah Hodges, "Second Opinion: The Global Menace," *Social History of Medicine* 25, no. 3 (2012): 719–28.

Several works range across diseases and themes: Peter Baldwin's government-oriented *Contagion and the State in Europe, 1830–1930* (Cambridge: Cambridge University Press, 1999); Sheldon J. Watts's extended critique of Western imperialism, *Epidemics and History: Disease, Power and Imperialism* (New Haven: Yale University Press, 1999); and Mark Harrison, *Contagion: How*

Commerce Has Spread Disease (New Haven: Yale University Press, 2012). For recent thematic discussions: Robert Peckham, *Epidemics in Modern Asia* (Cambridge: Cambridge University Press, 2016); and Randall M. Packard, *A History of Global Health: Interventions in the Lives of Other Peoples* (Baltimore: Johns Hopkins University Press, 2016). Older, but insightful and fascinating is Laurie Garrett, *The Coming Plague: Newly Emerging Diseases in a World Out of Balance* (New York: Farrar, Straus and Giroux, 1994).

For a history of medicine, consult Jacalyn Duffin, *History of Medicine: A Scandalously Short Introduction*, 2nd ed. (Toronto: University of Toronto Press, 2010); and W.F. Bynum et al., *The Western Medical Tradition: 1800–2000* (Cambridge: Cambridge University Press, 2006). For the development of history of medicine as a discipline, numerous topics are discussed in Frank Huisman and John Harley Warner, *Locating Medical History: The Stories and Their Meanings* (Baltimore: Johns Hopkins University Press, 2004). See also Charles E. Rosenberg, "Erwin H. Ackerknecht, Social Medicine, and the History of Medicine," *Bulletin of the History of Medicine* 81, no. 3 (2007): 511–32; and Naomi Rogers, "Explaining Everything? The Power and Perils of Reading Rosenberg," *Journal of the History of Medicine and Allied Sciences* 63, no. 4 (2008): 423–34.

The US National Library of Medicine hosts a large website with numerous scientific and historical resources. Digital collections, online exhibits, and other historical materials are available at https://www.nlm.nih.gov/hmd/index.html.

At Harvard University, the online collection *Contagion: Historical Views of Disease and Epidemics* presents hundreds of full-text historical works: https://library.harvard.edu/collections/contagion-historical-views-diseases-and-epidemics.

For resources particular to Canada, finding guides for online resources are available at the websites for the College of Family Physicians of Canada: https://www.cfpc.ca/ProjectAssets/Templates/Resource.aspx?id=1508&langType=4105.

Chapter 1

The articles in Volume 1 of *The Medieval Globe* (2014), especially the introduction by Monica Green, offer a good starting point for this large literature. They are archived at https://scholarworks.wmich.edu/medieval_globe/1/. See also Bruce M.S. Campbell, *The Great Transition: Climate, Disease and Society in the Late-Medieval World* (Cambridge: Cambridge University Press, 2016). For the earlier Middle Ages consult Peregrine Horden, "The Millennium Bug: Health and Medicine around the

Year 1000," *Social History of Medicine* 13, no. 2 (2000): 200–19; and Faith Wallis, "Disease 1000–1300," in *A Handbook of Medieval Environmental History, Vol. II: 1000–1350*, ed. P. Slavin and T. Newfield (Leiden: Brill, 2020).

For early modern Europe, classic studies include Anne G. Carmichael, *Plague and the Poor in Renaissance Florence* (Cambridge: Cambridge University Press, 1986); Paul Slack, *Impact of Plague in Tudor and Stuart England* (Oxford: Clarendon Press, 1985); and Carlo M. Cipolla, *Faith, Reason, and the Plague in Seventeenth-Century Tuscany* (Ithaca, NY: Cornell University Press, 1979). Edward A. Eckert, *The Structure of Plague and Pestilences in Early Modern Europe: Central Europe 1560–1640* (Basel: Karger, 1996) provides a quantitative regional study. For the eastern Mediterranean: Nükhet Varlik, *Plague and Empire in the Early Modern Mediterranean World* (Cambridge: Cambridge University Press, 2015).

For plague since the late nineteenth century see Myron Echenberg, *Plague Ports: The Global Impact of Bubonic Plague, 1894–1901* (New York: New York University Press, 2007); Guenter B. Risse, *Plague, Fear, and Politics in San Francisco's Chinatown* (Baltimore, MD: Johns Hopkins University Press, 2012); Nayan Shah, *Contagious Divides: Epidemics and Race in San Francisco's Chinatown* (Berkeley, CA: University of California Press, 2001); and, for recent developments, Paul S. Mead, "Plague in Madagascar—A Tragic Opportunity for Improving Public Health," *New England Journal of Medicine* 378 (January 2018): 106–108.

Chapter 2

For a comprehensive survey, one may still use Claude Quétel, *History of Syphilis*, trans. Judith Braddock and Brian Pike (Baltimore: Johns Hopkins University Press, 1990). For Europe, John Henderson, John Arrizabalaga, and Roger French, *The Great Pox: The French Disease in Renaissance Europe* (New Haven, CT: Yale University Press, 1997) focuses on learned medicine. Gender is a prominent theme in Laura J. McGough, *Gender, Sexuality, and Syphilis in Early Modern Venice* (New York: Palgrave Macmillan, 2010). Vivian Nutton, "The Seeds of Disease: An Explanation of Contagion and Infection from the Greeks to the Renaissance," *Medical History* 27, no. 1 (1983): 1–34, is a classic study of premodern medical theory. For treatment: John Parascandola, "From Mercury to Miracle Drugs: Syphilis Treatment over the Centuries," *Pharmacy in History* 51, no. 1 (2009): 14–23. For early modern England: Kevin P. Siena, *Venereal Hospitals and the Urban Poor: London's "Foul Wards," 1600–1800* (Rochester: University of Rochester Press, 2004).

For syphilis in the nineteenth century: Mary Spongberg, *Feminizing Venereal Disease: The Body of the Prostitute in Nineteenth-Century Medical Discourse* (New York: New York University Press, 1998); for a US history beginning in the colonial era: John Parascandola, *Sex, Sin, and Science: A History of Syphilis in America* (Westport, CT: Praeger, 2008). Susan M. Reverby, ed., *Tuskegee's Truths: Rethinking the Tuskegee Syphilis Study* (Chapel Hill, NC: University of North Carolina Press, 2000), includes a literature review and essays on the topic. Non-Western regions are discussed in the essay collection edited by Milton Lewis, Scott Bamber, and Michael Waugh, *Sex, Disease and Society: A Comparative History of Sexually Transmitted Diseases and HIV/ AIDS in Asia and the South Pacific* (Westport, CT: Greenwood Press, 1997); Megan Vaughan, *Curing Their Ills: Colonial Power and African Illness* (Stanford: Stanford University Press, 1991), 129–54; and Karen Jochelson, *The Colour of Disease: Syphilis and Racism in South Africa, 1880–1950* (New York: Palgrave, 2001).

Paul Ehrlich's biography is depicted in the film *Dr. Ehrlich's Magic Bullet* (directed by William Dieterle, 1940). The made-for-television film *Miss Evers' Boys* (directed by Joseph Sargent, 1992) chronicles the Tuskegee Syphilis Experiment.

Chapter 3

Donald R. Hopkins, *The Greatest Killer: Smallpox in History* (Chicago: University of Chicago Press, 2002 [1983]), provides an overview. The causes of mortality among Indigenous American peoples after the arrival of Europeans has been a topic of enduring interest. James C. Riley, "Smallpox and American Indians Revisited," *Journal of the History of Medicine and Allied Sciences* 65, no. 4 (2010): 445–77, reviews theories for Indigenous demographic decline. Catherine M. Cameron, Paul Kelton, Alan C. Swedlund, eds, *Beyond Germs: Native Depopulation in North America* (Tucson: University of Arizona Press, 2015), presents essays that highlight social factors. See also Paul Kelton, *Cherokee Medicine, Colonial Germs: An Indigenous Nation's Fight against Smallpox* (Norman: University of Oklahoma Press, 2015). David S. Jones explores the colonizers' perspective on Indigenous diseases over the long term in *Rationalizing Epidemics: The Meanings and Uses of American Indian Mortality since 1600*. Elizabeth A. Fenn, "The Great Smallpox Epidemic of 1775–82," *History Today* 53, no. 8 (2003): 10–17, concisely introduces the smallpox outbreak during the US Revolutionary War.

Elsewhere, for smallpox in the Atlantic World consult Dauril Alden and Joseph C. Miller, "Out of Africa: The Slave Trade and the Transmission of

Smallpox to Brazil, 1560–1831," *Journal of Interdisciplinary History* 18, no. 2 (1987): 195–224. David Arnold, "Epidemic Smallpox in India," *Historically Speaking* 9, no. 78 (2008): 31–33, offers a concise discussion. Akihito Suzuki, "Smallpox and the Epidemiological Heritage of Modern Japan: Towards a Total History," *Medical History* 55, no. 3 (2011): 313–18, offers a brief, instructive comparison.

Edward Jenner's smallpox vaccine and later vaccines (BCG, influenza, polio) are addressed in an essay collection edited by Stanley Plotkin, *History of Vaccine Development* (New York: Springer, 2011). For an engaging account of the eradication campaign from the 1950s, see the World Health Organization, *Bugs, Drugs and Smoke* (Geneva: WHO Press), 1–22. More critical is Sanjoy Bhattacharya, "Uncertain Advances: A Review of the Final Phases of the Smallpox Eradication Campaign in India, 1960–80," *American Journal of Public Health* 94, no. 11 (2004): 1875–82.

Chapter 4

J.R. McNeill, *Mosquito Empires* (Cambridge: Cambridge University Press, 2010), is an excellent account of yellow fever in the early modern Caribbean. McNeill provides a brief sketch of his argument in "Yellow Jack and Geopolitics: Environment, Epidemics, and the Struggle for Empire in the Caribbean, 1650–1825," *OAH Magazine of History* 18, no. 3 (2004): 9–13. For the literary resonance of disease during the era, see Emily Senior, *The Caribbean and the Medical Imagination, 1764–1834: Slavery, Disease and Colonial Modernity* (Cambridge: Cambridge University Press, 2018). Yellow fever's formative influence upon European disease surveillance is discussed in William Coleman, *Yellow Fever in the North: The Methods of Early Epidemiology* (Madison: University of Wisconsin Press, 1987). For the United States in the nineteenth century: Margaret Humphreys, *Yellow Fever and the South* (Baltimore: Johns Hopkins University Press, 1999).

For Latin America in the twentieth century see Paul Sutter, "'The First Mountain to Be Removed': Yellow Fever Control and the Construction of the Panama Canal," *Environmental History* 21, no. 2 (2016): 250–59. A more pointed analysis of public health's role in US imperialism and social control is offered by Warwick Anderson, *Colonial Pathologies: American Tropical Medicine, Race, and Hygiene in the Philippines* (Durham, NC: Duke University Press, 2006). Essays on yellow fever and other diseases are included in Alison Bashford, ed., *Medicine at the Border: Disease, Globalization and Security, 1850 to the Present* (New York: Palgrave Macmillan, 2006).

Chapter 5

The literature concerning various aspects of cholera in Europe is very large. Richard J. Evans, *Death in Hamburg: Society and Politics in the Cholera Years, 1830–1910* (Oxford: Clarendon Press, 1987), is a classic social history, as is Frank M. Snowden, *Naples in the Time of Cholera* (Cambridge: Cambridge University Press, 1996). Christopher Hamlin's *Cholera: The Biography* (Oxford: Oxford University Press, 2009) pursues the topic to the present and deals principally with questions concerning the perception of cholera.

Public health developments in mid-nineteenth-century London are extensively researched. See Christopher Hamlin, *Public Health and Social Justice in the Age of Chadwick: Britain, 1800–1854* (Cambridge: Cambridge University Press, 1998). For William Farr's contribution to medical statistics: John Eyler, "The Conceptual Origins of William Farr's Epidemiology," in *Times, Places, and Persons: Aspects of the History of Epidemiology*, ed. Abraham Lilienfeld (Baltimore: Johns Hopkins University Press, 1979), 1–21; and Ian Hacking, *The Taming of Chance* (Cambridge: Cambridge University Press, 1990), 47–54. Among many accounts of John Snow, a wide-ranging co-authored volume merits attention: Peter Vinten-Johansen et al., *Cholera, Chloroform and the Science of Medicine* (Oxford: Oxford University Press, 2003).

For cholera in India, see David Arnold, *Colonizing the Body: State Medicine and Epidemic Disease in Nineteenth-Century India* (Berkeley, CA: University of California Press, 1993), 159–99. For Iran: Amir J. Afkhami, *A Modern Contagion: Imperialism and Public Health in Iran's Age of Cholera* (Baltimore: Johns Hopkins University Press, 2019). For Africa: Myron Echenberg, *Africa in the Time of Cholera: A History of Pandemics from 1817 to the Present* (New York: Cambridge University Press, 2011). Although polemical, Ralph R. Frerichs, *Deadly River: Cholera and Cover-Up in Post-Earthquake Haiti* (Ithaca, NY: Cornell University Press, 2016), is the best account of a major recent epidemic.

Chapter 6

Helen Bynum's *Spitting Blood: The History of Tuberculosis* (Oxford: Oxford University Press, 2012) is a well-written recent survey; recent European studies include David S. Barnes, *The Making of a Social Disease: Tuberculosis in Nineteenth-Century France* (Berkeley: University of California Press, 1995). For the United States, Sheila M. Rothman's *Living in the Shadow of Death: Tuberculosis and the Social Experience of Illness in American History* (New York: Basic Books, 1994) focuses on sick people's experiences and frequent loss of autonomy in institutions.

The scientific and cultural shift from consumption to tuberculosis has elicited considerable scholarly interest. Documents related to the transition are collected in Barbara Gutmann Rosenkrantz, ed., *From Consumption to Tuberculosis: A Documentary History* (New York: Garland Publishers, 1994). Robert Koch's biography and the early development of microbiology are woven together in Christoph Gradmann, *Laboratory Disease: Robert Koch's Medical Bacteriology* (Baltimore: Johns Hopkins University Press, 2011). Social control and border control are considered in Amy Fairchild, *Science at the Borders: Immigrant Medical Inspection and the Shaping of the Modern Industrial Labor Force* (Baltimore: Johns Hopkins University Press, 2003).

For two generations, scholars have debated the causes of mortality decline and the respective roles of nutrition and living standards, medical treatments and vaccines, and sanitary measures. Bill Bynum neatly summarizes the issues and the career of the main disputant, Thomas McKeown, in "The McKeown Thesis," *The Lancet* 371 (2008): 644–45. The significance of tuberculosis for Native American communities is discussed in Mary Ellen Kelm, *Colonizing Bodies: Aboriginal Health and Healing in British Columbia, 1900–50* (Vancouver: UBC Press, 2011). Reflections on the resurgence of tuberculosis are collected in Matthew Gandy and Alimuddin Zumla, eds, *The Return of the White Plague: Global Poverty and the "New" Tuberculosis* (London: Verso, 2003). For Africa: Randall Packard, *White Plague Black Labor: Tuberculosis and the Political Economy of Health and Disease in South Africa* (Berkeley: University of California Press, 1989).

Katherine Byrne, *Tuberculosis and the Victorian Literary Imagination* (Cambridge: Cambridge University Press, 2011), discusses the disease in the works of Charles Dickens, Bram Stoker, the Brontë sisters, and others. The Canadian documentary film *Coppermine* (directed by Ray Harper, 1992) chronicles a 1929 outbreak of pulmonary tuberculosis in an Inuit community.

Chapter 7

The English literature concerning rinderpest is more modest than for other epidemic diseases. The requisite starting points are the large, encyclopedic work by C.A. Spinage, *Cattle Plague: A History* (New York: Plenum, 2003), and the essay collection edited by Karen Brown and Daniel Gilfoyle, *Healing the Herds: Disease,*

Livestock Economies and the Globalization of Veterinary Medicine (Athens, OH: Ohio University Press, 2010). For the European fourteenth century: Philip Slavin, "The Great Bovine Pestilence and Its Economic and Social Consequences in England and Wales," *Economic History Review* 65, no. 4 (2012): 1239–66. For rinderpest's nineteenth-century impact on European commerce, one may also consult Harrison, *Contagion*, chapter 8 (211–46). For British medicine and theory: Terrie M. Romano, "The Cattle Plague of 1865 and the Reception of 'The Germ Theory' in Mid-Victorian Britain," *Journal of the History of Medicine and Allied Sciences* 52, no. 1 (1997): 51–80.

For Africa, Waktole Tiki and Gufu Oba excerpt valuable oral history in "Ciinna—The Borana Oromo Narration of the 1890s Great Rinderpest Epizootic in North Eastern Africa," *Journal of Eastern African Studies* 3, no. 3 (2009): 479–508. C. van Onselen excerpts and cites useful printed primary sources in "Reactions to Rinderpest in Southern Africa, 1896–97," *Journal of African History* 13, no. 3 (1972): 473–88. The relationship of rinderpest and sleeping sickness is discussed in Daniel R. Headrick, "Sleeping Sickness Epidemics and Colonial Responses in East and Central Africa, 1900–1940," *PLOS Neglected Tropical Diseases* 8, no. 4 (2014): e2772. The end of rinderpest and the certification process for the eradication is recounted in Peter L. Roeder, "Rinderpest: The End of Cattle Plague," *Preventive Veterinary Medicine* 102, no. 2 (2011): 98–106; and Amanda Kay McVety, *The Rinderpest Campaigns: A Virus, Its Vaccines, and Global Development in the Twentieth Century* (Cambridge: Cambridge University Press, 2018).

Chapter 8

The best starting point is a wide-ranging essay collection—one of the few works that crosses national boundaries for this topic—with a comprehensive bibliography listed by country: Howard Phillips and David Killingray, eds, *The Spanish Influenza Pandemic of 1918–19* (London: Routledge, 2003). Many countries have one or more surveys. For the United States: Alfred W. Crosby, *America's Forgotten Pandemic: The Influenza of 1918* (Cambridge: Cambridge University Press, 2003) and Nancy K. Bristow, *American Pandemic: The Lost Worlds of the 1918 Influenza Pandemic* (Oxford: Oxford University Press, 2012). For Canada: Esyllt Jones, *Influenza 1918: Disease, Death, and Struggle in Winnipeg* (Toronto: University of Toronto Press, 2007); Mary Ellen Kelm, "British Columbia First Nations and the Influenza Pandemic of 1918–19," *BC Studies* 122 (Summer 1999): 23–48. For New

Zealand: Geoffrey Rice, *Black November: The 1918 Influenza Pandemic in New Zealand* (Christchurch: Canterbury University Press, 2005). For Britain: Mark Honigsbaum, *A History of the Great Influenza Pandemics: Death, Panic, and Hysteria, 1830–1920* (London: I. B. Tauris, 2013), usefully extends the time frame of the discussion backward.

The search for treatments and vaccines is addressed in John M. Barry, *The Great Influenza: The Epic Story of the Deadliest Plague in History* (New York: Penguin Books, 2005), and considered down to the twenty-first century in Gina Kolata, *Flu: The Story of the Great Influenza Pandemic of 1918 and the Search for the Virus That Caused It* (New York: Farrar, Straus and Giroux, 2011). Vaccines are discussed in John M. Eyler, "De Kruif's Boast: Vaccine Trials and the Construction of a Virus," *Bulletin of the History of Medicine* 80, no. 3 (2006), 409–38. David M. Morens and Anthony S. Fauci discuss mortality and morbidity in historical perspective in "The 1918 Influenza Pandemic: Lessons for the 21st Century," *Journal of Infectious Diseases* 195, no. 7 (2007): 1018–28.

Katherine Anne Porter's short novel *Pale Horse, Pale Rider* (1939) depicts the acute crisis of sickness, while William Maxwell's *They Came Like Swallows* (1937) explores pain and guilt in a family that loses a mother in the pandemic.

Chapter 9

James L.A. Webb Jr, *Humanity's Burden: A Global History of Malaria* (Cambridge: Cambridge University Press, 2009), provides a useful overview. For the twentieth century, Randall Packard's survey *The Making of a Tropical Disease: A Short History of Malaria* (Baltimore: Johns Hopkins University Press, 2007) argues that efforts to subdue mosquitoes overrode other positive measures. This argument is largely echoed by Frank M. Snowden, "The Use and Misuse of History: Lessons from Sardinia," in *The Global Challenge of Malaria: Past Lessons and Future Prospects*, eds Frank M. Snowden and Richard Bucala (New Jersey: World Scientific, 2014), 57–82.

For the early modern era, see Mary Dobson's authoritative *Contours of Death and Disease in Early Modern England* (Cambridge: Cambridge University Press, 1997), which discusses several diseases and many issues. For India: Mark Harrison, *Public Health in British India: Anglo-Indian Preventive Medicine, 1859–1914* (Cambridge: Cambridge University Press, 1994). Frank M. Snowden, *The Conquest of Malaria: Italy, 1900–1962*, traces the complementary effects of public health education, quinine, and pesticides. Ronald Ross's correspondence with Patrick

Manson is available in W.F. Bynum and Caroline Overy, eds, *The Beast in the Mosquito: The Correspondence of Ronald Ross and Patrick Manson, Clio Medica* 51 (Amsterdam: Editions Rodopi, 1998).

For the DDT controversy, useful primary sources are available in Thomas R. Dunlap, ed., *DDT, Silent Spring and the Rise of Environmentalism* (Seattle: University of Washington Press, 2008).

Chapter 10

Matthew R. Smallman-Raynor and Andrew D. Cliff provide an encyclopedic overview with eclectic data in *A World Geography. Poliomyelitis: Emergence to Eradication* (Oxford: Oxford University Press, 2006). For the United States, David Oshinsky, *Polio: An American Story* (Oxford: Oxford University Press, 2005), is an excellent single-volume history. Naomi Rogers, *Dirt and Disease: Polio before FDR* (New Brunswick, NJ: Rutgers University Press, 1996), is useful for the early twentieth century. Tony Gould, *A Summer Plague: Polio and Its Survivors* (New Haven: Yale University Press, 1995), covers similar territory to Oshinsky but also has seven substantial biographical sketches and his own recollections. A volume edited by Thomas M. Daniel and Frederick C. Robbins, *Polio* (Rochester, NY: University of Rochester Press, 1997), presents autobiographical essays from researchers, physicians, and polio survivors. For an account of a major Canadian epidemic, see Christopher J. Rutty, "The Middle-Class Plague: Epidemic Polio and the Canadian State, 1936–37," *Canadian Bulletin of Medical History* 13, no. 2 (1996): 277–314. The controversy that surrounded Elizabeth Kenny is used to shed light on the politics of US medicine in Naomi Rogers, *Polio Wars: Sister Kenny and the Golden Age of American Medicine* (Oxford: Oxford University Press, 2014). Recent conflict over polio vaccination in Nigeria is explored in Ayodele Samuel Jegede, "What Led to the Nigerian Boycott of the Polio Vaccination Campaign?" in *PLOS Medicine* 4, no. 3 (2017), https://doi.org/10.1371/journal.pmed.0040073.

Chapter 11

Although somewhat technical, Jacques Pepin's *The Origins of AIDS* (Cambridge: Cambridge University Press, 2012) is an absorbing reconstruction of the disease's emergence in the twentieth century. John Iliffe, *The African AIDS Epidemic:*

A History (Athens, OH: Ohio University Press, 2006), adds to his book's value with abundant citations from many disciplines. Now of historiographic interest is a presciently titled (for its time) essay collection: Elizabeth Fee and Daniel M. Fox, eds, *AIDS: The Making of a Chronic Disease* (Berkeley: University of California Press, 1992). One of the earliest works to engage AIDS in historical perspective is Elizabeth Fee and Daniel M. Fox, eds, *AIDS: The Burdens of History* (Berkeley: University of California Press, 1988). Simon Garfield, *The End of Innocence: Britain in the Time of AIDS* (London: Faber & Faber 1995), charts the early history of HIV/AIDS in Britain. Richard A. McKay, *Patient Zero and the Making of the AIDS Epidemic* (Chicago: University of Chicago Press, 2017), unravels how one man was falsely held to account during the initial epidemic in North America.

Three leading researchers reflect on the first three decades of the pandemic in Kevin M. De Cock, Harold W. Jaffe, and James W. Curran, "Reflections on 30 Years of AIDS," *Emerging Infectious Diseases* 17, no. 6 (2011): 1044–48. See also Michael Hobbes, "Why Did AIDS Ravage the US More Than Any Other Developed Country?" *The New Republic*, 12 May 2014.

Among many AIDS-themed artistic works, the filmed musical *Rent* (directed by Chris Columbus, 1996) depicts bohemian New Yorkers struggling with AIDS in a plot adapted from Puccini's opera *La Bohème*. In 1993, *The Philadelphia Story* (directed by Jonathan Demme) was among the first Hollywood films to acknowledge the AIDS epidemic. The Canadian film *Three Needles* (directed by Thom Fitzgerald, 2005) interweaves stories from rural China, a South African plantation, and Montreal to explore the global impact of AIDS.

IMAGE CREDITS

INDEX